Governing Health

Governing Health

The Politics of Health Policy

Carol S. Weissert
Associate Professor, Department of Political Science
Michigan State University
East Lansing, Michigan

and

William G. Weissert
Professor, Department of Health Management and Policy
University of Michigan School of Public Health
Ann Arbor, Michigan

The Johns Hopkins University Press
Baltimore and London

© 1996 The Johns Hopkins University Press
All rights reserved. Published 1996
Printed in the United States of America on acid-free paper
05 04 03 02 01 00 99 98 97 96   5 4 3 2 1

The Johns Hopkins University Press
2715 North Charles Street
Baltimore, Maryland 21218-4319
The Johns Hopkins Press Ltd., London

Library of Congress Cataloging-in-Publication Data will be found
at the end of this book.
A catalog record for this book is available from the British Library.

ISBN 0-8018-5265-X
ISBN 0-8018-5266-8 (pbk.)

Contents

Acknowledgments

We are grateful to our doctoral students who served as our research assistants, including Brian Janiske, Susan Silberman, Ellen Averyt, and Madeline Pfahler, as well as those who read some or all of the manuscript, including James Morone at Brown University; Dave Rohde, Bob Lowry, and Jim Granato at Michigan State; John Tierney at Boston College; and Thad Beyle at the University of North Carolina at Chapel Hill.

Bill's students at the University of Michigan School of Public Health graciously suffered through early drafts of the manuscript as their health politics text. They provided support and useful comments, which were much appreciated. The Kellogg Foundation's Community Partnership leadership fellows and their mentor provided feedback and encouragement to Carol in the early stages of the project. Thanks to all who read these drafts and found them valuable.

Thanks to our departments for professional support and released time for Carol, and to Gail Pienick for her tireless, and always cheerful, word processing efforts. Deepest gratitude goes to Terry and Chris Smith and to Roberta Pruitt for life-long support. Finally, we must acknowledge our sons, Will and Rob, who were more patient than we had any right to expect. It is still not clear to us why they did not find Certificate of Need and ERISA stimulating dinner conservation. Nonetheless, for their patience, support, humor, love, many other joys, and especially their willingness to accept responsibility for all errors in this book, we are eternally grateful.

Governing Health

Introduction

FEW ISSUES HAVE the persistence, economic significance, and personal consequences of health care policy. Its origins harken to the earliest days of the nation, when the federal government extended its reach up the rivers and into port cities to control infectious disease. Democratic and Republican presidents since Truman have moved one or more proposals to the national agenda to expand Americans' access to health insurance or improve their coverage. Though each acted as if theirs was the first plan to offer a given set of reforms, more often than not, the solutions designed after anxious nights of midnight oil turned out to mirror, in many respects, proposals made and rejected decade after decade. Often the most significant change was in the party making the proposals, as ideas once viewed as too limited and conservative become in the next iteration the fond hopes of liberals—the conservative position having moved to the right.

Comprehensive health care reform has proved elusive in part because of the differences in how the two parties and their supporters view the role of government. Many see public tampering in dictating the scope of coverage, or health professionals' fees, or performing the insurance risk-pooling function as inappropriate at least and for some, bordering on socialism. Americans inherently fear services provided, authorized, or subsidized by government, sure they will result in poor quality, long queues, and restricted access, despite many examples to the contrary, including Medicare. Payment sources have always been elusive: small and some large employers, especially those in the growing service industry, do not want to pay premiums for their workers, even though economists argue that it is the workers who really pay the cost through foregone wages. Few Americans—especially the 85 or so percent who have health insurance—are willing to pay substantially higher taxes to ensure access to others. Most middle-class Americans are well protected against the costs of health care, and their access to providers is largely unfettered. Strong interest groups resist change from the status quo for additional reasons; they profit under the existing system. Health care providers are well paid; research is lavishly supported. Technology developments proffered by the extensive health equipment industry foster demand, further aggravating utilization rates and costs per visit. Employers with enough clout can reduce their outlays by demanding discounts that shift costs to other payers. The practice of care itself and choices of intervention are largely unstandardized, varying with the physician's knowledge and style of practice, subject to few external controls on type or amount of care prescribed even though the physician clearly has an incentive to overprescribe in the most widespread payment systems—fee for service. Seldom does anything limit the extent to which Herculean efforts are mounted at great cost to extend life, often at poor quality. Prevention gets short shrift.

For most politically significant constituencies, the systems—both health care and political—are working well enough to make major change an unacceptable risk. As long as one is willing to ignore some continuing access barriers, meager outcomes among the poor, neglect among elderly nursing home residents, and too little effort preventing unhealthy behaviors, the widely held conviction that America has the best health care available in the world rings true.

While many experts and pundits feel that the health care market should be allowed to operate without governmental direction, the system's complexity and embedded governmental role make these positions seem overly simplistic, if not downright wrong. State and federal regulatory power remains the main tool of health professionals intent on improving quality and limiting cheaper competition for their services. Federal and state training and facilities subsidies for decades have dictated the bed supply and composition of the health workforce, distorting supply in relation to demand—often at great public expense. Subsidies for health insurance and subsidized insurance and care remove normal price rationing. Growth in federal expenditures for health care dwarf other priorities in federal and state governments. Per-capita spending in the United States vastly exceeds that of any other country. Complexity makes reform proposals easy targets for critics charging unworkability. Worse, few feel sure, even among supporters, that critics may not prove correct. A steep learning curve confronts those who tackle the issue's many facets. Periodic bursts of saliency and public support for real change tend to be temporary and waning. The crest of the wave passes before solutions can be formulated and ideological differences over the role of government in a reformed system become "sound bites" of partisan warfare in election years. Even if that were not the case, comprehensive change is especially hard because it concentrates costs on many separate interests, large and small, while thinly spreading the benefits to taxpayers and the insured in general. Fears of adverse selection (only the sickest will rush to sign up) make piecemeal solutions unstable, risky, and expensive.

Undaunted, some believe that health care policy reform cannot be avoided. Rising costs and declining coverage are said to demand it. Others argue that rapid churning of ownership, altered delivery systems, new provider-payer relationships, and business and industry unwillingness to simply continue paying higher and higher premiums may obviate the need for government takeover of the health care industry. Optimistic or not, this view may be the only ray of hope for those who want change but reasonably conclude from the past half-century of national health insurance policy that it may not be accidental that compromise has been elusive. Solutions have proved hard to find, sometimes producing as many problems as they solve.

Absent any clear vision, the American system is designed to default to inaction. A decentralized Congress, an overrated and weakened presidency, budget deficits, distrust of bureaucracies, erosion of state budgets, and federal preemption of state regulation merely aggravate the problem and dictate policy gridlock. States that try to ignore budget implications and forge ahead find themselves stymied by federal laws prohibiting them from exacting participation in reform plans from employers. Market-oriented strategies for making the health care system more efficient and narrowing the scope of public subsidy to those who cannot pay may have to precede taking on substantial new public initiatives in health care policy. The divisive and unrewarding politics of redistribution seem unavoidable. Incremental change may be all that can slip through the narrow policy window that sometimes opens for health reform.

Though we have been governing health for decades in this country, the form and scope of governance are regularly under public scrutiny. A crisis has been declared. Policies and the institutions that produced them are routinely scourged. Has governance gone amuck? Can we fix it? Should we? Or is it working as it should, and we are just not taking a long enough view? This book examines our experience with governing health. It is a political science book about health care policy. As such, it presents health care policy as the product of the American system of government, combining the many forces of the

—persistent power of ideological polarization and party politics;
—dominant need for members of Congress to constantly seek reelection;
—discretion of the bureaucracy;
—pervasive and well-financed influence of the burgeoning army of health interests;
—challenge of effective problem definition so that solutions to problems of the poor are also appealing to the middle class;
—ebb and flow of issue cycles;
—limited choice of policy options, constrained by the unwillingness of employers or taxpayers to pay much more for reform.

This book grew from frustration with finding a text written by political scientists for use in health politics classes. Sociologists and economists have authored or contributed to a small number of worthy volumes bringing their disciplines' perspectives to the topic of health politics and policy. While they have much to offer, a gap remains. Politics is more than the sociology of institutions or economic self-interest. Health care policy is politics at its richest and fullest.

The intended audience is health policy analysts who want to become more adept at gauging the political feasibility of their proposals, health professionals who seek a better understanding of how policy is made and how they might alter it, and political scientists who seek illustrations of how the principles of government work in a policy arena with all the magic ingredients of political conflict—saliency, huge stakes, powerful interests, and venues in all the institutions of government. *Governing Health* is a comprehensive synthesis of political science research on the institutions of government and the policy process, and an extensive review of the policies that have governed health care for a generation and more.

A central focus of the book is documenting change in the nation's chief political institutions over time. Each chapter in part 1 begins with a comparison of how differently the institutions under study confronted three presidents when they began the policymaking quest:

—President Johnson in 1965 rode the crest of a Democratic wave of power and ideas, and a growing consensus that the elderly poor at least deserved public health care subsidy, only to stretch the compromise to include all elderly by eliminating means testing from his Medicare proposal;

—President Reagan in 1981 was ushered in with a mandate to shrink and constrain government-supported health care, welfare, and social services, only to pass and then repeal expansion of the Medicare program modified by the Democrats by adding new coverages to a catastrophic coverage bill;

—President Clinton in 1993 interpreted Americans' concerns that their insurance might be canceled as a mandate for employer-subsidized universal coverage, only to have his congressional supporters punished at the next election, sweeping in the first Republican House of Representatives in forty years.

Each chapter relates changes in the institutions to these touch points and others, illustrating the conviction that only through a longitudinal view of policymaking can one accurately distinguish aspects of institutional features and norms that are unchanging from those that reflect present practice.

Part 1 of the book describes the institutions of government, reflecting the insights of political science research into the interaction of structures and motivations influencing members.

Chapter 1 describes the structures and functioning of Congress and the motivations of members. Its theme is that Congress was intended and has continued to be the dominant branch of government, but the norms have changed in ways that make it difficult to fulfill that responsibility. The chapter begins with a review of the motivations and sources of ideas of the framers who conferred enormous powers and many binding constraints upon the legislative branch.

Power shifts in party and institutional leadership relative to committee and subcommittee chairs are described in the context of their roles, responsibilities, and sources of power, including personality and institutional norms. Committees and subcommittees of special importance to health care policymaking receive the most attention and are used as examples of how committees work on issues of membership and jurisdiction, and with the rest of their houses. Conference committees, a central source of health care policymaking but little understood, are described with examples of how they rewrite legislation, often on the fly.

Budgeting, the increasingly dominant task of a deficit-ridden Congress, is closely examined, stepping carefully between the concepts that are likely to continue to characterize the process and the changing rules and terms that complicate its understanding.

A section devoted to legislative parties imparts an understanding of the paradox of their uncertain importance in the nation at large contrasted with their increasingly powerful role in the Congress. Incumbency, its benefits, liabilities, and persistent reelection statistics highlight the discussion of congressional motivations and introduce a review of the considerable political science literature on congressional norms and their evolution. The role of congressional staff and the growing number and size of congressional support agencies are important aspects of the section on the congressional enterprise; it provides contextual perspective for discussion of how members of Congress make decisions, and the role of saliency, the press, interest groups, and constituent concerns. The chapter concludes with a brief examination of the difficulties of making health care policy in the face of a decentralized, entrepreneurial congressional policymaking process, highlighting the sources and consequences of decentralization of power.

Chapter 2 examines the presidency, starting with the sources and scope of presidential power and the high stakes but sibling-like rivalry that characterizes the relationship of that office with the Congress even in the best of times. Focused as the book is on health care policymaking, it is the domestic president who is the subject of this chapter, and it is how he makes choices about proposals and solutions for domestic problem solving that is of concern. While his role in agenda setting, proposing, and monitoring the progress of proposed solutions is closely examined, a theme of the chapter is that there is truth to the axiom that a president proposes but Congress disposes. He is much more influential than any of the 535 members who work for or against him, but he is not, in the final analysis, a legislator. Measures of presidential legislative success are examined and lend credence to the view that presidential power is generally overrated, especially in the face of divided power when Congress is half or fully controlled by the other party. Such circumstances often lead presidents to "go public," a strategy of mixed success practiced with differential skill by presidents. Managing the press is also part of the job, done moderately well by those who figured out how to manage it and tragically by others who did not.

Bureaucracy nominally reports to the president too, though few have found effective ways to use it, leaving its direction more to Congress than suggested by the government manuals' organization charts. That other bureaucracy, the White House staff, is more likely to consume the managerial talents of most presidents. The chapter concludes with a reprise of the presidential role in health policymaking—a spotty record of mixed success and many notable failures, especially by those who, like President Clinton, really tried to fix the whole thing at once.

Chapter 3 describes the zealous hucksterings of that diverse congeries of niche groups, coalitions, political action committees (PACs), and ground-swell participants who engage in lobbying, campaign giving, and grass-roots organizing to try to keep things off the public agenda or shape them to their liking when they cannot. One theme is that interest groups are extremely influential in health care policymaking and in many instances, the controlling influence. With their money, organizing skills, and singularity of purpose, they are only too happy and altogether competent to show a legislator the correct path toward constituent service and comfortable reelection margins. But are they necessarily deserving of their vilification as "special interests?" Another theme is that interest groups have long been one of the key institutions of government. While there is no suggestion that groups always or even usually act in the public interest, a point made is that they are undeniably part of the way in which American government is made so broadly participatory. Those special interests they represent often correspond to a members' priorities for their districts.

How interest groups form and stay together is examined, including the role of economic self-interest, selective benefits, entrepreneurs, the dominant role of occupational alliances, and the deliberate or inadvertent role of government itself in sometimes spawning groups.

The interest group world is described as much more complex than it was in the 1960s or earlier. It is characterized by permanent and temporary coalitions that share and complement the other's strengths and resources. Charts show a huge increase in the number of health interest groups, which generally find they agree more than fight with one another. Interest groups' unglamorous daily ardor of monitoring legislation and providing information is shown to be the essential ingredient in that magic elixir of influence—access—which must precede their ability to provide a pearl or two of information that may sway a critical decision. The ways in which they alter strategies as they move through the many venues of government is described, as well as the strategies they employ in campaign giving and grass-roots campaigning. The link, or lack of it, between money giving and vote casting is examined, but little doubt is raised that coupled with features of congressional decision-making described in Chapter 1, the role of interest groups makes health reform all that much harder. Since most people are in groups, however, we are loathe to conclude that Americans are not getting what they want.

Chapter 4 takes a sympathetic view of public bureaucracy, arguing that its considerable power is underrated, on the one hand, while on the other its responsiveness to Congress makes it the fall guy for much that is beyond its control.

Bureaucracy here is viewed as a repository of expert, detail-oriented people who bring the long view to the policy process and stand ready to serve their multiple masters—Congress, the president, the courts, their beneficiary constituents, and their regulatory foes—but suffer when pulled in multiple directions as much as when they are ignored. Careerists' differences from politicos, the nature of the agency's political environment, and the importance of the agency's mission are highlighted in a comprehensive review of the fascinating literature describing how bureaucrats function, their relationship to the other branches of government, and the incentives and constraints governing their behavior.

Both sides of the argument over whether bureaucrats are getting weaker or stronger are advanced. Though neither side is chosen as more correct, a rich array of examples from health care policy leaves the clear impression that bureaucrats influence all aspects of the process, especially their special province: implementation. A substantial portion of the chapter is devoted to regulation and the factors modulating the degree of success that agencies enjoy or suffer in gaining industry compliance. An overarching point is that no matter how green the eye shades, regulation is political, and evaluation of the agency's performance is gauged with a political yardstick. Health agencies are examined, their turf described, and their political fortunes weighed in light of past performance and as viewed by important beholders.

Chapter 5 traces the evolution of state government from the good old days of the good old boys in the 1950s and 1960s through their awakening and federalism's many redefinitions. The case is easy to make that most states today are modern, savvy, lean, innovative, socially responsible, and politically independent power centers—with huge differences in resources to be sure—but determined not to lose their identity and to regain their autonomy. States still want all they can get from the federal domestic budget, but they have grown weary of the federal government presuming that Washington knows better how to spend it to solve problems.

While no one was watching, the states have reformed their governance and become important players on the health care provision and policy scene. One major section of the chapter recounts the long list of state health innovations, suggesting that most health policy reform ideas offered by the federal government began first as a state initiative. The future is likely to see more of the same, especially if the federal government removes some of the barriers it has erected to state innovation.

Institutions are again a central focus of the chapter, highlighted by close examination of differences and similarities among the states and compared to the federal government. Comparisons include budgets, spending, revenues, and documentation of the rapacious effects of Medicaid and other health spending on states' ability to set their own agendas. The uniquely state feature known as direct democracy—initiative, referendum, and recall—is examined, and its benefits and liabilities considered.

Part 2 of the book describes the policy process. Chapter 6 defines public policy, its evolution, unintended consequences, and demands. It describes various attempts to categorize public policies and their value in understanding the effect of the type of policy on its politics, and vice versa. Health policies are used as examples of regulatory, distributive, and redistributive policies, and highlight the political ease or difficulties encompassing policies designed to do different things in different ways.

The chapter also describes several models of the policy process (the heuristic model, the garbage can and Kingdon's refinements, Downs, Lindbloom, and others). It provides a compendium of examples of the political ways in which health care problems get defined as part of the effort to widen the scope of conflict and interest the disinterested so that topics move to the public agenda. Problems do not just emerge; they are carefully nurtured, defined, framed, and often exaggerated to promote a desired policy solution. Ultimately, a decision must be made whether a problem augurs for a public or private solution—a choice inevitably tied to the often-controversial concern about the role of government.

Chapter 7 treats criteria solutions. It reviews the solutions to which Congress has resorted, or struggled to resort to, over the past several decades of health policy choices:

—providing national health insurance;
—subsidizing the supply of facilities, personnel, and services to poor people;
—containing costs.

This chapter is the product of an original research effort that traced the health policy actions of Congress year by year, issue by issue from the mid-1940s to the mid-1990s through the annual blow-by-blow chronicle of the *Congressional Quarterly Almanac*. Issues the subcommittees, committees, and houses considered; criteria applied in their search for solutions; and the variety of solutions they considered are synthesized and chronicled to describe the scope and flavor of health policymaking during a half-century of massive growth, expansion of the public role, and the retrenchment that began under President Reagan and was revitalized under Newt Gingrich, Speaker of the House.

The chapter shows both what happened in health care policy during a critical half-century and how Congress made the choices it made. It ties together the policy literature of political science research with examples of the legislative process, including coalition building; partisanship in committees and caucuses; policy entrepreneurship; interaction among committees and turf battles between them; deference to and defiance of the executive branch by the legislative branch; the influence of the Office of Management and Budget (OMB) and Congressional Budget Office (CBO) on committee decisions; the power of persistence, determination, personality, and self-interest; the free-wheeling power of conference committees and their domination by the money committee chairs; the influence at every level of the policy process of the American Medical Association (AMA); the distaste legislators have for cutting hospital payments; and the tempering of interest group influence by the inexorable wearing down of resistance to good ideas until crisis punctuates the process and produces change. The body of actions that constitutes American health policy is all here, categorized, chronicled, synthesized, and summarized, along with many of the positions taken by a large sampling of those in the cast of characters who have dominated health care policy for a generation: Mills, Johnson, Nixon, Long, Ted Kennedy, Waxman, Bentsen, Stark, Clinton, Dole, and many others.

Chapter 8 concludes with a prognosis for health care policy. It predicts an era of vigorous efforts by both federal and state governments to control their financial obligations through much tougher payment and subsidy policies, and a redefined and broadening role in monitoring and enforcement.

Part I

Health Policy and Institutions

1

Congress

A LOOK BACK

1965

DEMOCRATS SEEMED to be everywhere when the first roll of the Eighty-ninth Congress was called on 4 January 1965. So tightly squeezed in were House members that many found it more comfortable to stand at the railing around the back of the chamber. There were 155 more Democrats than Republicans in the House and 36 in the Senate, the product of a Democratic landslide victory that would make possible feats of legislative legerdemain seldom seen in the almost-always fractious Congress. There was the usual splintering of Democrats, which typically separated Northerner from Southerner and big-city from small-town Democrat, but when enough Democrats stuck together, they could pass almost anything. Their newly elected president, Lyndon B. Johnson, meant to take full advantage of the majority held by his party to tackle a huge legislative agenda: Medicare, Medicaid, maternal and child health programs, health planning, regional medical programs, physician training programs, specific disease research (including cancer and heart disease), not to mention civil rights, education, economic opportunity, model cities, urban mass transit, nutritional programs for the poor, and more. Though some of these subjects—civil rights and Medicare, for example— were among the most divisive issues in American politics, this Congress would tackle them all and pass most of them.

In 1965 John McCormack was the Speaker of the House and Mike Mansfield the majority leader of the Senate. While both were well-respected and talented legislators, their powers were constrained by the strength of the committees, headed by Southerners. The North-South split was the greatest source of conflict within the Democratic party. The 1964 Johnson landslide brought forty-two new Northern Democrats into the House and forced a change in the balance of party power. The Ways and Means Committee was transformed; a bare majority of curmudgeons had steadfastly refused to allow a payroll tax to finance Medicare. Legislative leaders urged by the president took every opportunity to replace them one by one.

Medicare, in its broader incarnation usually called national health insurance, had been the subject of bitter debates, media fear campaigns, and committee-blocking tactics for two decades. With its decisive majority, the eighty-ninth Congress would (after considerable bargaining and compromises aimed at splitting interest group opposition) roll over its opposition. As the final vote on Medicare was being tallied and the outcome became clear, one member of the Republican leadership stormed out of the House center aisle doors, turned to the pages and doorkeepers gathered to watch the show, and in exasperation exploded, "We've got Goldwater to thank for this." He was referring to the fact that the defeat of the 1964 Republican presidential candidate Barry Goldwater had been so decisive it swept in the large Democratic majority, which could now run roughshod over the shrunken Republican minority.

1981

Contrast this bold, decisive, ideologically unalloyed Democratic juggernaut and its massive show of party strength to the Congress of 1981, a time when the seeds of conservatism and antigovernment sentiment growing in the late 1970s had flourished to produce a Republican landslide presidential election and the first Republican majority in the Senate in a quarter-century (table 1.1).

Republicans picked up thirty-four seats in the House and twelve in the

Table 1.1. Congressional Parties and Leaders in 1965, 1981, and 1993

Year and Congress	House of Representatives	Senate
1965, 89th Congress	295 Democrats	68 Democrats
	140 Republicans	32 Republicans
	Speaker: John McCormack (MA)	Majority Leader: Mike Mansfield (MT)
1981, 97th Congress	243 Democrats	46 Democrats
	192 Republicans	53 Republicans
	Speaker: Thomas P. "Tip" O'Neill (MA)	Majority Leader: Howard Baker (TN)
1993, 103rd Congress	258 Democrats	57 Democrats
	176 Republicans	43 Republicans
	Speaker: Thomas Foley (WA)	Majority Leader: George Mitchell (ME)

Senate. Republicans relished their new leadership role in the Senate. Liberal critics said they had been put in charge only because the voters were dominated by the "me" generation, so-called yuppies who had lost faith in, or could no longer see themselves benefiting from, public programs. Republicans retorted that liberals had had their chance. Health care reforms would take the shape of reduced spending, prospective budgets, and narrowed eligibility rules for subsidized services. This was nothing short of a sea change in the role of government, made possible because of the Republicans' majority in the Senate, a large enough minority in the House to forge a majority with Democrats who strayed from their party's dominant positions, and for a time, Democrats' fear that the popular Republican president could hurt them in the next election.

But the Democrats had a few resources of their own. They were not so easily split as in the old days, when quarrels over racial policies sent Southerners across the aisle looking for allies. Party leaders were stronger. No longer could they be held hostage by feudal committee chairs who bottled up legislation they did not favor, snubbing their noses at their party's majority. Leaders had been given their own weapons by a series of reforms in the early 1970s, which were gleefully used by the large first-year class of 1974 elected on the heels of Watergate. The party's leaders now appointed members of the Rules Committee, which set the rules for floor debate on most bills; leaders could refer bills to multiple committees, virtually ensuring that at least one committee would report a bill; and leaders played a crucial role in awarding committee assignments by appointing a majority of the members of the Steering and Policy Committee, which made appointments. Leaders were "more aggressive and more willing to use institutional resources" to a greater extent than those who had served in previous Congresses (Herrick and Moore 1993, 4).

One price of clipping the committee chairs' wings was fragmentation. Subcommittees had filled the power vacuum, and with their own staffing and considerable autonomy, subcommittee chairs and members could become expert in health policy and use their influence to profoundly shape the legislative proposal that went to the full committee (Bowler 1987). House Energy and Commerce Health Subcommittee chair Henry Waxman embodied this new, entrepreneurial subcommittee chair. Accepting the reality that no comprehensive health care program would see the light of day in the near term, he adopted an incrementalist approach: gradual expansion of Medicaid to cover more and more near-poor individuals, starting with children and their mothers. This approach worked for eight years. Every year between 1984 and 1991, at least one federal law expanding Medicaid eligibility or services was enacted, until opposition from state governors finally succeeded in putting an end to Medicaid mandates in 1991 (Weissert 1992).

1993

The Congress faced by President Bill Clinton in 1993 was different again. The 1992 elections brought in the largest first-year class in the House since 1949—sixty-three Democrats and forty-seven Republicans—but these newcomers were not political neophytes. Many had come up through the political ranks, including state legislative stints. Along the way they lost the patience and humility usually expected of first-year representatives. After five months of toeing the line, they began showing their independence. With eighty-two more Democrats than Republicans in the House, the president's hallmark budget and tax package passed with only two votes to spare. Was this the party that would overhaul a health system comprising more than one-seventh of the economy and potentially displace 3.1 million workers?

Leadership had also changed. Though powerful on paper, the current crop of leaders had a more mellow style than their predecessors. Rather than commanding their troops, modern leaders had learned to act as "agents in pursuing the party's legislative agenda" (Rohde 1991, 35). Their job had become more collegial, using the powers granted to them to accomplish goals they held in common with other Democratic members. Rather than raw power, leaders counted on homogeneity of values. Where it existed, leadership could be granted discretion and expect to be followed; where it did not, members would go their own way. Since the late 1970s, Speakers have relied heavily on the party whip organization to enhance morale, build support for party positions, and poll members. Since the 1980s, approximately 20 percent of Democratic House members were part of the whip "organization," which meets weekly with leadership to "enhance their two-way communication with members" (Rohde 1991, 93) and make the leadership more effective in advancing its program.

Tom Foley (D–Wash.), Speaker of the House, showed his distaste for bare knuckles early in the session. Eleven Democratic subcommittee chairs voted with the Republicans against the administration's budget. Some in the party wanted to "strip" the chairs of their subcommittees, but Foley demurred, preferring instead to share the tasks of reprimanding recalcitrants by forcing caucus elections of all subcommittee chairs.

The president had even less power to force compliance with his program. Thanks to independent candidate Ross Perot, the president had been elected with only 43 percent of the popular vote—a smaller margin than any member of either house. Clinton would be of limited use at reelection. This would become important when members of his party splintered in their support for health reform: one gaggle demanding complete government takeover of financing while, at the other extreme, another group pressed for everything to be voluntary. In short, the Democratic Party controlling the House lacked the discipline required to produce a legislative program.

POWERS AND CONSTRAINTS

Many people forget that for its first thirteen years, this country operated under the Articles of Confederation, that set up a weak national government and strong states. The experiment failed, and a convention ostensibly called only to modify the Articles of Confederation took the opportunity to rewrite the institutional power structure in significant ways. When the debate ended, a national government had been designed that placed primary power in a legislative body split between a popularly elected House of Representatives and an elitist Senate elected by the state legislatures, which was further checked by the powers of an energetic executive with veto power and a strong appointed judiciary. Any tendencies central government officials might have had to wield power with a heavy hand would be checked by their own structure. In turn, democracy running amuck in the states could be restrained by the powers granted to the national government.

The constitution, like the country it reflects, is far from static; the carefully balanced power relationships of 1789 have been skewed over the years. Thanks in part to some key Supreme Court decisions, the national government is the most important player in federalism. The Congress is the dominant player among the three co-equal branches. Such dominance would have suited at least one of the founding fathers, James Madison, just fine: "In republican government, the legislative authority necessarily predominates" (Oleszek 1989, 1). Two hundred years have proven him correct.

CONGRESSIONAL STRUCTURE

The bicameral nature of the congressional structure, carefully designed by the framers, is an important element in national policymaking. Political scientists have studied the effect of bicameralism and concluded that the presence of a second chamber tends to provide a check on potentially volatile and misled majorities in one house (Janiskee 1995). In 1995, Americans witnessed what has been dubbed "cooling the coffee," as the Republican-led House passed twenty-seven out of twenty-nine elements of their "Contract with America" in the first 100 days of the session; the Senate, in contrast, passed only five and rejected one of the measures.

Both the institutions and those who serve in them are vastly different. U.S. senators serve six-year terms, are elected statewide (thanks to a constitutional amendment), and tend to have a broader, longer-term focus than their colleagues who work on the other side of the Capitol. The Senate has 100 members, two from every state regardless of population. The House has 435 members allocated on a state's relative population. Delegation sizes vary from one member from the Dakotas, Alaska, Montana, Wyoming, Delaware, and Vermont to fifty-two from California. Since the size of the House remains stable, population shifts cause changes in the distribution of members every ten years following the Census. For example, in 1992 Michigan lost two members and California added seven.

In recent years the Senate has attracted extremely wealthy people, often without prior political experience, who use their own resources to fund their campaigns. Few are women, and far fewer are African Americans or other minority group members. The House is more representative, but only in comparison to the Senate. In good years 10–15 percent may be women and perhaps another 10–15 percent members of a minority group.

Newspaper columnist and commentator David Broder (1993b) contended that the compromise that made the Senate a smaller and more lordly body than the House has run amuck in recent years: a majority of senators come from states that collectively elect only 20 percent of the members of the House, and Senate leaders typically come from smaller states, such as Maine, Kansas, Kentucky, Wyoming, West Virginia, and Mississippi. In 1995 the two senators from Oregon—a state with a population approximating that of the metropolitan area of Atlanta, Georgia—chaired the two key money committees—the Appropriations Committee and the Finance Committee. The Senate majority leader that session was from Kansas and the minority leader from South Dakota. The leaders of the House tend to come from large and medium-sized states like Texas, Illinois, Michigan, Washington, Missouri, and Georgia. A similar disparate domination of state legislatures by rural members in the 1950s made it impossible to pass progressive legislation for cities and suburbs until the U.S. Supreme Court ruled that state legislators had to be apportioned on the basis of population, not geographic area (*Reynolds v. Simms* 1964). Is such a reform possible for the Senate? No, the U.S. Constitution precludes amendments that strip away the geographic basis of Senate membership. Perhaps populous states should seek permission to split into several states to gain more equitable representation. Or the nation might follow the extreme remedy of one prominent congressional scholar, whose advice regarding the Senate was "Close it down. Put it out of its misery. It's just a bunch of egomaniacs looking around for people to fawn over them."

No wonder they feel important. Senators have a greater chance of serving on desirable committees and achieve chair status more quickly than their House counterparts. The Senate has fewer rules of procedure to restrict individuality. Amendments do not have to be germane to the subject of a bill. One senator can temporarily halt floor action with a filibuster, which can be stopped only with sixty votes. And senators are no longer shy about using it. Once a rarity, the filibuster has been used an average of twenty-two times per year since 1990, compared to close to a dozen times per year between 1968 and 1989 (Flemming and Marshall 1994). C-Span devotees are familiar with the variety of procedural tricks to slow things down and prevent legislation from coming to a vote—quorum calls, roll call votes on motions to take up a bill, and demands for long amendments to be read in their entirety. Unless a bill has sixty aggressive supporters who are willing to stay up late, a small group can defeat a bill in the Senate. No wonder that barely more than 10 percent of the bills introduced in a given session ever become law (Ornstein, Mann, and Malbin 1994).

Leadership

Both houses are organized by the political parties. The majority party selects the Speaker (majority leader in the Senate), who makes decisions on scheduling, committee membership, which committees bills get referred, who sits on the "conference committees" to resolve differences in legislation passed by the two houses, and more (box 1.1).

Not surprisingly, the strength of party leadership is affected by party unity and the personalities of those chosen as leaders. Where party leadership is weak, committee chairs often gain in power. Congressional history is replete with pendulum shifts in the predominant source of power. In the 1890s the Speakers were so strong they were dubbed "Czar" Reed and "Boss" Cannon. The Speaker's powers were curbed shortly after the turn of the century, and for decades the power of committee chairs and later the subcommittee chairs increased in the 1970s and 1980s. In 1995, when the Republicans gained control of the House after four decades in the minority, they set up a more centralized leadership system, providing the Speaker with more power than had their compatriots across the aisle. Speaker of the House Gingrich named the committee chairs (passing over more senior members on three key committees—Appropriations, Commerce and Judiciary) and set up computer systems to keep track of scheduling and legislative progress. The new Speaker set about to avoid disagreements among committees or between committees and the leadership by establishing task forces and regular meetings with committee members and aides to make certain legislation is moving apace and with the content desired by the leadership. No better example can be found than in the health subcommittee of the Ways and Means Committee where the new chair was discouraged from drafting legislation on Medicare until the leadership had "set its course" (Serafini 1995, 1712).

Committees

To Woodrow Wilson, writing in 1885 (79), "Congress in its committee-rooms is Congress at work." More than a century later, Wilson is still right. Standing committees, about twenty in each house—down in recent years from more than twenty in the House—are "the main paths along which Congress moves [and] all lead through the committee system" (Keefe 1984, 92). They are the workhorses of the legislature, considering legislation, holding hearings (often outside of Washington), amending legislation, and supporting

Box 1.1 Party Leadership in the U.S. Congress

The main leadership positions in Congress are the Speaker of the House, the House majority and minority leaders, the House majority and minority whips, and the Senate majority and minority leaders.

The House of Representatives

The Speaker of the House is formally elected by the chamber as a whole, though really chosen by majority caucus. The Speaker presides over the House, shapes the agenda by deciding which bills have priority and on which calendar they appear, refers bills to appropriate committees, and designates members of joint and conference committees. The Speaker is the majority party spokesperson in the House, assisted by a number of party leaders, including

—the majority leader, who formulates that party's legislative program in cooperation with the Speaker and other party leaders, helps steer the program through the chamber, and assists in establishing the legislative schedule;

—the minority leader, who has the top leadership position for the minority party, formulates the party's legislative program in conjunction with other leaders, helps steer the program through the chamber, and serves as the party spokesperson for that chamber;

—party whips, who assist both the majority and the minority leaders, mobilize party members behind legislative positions that the leadership has decided are in the party's interest, and keep an accurate count of the votes and preferences of members on bills.

The Senate

According to the U.S. Constitution, the vice president of the United States assumes the post of president of the Senate and presides over it. In the vice president's absence, the president pro tempore, a powerless, honorific position, generally presides over the Senate.

The primary leadership duties are performed by the majority leader, who is the spokesperson for the party, affects the assignment of members to committees, schedules floor action, formulates the party's legislative program, schedules bills, works with committee chairs on action of importance to the party, and directs strategy on the floor. The minority leader is the spokesperson for the party, mobilizes support for minority party positions, and directs the minority party's strategy.

The role of Senate whips is similar to that of House whips: aiding party leadership in developing a program, transmitting information to party members, conducting vote counts, and persuading members.

their "product" on the House floor. Conference committees are temporary, created to adjust differences between the chambers when the two houses pass different versions of legislation.

Standing Committees

Standing committees are those with stated jurisdictions, created by the rules of the House, permanent (unless rules are changed), and responsible for screening, examining, and reporting on legislation referred to them. Box 1.2 provides an overview of the jurisdictions and functions of standing committees. Committees are where ideas are debated, deals are cut, interest groups ply their trade, and partisanship is paramount. The stakes are high in committees, and members know it.

The influence of committees extends beyond Congress. They wield considerable clout over the bureaucracy, conducting oversight or congressional review of the actions of the federal departments, agencies, and commissions, and of the programs and policies they administer. When the other party is in the White House and charged with overseeing administrative agencies, the committees turn up the heat. But even a president of their own party does not go unwatched. Cabinet officers say they spend one-third of their time on Capitol Hill testifying before committees and meeting informally with staff. Bruce Babbitt, Interior Secretary under Clinton, said he was "astonished at the degree to which Congress is present in my daily life and shares at every level" in the direction of his department (Broder and Barr 1993, 31).

The "despotic" committee chairs of the 1950s and 1960s (Clapp 1963) have been replaced by committee chairs better described as diplomats. John Dingell, of Michigan, chair of the House Energy and Commerce Committee for years, was long known for his legislative imperialism. But with the passing years, he had to learn to seek compromise on Clean Air Act reauthorization and other bills. In trying to push health reform through his major health committee in 1994, Dingell made it plain that everything was "negotiable" (Weisskopf 1994, 14). That included voluntary rather than mandatory insurance-buying cooperatives, grants to tobacco farmers to help them develop alternative crops, and protection from proposed federal review of new drug prices. He failed nonetheless to reach agreement and his committee produced no bill.

Committees are not equal in power or popularity among members. The House Ways and Means, Senate Finance, House Rules, and House and Senate

Box 1.2 Congressional Standing Committees

There are thirty-five standing committees (nineteen in the House and sixteen in the Senate). Their role is pivotal to the workings of a legislative body; approximately 8,000 bills are introduced in a two-year session. Committees speed the work load; facilitate meaningful deliberations on important measures and issues; develop and nurture expertise among members and staff; and serve as the final resting place for inept or inappropriate proposals (Bailey 1970). Debate and procedures are more informal than in the whole House, and partisanship is often restrained. As Manley (1965) put it, partisanship should not interfere with a thorough study and complete understanding of the technical complexities of the bills considered by the committee.

The committee that drafts and reports a bill also manages it on the House floor. It does most of the wheeling and dealing with White House staff, lobbyists, and others who reshape major provisions to win enough votes for passage. Should the legislation pass, the committee keeps responsibility for the issue in future years. It holds the hearings for renewal and amendment, and makes the bid for it each year in budget committee negotiations.

Floor procedures, information advantages, the norm of reciprocity among committees, and daunting power of a united committee front make committees' recommendations likely to prevail on the House floor. Since committees provide careful scrutiny of measures and have members knowledgeable on the subject, such deference by members who are not so expert and who have not devoted much time to the issue makes sense. As an illustration of the power of committees, consider that every health bill moved by the Senate Labor Committee in the Ninety-ninth Congress was passed on the Senate floor without debate or opposition (Nexon 1987, 74).

On highly salient bills or when the committee's interests may not mirror the House, floor amendments may be offered and can pass with a simple majority vote. The whole process is repeated in the other house, sometimes sequentially, sometimes more or less simultaneously. If one house completes action first, it may wait to see whether the bill passed in the other house differs. Differences may be resolved by the first house passing the revised bill or encouraging the second house to redo theirs. Less frequently, a conference committee is appointed to strike a compromise bill, which both houses then must pass.

Although expertise is a key factor in the committee's value to the House, some bills cut across areas of committee expertise and are sent to more than one committee. At the peak of this practice, some 20 percent of bills were referred to more than one committee (Young and Cooper 1993). Included in that tally were bills for which party leadership used the multiple referral process to advance its own agenda. An example was a trade bill referred by the Speaker to six different committees—his way of making sure that what came to the floor for a vote had broad Democratic support (Rohde 1991). Republicans who took over the House in 1995 changed this rule, prohibiting simultaneous multiple referrals in favor of sequential referral—first to a primary committee, then to a secondary committee.

Senate committees tend to be about half the size of the House committees, averaging close to twenty members, compared to the House average size of nearly forty members. The Appropriations Committee in the House is usually largest, with about sixty members, followed by the National Security and the Banking and Financial Service Committees. In the Senate, the Appropriations Committee is also the largest committee with close to thirty members.

Appropriations and Budget committees have been called "power committees" (Loomis 1984). Membership on them is very competitive and highly prized by members who want to make a name for themselves in Congress. Leaders usually get their training in committee, learning to cut deals, avoid minefields, and work to balance the conflicting pressures of other committees, lobbyists, and the broader house membership.

Policy committees are responsible for authorizing legislation and are organized by subject area. Some policy committees are more attractive than others. Popular House policy committees include the Commerce, Education and Labor, and Banking and Financial Services committees. Losers are the House oversight and veterans' committees, though some are quite happy to be members and have found those committees a source of influence and constituent-pleasing jurisdiction. Committee attractiveness can wax and wane, with changing policy priorities and recent esteem or repute in which a committee comes to be held. During the 1980s, the House Judiciary Committee's popularity plummeted; in the 1990s, following its embarrassing racially tainted and gender-biased hearings over the Supreme Court nomination of Clarence Thomas, the Senate Judiciary Committee found itself for a time unable to find enough members to fill all its slots.

The two policy committees that have primary jurisdiction over health are the Senate Labor and Human Resources Committee and the House Commerce Committee. These committees, along with relevant subcommittees, and six other important committees are listed in box 1.3. However, it is important to keep in mind that a number of committees have some interest in health, particularly some specific aspects of it. For example, Veterans' Affairs, Government Operations, Science, Space and Technology, and Small Business Committees in the House often hold hearings on health issues. One recent count of hearings on health care between 1980 and 1991 (Baumgartner and Talbert 1995) found that the committee that held the most hearings was the House Select Aging Committee, a committee with no statutory responsibility (it cannot write bills). In spite of the spate of committees with some stake in health, the two policy committees and the House Ways and Means Committee and Senate Finance Committee are generally viewed as the dominant health legislative players. In 1991 the House Health and Environment Subcommittee had jurisdiction over roughly 85 percent of the nearly fifty major health programs identified by the National Health Council.

The jurisdictions of major health programs in the Senate are more diffuse, with the Labor and Human Resources Committee responsible for barely more than half of these major programs. Finance Committee and Ways and

---

Box 1.3 Key Health Committees and Subcommittees

1. Senate Finance Committee
   Subcommittee on Medicaid and Health-Care for Low-Income Families
   Subcommittee on Medicare, Long-Term Care, and Health Insurance

2. House Ways and Means Committee
   Subcommittee on Health

3. Senate Labor and Human Resources Committee

4. House Commerce Committee
   Subcommittee on Health and the Environment

5. Senate Appropriations Committee
   Subcommittee on Labor, HHS, and Education

6. House Appropriations Committee
   Subcommittee on Labor, HHS, and Education

7. Senate Budget Committee

8. House Budget Committee

Means Committee subcommittees are also important, usually wielding jurisdictional power over roughly a quarter of the health programs in the House and a third in the Senate. These committees plus a few others try to carve out a piece of any major health reform proposal. The House Rules Committee and the leadership must then find a way to put the pieces together.

Membership choices are always a tension when an individual's expertise and interest are not the same as that of the constituency the member represents. Members whose constituents are farmers are likely to feel they must be members of the Agriculture Committee even if their real interest is in health. They will seek to join both committees but are likely to spend their time and energy where their personal interests lie unless they are lucky enough to actually feel passion for the topic of paramount interest to their constituency. Former Portland, Oregon, Representative Edith Green, a one-time teacher, served on the Education and Labor Committee out of passion and on the (now defunct) Merchant Marine and Fisheries Committee out of a sense of duty and electoral advantage. She seldom attended meetings of the fisheries committee but was a key subcommittee chair and major mover and shaker on the Education and Labor Committee.

One result of the passion and district-interest motivations of committee members is that they are not typical of the Congress as a whole. Shepsle and Weingast called committee and especially subcommittee members "preference outliers" (1984, 345). Not surprisingly, this puts committee and subcommittee members in a difficult position. If they draft legislation to their own liking, it may not pass the house. The result: committees are often constrained in their actions by the expected reception on the house floor. They risk rejection if they report bills that deviate substantially from the majority's values. One of the jobs of an astute representative or senator is to become expert at anticipating the reactions of the chamber (Shepsle and Weingast 1987; Kiewiet and McCubbins 1991). Committees that too frequently do not correctly adjust to the prevailing political winds lose power (Fenno 1973). That some committees are more responsive to outside forces than others is usually explained by the salience or visibility and level of conflict of the issues assigned to them (Price 1978).

The observation that although "money isn't everything, it can be exchanged for everything" works in Congress, too. Those who play an important role in spending or appropriating federal dollars command power and respect. Most federal spending must be appropriated annually by the House and Senate Appropriations committees. The House Appropriations Committee usually takes the lead on budget actions, and even though its power was reduced in the 1970s with the establishment of the Budget Committees and the consolidated budgeting process, it is still a highly desirable committee. It offers opportunities for members to "bring home the pork" in the form of appropriations targeted to benefit programs and projects in their home districts.

Writing the Rules

Bills that make it out of Senate committees go directly to the floor, but most major House bills need an additional stop: the House Rules Committee. This committee decides the rules of floor debate for the bill, including whether or not amendments will be allowed, the level of detail at which sections of the bill must be voted up or down, and other aspects of the amendment process. The rule adopted by the Rules Committee can help or hamper the passage of the bill. Once the Rules Committee was a formidable barrier to a bill's progress. Democrats on the Rules Committee—over the objections of the Republicans on the committee—allotted only ten hours to debate the original Medicare bill, permitted no amendments, and required an up or down vote on the entire complex bill rather than allowing section-by-section votes. Disallowed by that rule were votes on amendments that might have passed, such as relating premiums to income. Members who wanted the bill but with changes had to vote for it "as is," or go home and explain during reelection why they voted against a popular bill.

Since 1975 the committee has lost its autonomy and is under control of the Speaker, who uses it to help the passage of bills by restricting floor amendments and giving majority party leaders the "opportunity to structure floor consideration of legislation in a manner that meets the needs of the party and of the standing committees that the party controls" (Smith and Deering 1990, 185). For the majority party, which can order amendments and bar amendments that would cause political difficulties, the rules can eliminate political heat and reduce the possibility of embarrassing votes on the floor (Rohde 1991). In the early 1990s there was much grumbling about unreasonable rules, even by Democrats. In 1993 a group of conservative Democrats, calling themselves FROGS (Fair Rules and Openness Group), five times voted with Republicans to defeat a leadership-sponsored rule, previously an infrequent event (Carney 1994). But it was the Republicans who complained the most and the most vociferously. Some 150 lawmakers and 200 challengers included the pledge for an open rule on the package of ten bills they promised to bring to the House floor in their "Contract with America" if Republicans could get control of the House. The following year they did just that. Critics asserted, however, that the new rules are not all that open, suggesting that openness is a matter of some interpretation.

Subcommittees

Since the mid-1970s, subcommittees have played an increasingly important role in congressional decision making. Typically, the Senate has more than eighty subcommittees and the House well over 100. Appropriations committees in both houses have the most, usually more than a dozen. Recent House rules limit the number of subcommittees to six, except for the Appropriations and the Reform and Oversight committees.

The proliferation of subcommittees, spawned in part by the 1970s reforms in the House, has led to a dispersion of power that has been called "the rise of subcommittee government" (Davidson 1981, 102). These subcommittees exercise veto power over new policies that threaten current beneficiaries or constituents, and as such are powerful players in the policy debate. A subcommittee bill of rights guarantees them staffing, explicit jurisdictions, recorded committee votes, and open sessions. No longer can the committee chair use the entire staff allocation to take friends to a Caribbean island, leaving subcommittees to fend for themselves, as did a House Education and Labor Committee chair in the 1960s. In 1979 Henry Waxman took advantage of then new election rules to challenge a member of greater seniority for the chair of the Commerce Health and Environment Subcommittee. To sweeten the pot, he gave some of his considerable excess campaign money to committee Democrats. He won.

Not wanting to rush such things, the Senate took another decade to reform itself, in part because it had less to do. Select and special committees were abolished in the mid-1970s. Limits were placed on the number of committee assignments each senator could have and the number of chairs a senator could hold. Staffing for minority members and computerized scheduling made things more balanced and brought the Senate into the modern age.

The two houses vary in the ways they use subcommittees. House subcommittees are heavily involved in legislating: holding hearings and amending or "marking up" (writing) bills. Full committees conduct their own markup but generally do not hold additional hearings. Senate subcommittees often hold hearings but frequently do not mark up bills. Markup is usually the province of the full committee. The reality is, however, that the subcommittee role varies so much from committee to committee in the Senate that it is hard to generalize. Judiciary Committee rules send bills first to a subcommittee unless a majority votes or the chair and ranking member agree to do otherwise. Finance takes the opposite default position (Smith and Deering 1990). The Senate Labor and Human Resources Committee retains jurisdiction over twenty-six major health programs at the full committee level. Its health subcommittee, active in the 1970s under Senator Edward Kennedy (D–Mass.), was eliminated in 1981 when Republican Orrin Hatch (R–Utah) took over as chair of the full committee. When the Democrats regained the majority in 1987, Kennedy was the chair of the full committee and did not reconstitute the subcommittee. (Neither did the Republicans when they took over the Senate in 1995.)

In the House the responsibility for health care policy frequently lies with the Commerce Health and Environment Subcommittee, not the full committee. Under the long Democratic rule, that subcommittee traditionally set its own agenda and picked its own battles, usually winning them. One exception was the major health reform initiative of the Clinton years. Neither the subcommittee nor the full committee was able to reach consensus on a bill. When the Republicans took control in 1995, the subcommittees, including the Health and Environment Subcommittee, were less powerful. The Republicans gave committee chairs more control over subcommittee agendas and staffing. The new House Commerce Committee chair centralized staffing and discouraged the subcommittees from drafting legislation until the leadership decided the direction it wished to pursue.

The relatively larger clout of House versus Senate subcommittees can be quantified. Smith and Deering (1990) found that 85 percent of measures brought to the House floor were first referred to subcommittees, compared to only 42 percent in the Senate. Eighty percent of those brought to the House floor were reported from subcommittees, compared to only 46 percent in the Senate.

A 1965 House member had to wait several terms to take over as a subcommittee chair. Only one-third of those first elected in 1964 chaired subcommittees by their fourth term, and only 7 percent were members of a power committee. Thanks to the House reforms, the large Democratic class brought in a decade later fared much better. Two-thirds were subcommittee chairs by their fourth term, and more than one-quarter sat on power committees. Of the thirty-one members serving their fourth term in 1994, more than 35 percent were members of power committees. Advancement to subcommittee chair or power committee positions, along with increased personal staff resources mean that members can exercise "real power" relatively quickly after their elections (Loomis 1984, 190). The system also encourages specialization and expertise, but it is not without problems. Subcommittee hegemony makes the task of leading the Congress more difficult and the task of influencing it more time consuming (see Chapter 3, Interest Groups). Institutional fragmentation contributes to the difficulties of producing comprehensive, integrative legislation (Rabe 1990).

Committee Turf Battles

Turf is a big deal among the committees, and one job of the chair is to fight hard to maintain responsibility for the committee's issues. In 1993 House Judiciary Committee chair Jack Brooks (D–Tex.) would not stand for turning over medical malpractice to the Ways and Means Committee; no matter that Ways and Means had already drafted and passed a reasonable proposal. Lawyers were his committee's turf, and he got the issue back. New chairs often see their ascension as a time to expand turf. When Paul Rogers took over the chair of the health subcommittee of the House Interstate and Foreign Commerce Committee in 1971, he changed its name from the Public Health and Welfare Subcommittee to the Public Health and Environment Subcommittee. He argued persuasively that the committee should have jurisdiction over nonfinance issues on national health insurance, at that time, within the province of the House Ways and Means Committee (Iglehart 1971). Four years later his subcommittee garnered jurisdiction over Medicaid (again from the Ways and Means Committee) and agreed to share jurisdiction with Ways and Means over Part B (physicians) of Medicare. In the Senate the Finance Committee maintains sole jurisdiction over both Medicare and Medicaid.

Turf expands when new issues come along. When the 1970s oil embargo sent energy to the top of the domestic policy agenda, the number of committees and subcommittees claiming jurisdiction over energy soared. When health care became the number-one domestic policy issue in 1993, fifteen committees not only claimed jurisdiction but also argued that they had been experts on particular aspects for years. Before health was front-page news, the eight committees in box 1.3 had been the recognized experts. Caught in the middle, First Lady Hillary Rodham Clinton testified before five committees in a single week, starting off with the suddenly health-oriented Education and Labor Committee, which claimed that since the Clinton health plan included employer mandates, it had jurisdiction. Its work was subsequently ignored by the rest of the House.

Some referral decisions are obvious, others are not so easy, and some get very complicated by the clashing of committee agendas and members' egos. Take major health reform legislation, for example. The Senate Finance Committee would obviously have jurisdiction over any tobacco tax attached as a revenue source as well as the other favorite target of money to pay for new health care initiatives—Medicare and Medicaid cuts. Yet who wants to just pay bills? When the Clinton reform package came along, Senate Finance's new chair, Daniel Patrick Moynihan (D–N.Y.), could see no reason why his committee should not take jurisdiction of the whole bill. So he did, arguing that premiums paid by businesses and employees to finance health reform are a tax. But Senator Edward Kennedy had always been Mr. Health Reform in the Senate, and he was not about to sit out the big one. His Labor and Human Resources Committee, the traditional health-authorizing committee, claimed jurisdiction over all nontax health issues, including any employer mandate, premiums, insurance policy–buying cooperatives, or insurance reforms.

Turf was not the only reason for the dispute, however. Senator Kennedy has been a friend of health reform for three decades. Senator Moynihan has long been an advocate of welfare reform. Highly unpredictable, he is likely to speak his mind. On a national Sunday news show, he questioned whether

health care was really a crisis, a question his party's president had already answered with a resounding "Yes!" The White House was not happy, but nonetheless was deferential. A fight with the chair of Senate Finance they did not
need.

Turf also means publicity when an issue gets hot. The Federal Emergency
Management Agency (FEMA), the agency that provides relief for (and receives enormous publicity during) disasters, is responsible to sixteen committees and twenty-three subcommittees. Committees want jurisdiction over
FEMA because when disasters occur, they want to be the ones under the Kleig
lights claiming credit for "a massive relief effort." In fact, the agency's annual
budget (below $1 billion) is nearly trivial by Washington standards (Segal
1994).

A few committees enjoy "jurisdictional monopolies," or exclusive authority over an issue. Typically, these committees work on issues of low salience
(Jones, Baumgartner, and Talbert 1993, 660). In that sense, they are exclusive
in the way of the old adage about some newspapers' "exclusive" stories—exclusive because nobody else wanted them. But the power of such committees
is real. With no one watching, such nonsalient committees can do much for
their members' districts and favorite causes; for example, they can direct a
veterans' hospital to be built in a city already oversupplied with hospital beds.

Conference Committees

Conference committees are ad hoc congeries of representatives from both
houses charged with the responsibility of reaching a compromise version of
the bill. Membership in conference committees, dubbed by scholars as the
penultimate power (Shepsle and Weingast 1991), is prized because the decisions made in conference are usually final. Conference committee language
cannot be amended: the houses must vote the whole bill up or down. Conference committees can rewrite or change the legislation, for example, by
choosing to "give up" items passed in their own house in favor of the other
house's language. Sometimes they add provisions out of whole cloth. Conferees are named by House and Senate leadership based on recommendations from committee chairs. Conference committees are usually dominated
by members of the committees that originated the legislation. Thus, as Shepsle
and Weingast said, "the conference is often a gathering place of kindred spirits rather than an instance of bicameral conflict" (1991, 202). Exceptions can
occur. For example, Senator David Durenberger (R–Minn.), chair of the

Senate Finance Committee's Health Subcommittee, was not even a conferee at the Medicare subconference on the 1985 reconciliation bill. Senator John McCain (R–Ariz.), sponsor of the bill to repeal the Medicare catastrophic program in 1989, was not named to the conference committee reconciling his bill with its House counterpart.

Conference committees can be quite large, especially when bills were considered by more than one committee. The 1989 conference on the savings and loan bailout had eight members from the Senate and ninety-four from the House, including all fifty-one members of the House Banking Committee. Since any agreement must have the majority vote of both houses, such a mismatch in numbers is not problematic. Sheer mechanics, however, may be difficult. Sometimes subgroups are named to deal with specific issues; sometimes conferees are limited to discussing only certain parts of the measure on which they are most knowledgeable; sometimes informal rump groups evolve into preliminary negotiating panels. On large conference committees, much of the work is done by staffs that conduct major negotiations among members on key issues.

Most Americans do not appreciate the formidable power of conference committees. Few are aware, for example, that the conference committee on the Employee Retirement and Income Security Act (ERISA) of 1974 inserted a preemption clause that has proved a major impediment to state-level health care reform. A few House conferees inserted language that preempted state laws relating to "any employee benefit plan" to replace language that prevented states from legislating about subject matter regulated by the act. An additional phrase said that no employee benefit plan shall be deemed an insurance company. The result: state insurance regulation over self-insured or corporate health insurance plans was prohibited. Together, the two provisions—added ten days before the final passage of the law without the knowledge of many health insurers, the Department of Labor, or state government associations—have withstood efforts in Congress and the courts for change and have played a powerful constraining role in state health care innovations (Fox and Schaffer 1989).

Similarly, a last-minute "surprise" in the 1988 catastrophic health insurance conference bill was a mandate that state Medicaid programs must pay all Medicare premiums, deductibles, and copayments for beneficiaries with income below the federal poverty level (Torres-Gil 1989). This provision was one of only two major initiatives not repealed the following year.

Conference reports get special treatment in their houses. They cannot be amended once conferees agree on the content. An up-or-down vote must take place on the negotiated version. The conference process, drawing members from the committees and allowing them to amend or veto floor action, strengthens the committee role in Congress and serves as "one of the foundations" of committee power (Shepsle and Weingast 1991, 214).

BUDGETING, WASHINGTON STYLE

Under the U.S. Constitution, Congress has the "power of the purse" embodied in the language that gives it the power to "lay and collect taxes . . . to pay the debts and provide for the common defense and general welfare of the United States." The Congress can also borrow money. The congressional allocation of resources gets to the basic political question of who gets what and who pays. Further, the budget not only represents a document of government operations but also is a statement of government priorities.

The legislative process is defined by two types of bills: authorizations, which establish or continue an agency or program, and describe its operations; and appropriations, which provide the funding for the agency or program. The two-part system is designed to separate the policy from fiscal decision-making. The process is generally sequential, with the authorization preceding the appropriation. Appropriations are made annually in the form of thirteen general appropriations bills, considered by the thirteen appropriations subcommittees in each house. These appropriations generally specify the money to be provided and the use for that money. Unless a program is funded by appropriations, it ceases to exist. Congress must vote affirmatively to increase the funding level of a program each year; it cannot grow automatically (Gilmour 1990). A third type of program is a combination of authorization and appropriation: entitlements.

Entitlements

Entitlements are guaranteed services that are provided to all recipients who meet the specified qualifications for the program. Entitlements are funded automatically and do not require appropriations. Entitlement spending makes budget control difficult. With no overall spending limit, the spending is determined by the number of eligible beneficiaries of the program who are legally entitled to the program funds. Social Security, Medicare, Medicaid, Food Stamps, Aid to Families with Dependent Children (AFDC), and agricultural

price supports are entitlements and are exempt from the annual appropriations process. In recent years entitlement programs were sometimes enacted as
a way for the authorizing committees to circumvent the appropriations committees (Gilmour 1990). Entitlements were also strongly supported by interest
groups benefiting from a cordial relationship with the authorizing committee.
Once an entitlement program is enacted, it can escape yearly evaluations and
can operate (sometimes in relative obscurity) with little congressional scrutiny. Many entitlements are indexed to the cost of living, so payments are
increased automatically without congressional action. Entitlements can be
curbed only by changing the law setting up the program or the regulations
governing its implementation. Other uncontrollable elements of the budget
are interest on the debt and outlays from prior obligations, largely related to
defense spending. In 1992 the uncontrollables totaled some $1.2 trillion—
nearly 80 percent of the total budget (Ornstein, Mann, and Malbin 1994).

In part because of its uncontrolled nature, entitlement spending is the largest and fastest-growing part of the federal budget. In fiscal year (FY) 1964 entitlements made up 24 percent of federal spending; in fiscal year 1996 they accounted for half of the total. Since 1964, entitlement outlays have risen at an
average of 12 percent per year. While the 1974 budget reform bill put an end
to any new entitlement programs without consent of the appropriations committees, existing programs were "grandfathered in," meaning they do not have
to comply with the appropriations review. The largest entitlement programs
are Social Security, Medicare, and Medicaid. Social Security alone accounts
for more than one-fifth of total federal spending; Medicare and Medicaid are
the next largest spending category at 17 percent (figure 1.1).

Between 1980 and 1990, Medicare spending increased by more than 200
percent; between 1990 and 1994, spending grew by 55 percent, to more than
$160 billion. Medicaid spending was slower from 1980 to 1990, but its growth
escalated sharply in 1990. It grew from $26 billion to $72 billion in the 1980s,
but rose from $72 billion in 1990 to $118 billion (federal and state) in 1993—
a growth of more than 65 percent in four years. Stanley Collender, Price Wa-
terhouse's budget expert, summed up the role of Medicaid and Medicare in
the entitlement picture as follows: "When you look at entitlements, controlling Medicare and Medicaid are the top five priorities, period" (Ratan 1993,
102). While Social Security is growing as well, its growth is much slower than
that of the two health entitlements. The escalation of entitlement spending
can be attributed in part to demographic factors, including the aging of the
nation's population, increased utilization, and automatic cost-of-living adjustments. Another problem is political.

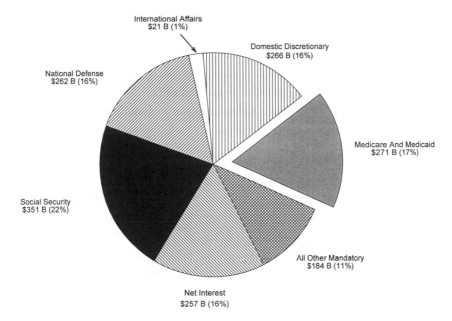

Figure 1.1 Federal Spending

Source: Data from Fiscal Year 1996 Budget of the United States.

Cutting entitlements is extremely difficult. Entitlements are popular programs, especially to the recipients. Elderly people, a major category of recipients, are well organized and quick to fight any possible cut in their programs. Means-testing Medicare, or requiring those who can afford it to pay a substantial portion or the full cost of their premiums, could save billions of dollars, but "no one wants to put them [elderly entitlements] on the table," said Representative Timothy Penny of Minnesota (Ratan 1993, 104). Nebraska Senator Bob Kerrey, cochair of a 1994 bipartisan commission on entitlement and tax reform, called entitlements "the political third rail" that politicians are afraid to touch (Shear 1994). Kerrey should know; his commission was split on what to do about entitlements and was unable to produce strong recommendations for reform.

The Congressional Budget Process

For the country's first 150 years, there was a surplus of funds, and federal spending—with the exception of military pay, equipment, and supplies—was relatively low. In the 1930s the federal budget began to grow as the government assumed new domestic responsibilities, including regulating business and providing for those temporarily or permanently disadvantaged. Presidential control over the budgetary process dates back to 1939, when the Bureau of the Budget (BoB) was made part of the executive office. In 1970 the BoB became the Office of Management and Budget, and its responsibilities expanded (see Chapter 2). The presidential budgetary power peaked in the early 1970s, when President Richard Nixon aggressively "impounded," or refused to spend, funds appropriated by Congress for programs he did not support. The 1974 budget act was passed in part as a response to congressional unhappiness over this increased presidential role. It was also enacted as a way to improve congressional control over the federal budget, thus allowing it to set fiscal policy and make choices among programs (Ellwood and Thurber 1977). The Congressional Budget and Impoundment Control Act of 1974 (Public Law 93-344) set up the House and Senate Budget committees and the Congressional Budget Office. It also mandated a concurrent budget resolution setting forth aggregate federal spending, which serves as a fiscal blueprint to guide authorizing, appropriating, and taxing committees. The act established a process known as reconciliation, designed to bring existing law into conformity with the budget plans. Table 1.2 outlines the congressional budget process in more detail.

The first decade of the new system was not generally viewed as a great success. Committees largely ignored the targets, and the Budget committees had little recourse to force compliance. In the early 1980s it became clear that something was needed to control governmental spending and reduce the burgeoning deficit. The deficit had doubled (from $1 trillion to $2 trillion) in the first term of the Reagan administration, thanks largely to a $600-billion reduction in taxes ($150 billion a year) and a $115-billion increase in defense spending.

The Balanced Budget and Emergency Deficit Control Act of 1985, better known as the Gramm-Rudman-Hollings act, was designed to force Congress to reduce the deficit. It mandated some $36 billion to be cut yearly from deficit ceilings until the deficit was zeroed out in fiscal year 1991. A new budget device, called sequestration, was developed that provides for across-the-board cuts, evenly divided between domestic and defense programs, to achieve the desired target if Congress fails to make these cuts on its own. One problem was that many large programs, such as Social Security, Medicaid, and AFDC, were excluded from the sequestration; others, such as Medicare, were subject to only limited cuts. The process could be "triggered" by the comptroller general of the General Accounting Office (GAO). When the U.S. Supreme Court declared this part of the law unconstitutional, Congress amended the

Table 1.2. The Congressional Budget Calendar

Date	Action
Between first Monday in January and first Monday in February	President transmits the budget, including a sequester preview report
Six weeks later	Congressional committees report budget estimates to budget committees
April 15	Action to be completed on congressional budget resolution
May 15	House consideration of annual appropriations bills may begin
June 15	Action to be completed on reconciliation
June 30	Action on appropriations to be completed by House
July 15	President transmits midsession review of budget
August 20	OMB updates the sequester preview
October 1	Fiscal year begins
15 days after the end of a session of Congress	OMB issues final sequester report, and the president issues a sequester order, if necessary

Source: Data from Fiscal Year 1996 Budget of the United States.

law to allow the OMB director to issue the sequestration trigger. The process set up by Gramm-Rudman-Hollings was the quintessential political answer to the problem of reducing the deficit because it did not rely on congressional action to reduce spending or raise taxes. Rather, the "process" caused the political pain, and no congressional vote could be pinpointed and used by opponents in later campaigns.

The budget process has been reassessed and revised several times since 1987, with presidential-congressional summits and several new provisions. The Budget Enforcement Act of 1990 established a binding five-year deficit-reduction plan, capped three areas of spending (domestic, defense, and international), and set up pay-as-you-go rules governing mandatory spending, including entitlements, and revenues. In 1993 the process was strengthened with the enactment of a "hard freeze" on spending, rigidly setting the amount of money that can be spent on nonentitlement, nondefense programs until 1998. The changes have produced a zero-sum situation for the Congress requiring those who want spending increases to offer counterbalancing cuts in other programs or new taxes. Those who want tax cuts must make cuts in entitlement programs because only entitlement cuts accumulate into future years to offset accumulation of revenue cuts. Campaign-promised tax cuts become very painful when victors realize they must first find offsetting savings by cutting fiercely guarded entitlements. The 1995 budget resolution, seeking to balance the federal budget by the year 2002 by cutting Medicare and Medicaid spending by $450 billion over seven years, was a case in point.

The Reconciliation Process

As it has evolved over the years, the budget process has weakened the power of authorizing committees and given more power to party leaders and members. Authorizing committees rarely have the opportunity to launch new programs, but rather must work hard to protect their programs from budget cuts. The appropriations committees have emerged strong in the 1990s, even though they have control over only about one-third of federal spending. In light of the spending caps, the appropriations committees are the venue for the tough decisions and as such have become the source of lobbying by interest groups and fellow members alike (Davidson and Oleszek 1994).

In the early 1980s the reconciliation bill, a compilation of legislative committee recommendations implementing the concurrent budget resolution, was used as a vehicle to enact new provisions and programs, and otherwise change policy. Its attractiveness was clear. Measures could become law with minimal attention and no hearings. They would likely sail through both houses, which were eager to vote to reduce the deficit. Thus, the FY 1982 reconciliation bill, known as the Omnibus Budget Reconciliation Act (OBRA), cut or eliminated more than 100 programs and formed six new block grants from existing programs. In FY 1983 the size and members' terms of the Interstate Commerce Commission were reduced. A 1987 rule, known as the Byrd rule (for the senior senator from West Virginia), limited inclusion in the reconciliation bill to revenue-related items. In 1993 ERISA waivers from several states were deleted from the reconciliation bill using the Byrd rule. Nevertheless, the system is far from airtight, illustrated by the fact that in 1989 a restriction on consumers' access to "dial-a-porn" services and a reinstatement of the broadcast fairness doctrine were included in the reconciliation bill.

The reconciliation bill is important to health policy. In the 1980s virtually every major piece of health legislation was in that bill. The formation of four new health block grants, changes in physician payment systems, expansion of home- and community-based care, and nursing home reforms were included in the reconciliation bill as a way to reduce spending. Interestingly, some provisions in reconciliation increased spending, especially Medicaid mandates to states to qualify women and children above the poverty level in the program. Representative Henry Waxman, then the chair of the Health Subcommittee of the Energy and Labor Committee, was a master at using the reconciliation process to achieve his goal of providing health care to near-poor women and children. Called the budgetary time bombs or, more poetically, the Waxman wedge, the strategy called for stretching out the spending so that it would fall mainly in later years not included in the budgetary ceilings (Morgan 1994, 8). For example, major changes liberalizing the coverage of pregnant women and children under the age of eighteen were phased in over a decade (budget resolutions typically project spending only three years).

Needless to say, the use of the reconciliation bill as a replacement for the authorization-appropriations process with extensive hearings and open sessions has changed the nature of health policymaking. Fuchs and Hoadley (1987) feel the reconciliation process has "quickened" the pace of deliberations, moved much of it behind closed doors, and curbed outside influence. They also note that as the decisions become more and more detailed and budget estimates more important, staff members have become increasingly important, especially the staff of the Congressional Budget Office, which provides the budget estimates now crucial to decision making. For example, second surgical opinions for Medicare were included in the 1985 reconciliation bill only after CBO provided an estimate that such a provision would save money.

The effect of the budget reconciliation process on congressional members is disputed. Fuchs and Hoadley (1987) believe that the process has given more power to the health experts, especially those on subcommittees who can use the expedited process of reconciliation to pursue their agenda. Certainly, using the reconciliation bill to impose mandates on states to expand the Medicaid program to pregnant women and children would support this view. On the other hand, Gilmour (1990) believes the process has taken away power from committee chairs and members, and given power to congressional members, through floor votes on reconciliation, and to party leaders, who work with committee chairs to formulate the budget targets. He argues that the budget process gives floor managers more control over committee chairs, who are forced to negotiate with party leadership and others. He points out that "the most important decisions made each year in Congress—about the nature of the budget policy and means of attaining it—have been made essentially outside the regular committee system, by the parties, caucuses, and bipartisan coalitions" (94). Gilmour says that budget politics is floor centered, in the sense that mobilizing a floor majority to pass a comprehensive budget resolution has become the most important action each year in Congress; moreover, this majority does not accept the choices presented to them by the committees. Rather, the resolution emerges from negotiations that involve large numbers of members.

Can both Fuchs and Hoadley and Gilmour be right? Yes, probably. Both sides agree that committees have been weakened. It is feasible that a few health experts (such as Henry Waxman) can use the system to get through seemingly incremental proposals with little scrutiny or public attention, and that the importance of the budget resolution is so great that all members can participate in coalitions to shape the final product passed on the House floor.

Most observers and scholars agree that the changes in the budget process coupled with the increasing size of the federal deficit have changed the focus of congressional priorities, to the point that one scholar says, "Congress has had little time to consider anything else" (Shepsle 1989, 260). Shepsle believes that assessing the various budget resolutions, reconciliation acts, proposals for deferrals and rescissions, and coordinating these moves with authorizing, appropriating, and revenue-raising actions, has "stretched Congress's capacity to act" (260). Ironically, Congress may be working harder and producing less. The odds that an introduced piece of legislation will pass have declined over the past half-century. A bill introduced today has about half the chance of success it would have had in the early 1950s (Ornstein, Mann, and Malbin 1994). Many factors go into explaining that statistic—rules changes, such as permitting co-sponsorship of bills, for example—but budget constraints are very limiting.

The new budget process may also have given more power to the executive branch, particularly in its ability to sequester funds. Many in political science would agree that executive control over the budget is an important and appropriate function. Yet the extent of the control and absence of public debate over important policy issues it entails affect the power balance between the branches (Spitzer 1993).

Finally, the 1993 "hard freeze" on spending put a major constraint on congressional policy options. No new spending can be undertaken without new taxes or cuts in an existing program. Many a "good" idea was abandoned in the health care debate of 1994 simply because it involved more spending. While many citizens might welcome such constraint, the members find that the budget rules dramatically restrict their room to negotiate and their ability to respond to constituents' needs.

LEGISLATIVE PARTIES

Few people argue with the statement that political parties in this country are weak. Crossover voting, split tickets, and the growth of voters calling themselves independent provide evidence that voters can no longer be considered stalwart partisans. Direct primaries, growth in PACs, and the increased role of media in campaigns have contributed to the weakened position of parties in recruiting candidates, and in funding and guiding their campaigns. The party in government—the role of the political party in organizing and overseeing legislative action—has also often been characterized as weak (Schlesinger 1966; Scott and Hrebenar 1979; Burns 1984). In comparison with their counterparts in the British House of Commons, for example, members of Congress do not vote in unified blocks to enact policies espoused in the previous election; majorities that coalesce are fleeting and ad hoc; and action can be stymied by small groups or strategically placed opponents.

Nevertheless, evidence exists that parties play an important role in defining and shaping the legislative product. Figure 1.2 provides a longitudinal look at party loyalty through legislative voting since 1965. Party votes, the percentage of votes on which a majority of Democrats opposed a majority of Republicans, are a measure of conflict or interparty disagreement. As figure 1.2 illustrates, party loyalty in the House has risen sharply since 1970. In 1992 a majority of voting Democrats opposed the majority of voting Republicans on 64 percent of the votes, a jump of 23 percent over the 1965 percentage. The Senate unity votes similarly increased substantially, from 42 percent of the time in 1965 to 53 percent in 1992 (Ornstein, Mann, and Malbin 1994). Overall, the partisanship in the Senate is lower than in the House. Recent party influence in committee votes surpasses that on the floor (although some committees are much more partisan than others) (Ward 1993).

The party unity trends can be explained by a variety of factors, including the increasing homogeneity of the population, effects of legislative reforms strengthening the role of party leaders, and the personalities and persuasiveness of party leadership. In fact, an argument can also be made that the disdain for electoral party loyalty might well lead to strengthened parties in the House and Senate because candidates need all the help they can get, and they can often get that help from their fellow party members. Rohde argues that members of Congress are linked to their party through their constituency (170). Where party constituencies are similar across the country, the positions taken by their representatives become more similar.

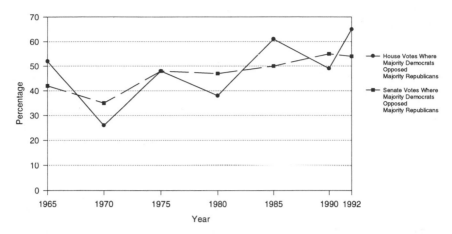

Figure 1.2 Party Unity Votes in Congress, 1965–1992

Source: Data from Ornstein, Mann, and Malbin (1994).

Wilson (1992) described three problems inherent in the congressional structure that political parties can help solve: problems of coordination, collective action, and collective choice. Parties and leaders can be focal points to coordinate individual members following sometimes similar, sometimes dissimilar interests. They can bind individual members to collectively desired goals that without parties would not be articulated or achieved. They can provide the stability necessary to prevent domination by individual members bound to highly variable districts. In short, parties can transform the actions of 535 independent agents into a workable, more focused institution with the opportunity to act in the public interest.

Party leaders in Congress play an important role in guiding the independent agents who make up the modern Congress. One proof is the time that party leadership spends conferring with members. According to the *New York Times,* Dick Gephardt, the House majority leader during the early 1990s, "does meetings." He meets with small groups of Democrats, large groups of Democrats, and individual Democrats. By meeting, and listening, he understands the positions of the members and is in a good position to build consensus and develop a meaningful political strategy (Toner 1994b, A7). Members who wish to be involved in party leadership can volunteer to be a party whip or to be active in the Democratic caucus; many are actively engaged in such activities. Most members' daily activities are much more dominated by party activities than in the 1970s when committee work occupied most of their time. In 1995,

Republican party leadership was more directive but still relied on task forces and informal groups of members for policy guidance and coordination.

What is the effect of this party resurgence? The effect is probably at the margins—but the margin is important because parties tend to take positions on major bills, and votes on those bills are more important than on more narrowly construed, less-salient measures (Sinclair 1989).

Legislative Behavior

Fenno's research on congressional motivations (1973) found that members of Congress strive to meet three goals: reelection, influence within the house, and good public policy. Individuals differ in how much importance they place on each. Someone secure in her district may prefer to try to gain influence or promote her idea of good policy. Mayhew (1974) argued that of the three, reelection underlies everything else. It keeps members accountable, and without reelection, the other goals mean nothing.

Members can, if they choose, focus on producing particularized benefits to their districts in the form of casework and federal funding for projects ("pork"). Or they can take the high road, trying to help enact good public policy that produces collective or generalized benefits. They can choose a committee membership that best meets their electoral needs, either a constituency-responsive, reelection-oriented committee (Agriculture or Interior and Public Works), a policy committee (International Relations, Energy, or Commerce), or a power committee (Appropriations, Rules, or Ways and Means) (LeLoup 1979).

For most, reelection is their proximate goal; in Mayhew's (1987) terms, a goal that must be achieved over and over to make everything else possible. Incumbency helps make that happen. Incumbents are overwhelmingly re-elected with margins that have grown increasingly larger in most elections in recent decades. From the mid-1960s through the early 1990s and beyond, members were rarely defeated, and changes were usually instigated only by retirement (Fiorina 1977)—reminiscent perhaps of Robert Audrey's dictum: "Where there's death, there's hope." Table 1.3 shows the percentage of incumbents elected in both houses and the margins of victory since 1965. Compared with the mid-1960s, reelection had been the expected outcome of House races—and with larger margins—until a recent downturn in the early 1990s, probably as a result of redistricting, anti-incumbent feelings, and fewer uncontested seats (Ornstein, Mann, and Malbin 1994). Even the 1994 election

Table 1.3. House Incumbency Trends and Reelections

Year	Number of Incumbents Running	Percentage Reelected	Percentage Reelected by at Least 60 Percent
1964	397	86.6	58.5
1966	411	88.1	67.7
1968	409	96.8	72.2
1970	401	94.5	77.3
1972	390	93.6	77.8
1974	391	87.7	66.4
1976	384	95.8	71.9
1978	382	93.7	78.0
1980	398	90.7	72.9
1982	393	90.1	68.9
1984	411	95.4	74.6
1986	394	97.7	86.4
1988	409	98.3	88.5
1990	406	96.0	76.4
1992	368	88.3	65.6
1994	382	90.8	62.2

Source: Data through 1992 from Ornstein, Mann, and Malbin (1994). Data for 1994 taken or calculated from *Congressional Quarterly Weekly Report* 52, no. 44.

that turned the House over to the Republicans for the first time in 40 years defeated only Democratic incumbents. Not a single Republican incumbent was defeated, leaving the percentage of incumbents reelected still quite high.

Nonetheless, evidence abounds that even incumbents with seemingly healthy electoral situations remain worried about reelection and may continue to support their districts. John Dingell, a member of Congress for more than forty years, who has not faced a tough election since 1964, remains vigilant, making no apology for putting forth every effort to support the auto industry. "That's what I'm sent here to do," he said (Duncan 1993, 13).

Members must respect the prospect of being tossed out, because it does happen. The best example was the 1994 election, in which scores of incumbent Democrats (including Tom Foley, Speaker of the House) lost their seats as voter dissatisfaction culminated in a political takeover of both the House and Senate. It was the first time the Republicans had control of the Senate since 1986 and the House since 1954. The fear of electoral loss helps keep members accountable and ensures that they will carry out the duties associated with re-election: advertising, credit-claiming, and position-taking. Advertising promotes name recognition and plants an image of personal qualities without the distraction of policy content. Credit-claiming paints the member as personally responsible for some desirable policy or program, including individual casework assistance, that brings specific benefits to the district. Federal agencies announcing grants phone the good news simultaneously to members so each can claim credit. Position-taking can range from votes on issues to speeches on the floor or at the Rotary Club, to letters to the editor in the local newspaper. As Mayhew put it, "the position itself is a political commodity" (1987, 23).

Fiorina (1977) argued that one of the reasons incumbents win is that they have mastered the art of using the federal bureaucracy to make them look good on pork barreling, casework, and leaning on the agencies on their constituents' behalf. Compared with lawmaking, these tasks are a cakewalk. They make constituents happy, and they are rarely controversial. Lawmaking, on the other hand, invariably makes some constituents mad, even when it pleases others. Members from politically heterogeneous districts take the most heat for their legislative positions. Fiorina argued that smart politicians have figured this out and choose to duck the lawmaking part more and more. Many have become masters at bringing home the pork. Oregon Senator Mark Hatfield, ranking minority member of the Senate Appropriations Committee, earmarked $90 million in Department of Energy and Health and Human Services (HHS) appropriations for the Oregon Health Sciences University, allowing it to build new buildings, hire prestigious faculty, and become more competitive with other health sciences units across the country (Zachary 1994).

Agency oversight, another task in the member's job description, is even less fun and noticed by very few. Not surprisingly, it often goes overlooked—except in dramatic cases or those with photogenic causes. Political scientists call the process "fire alarm" oversight whereby Congress generally ignores day-to-day oversight until there is a fire, when they bring out the fire trucks of highly televised hearings and accompanied by (often) heavily exaggerated accusations about violations of the public trust (McCubbins and Schwartz 1984). Hold an oversight hearing on the evils of smoking with a teenage movie star talking about her personal conviction not to smoke and the session has to be moved to the Caucus Room to hold the crowd and network television. Similarly, taking the agency head to task for excess spending or an unflattering evaluation will often prove appealing, especially to those of the party opposite the president. Much of this oversight is carried out by staff. When the cameras leave, so do the members. Day-to-day oversight is boring and mundane, and not sought out by members, such as the one who described oversight to Segal (1994) as complex and not very "sexy." In part this reflects the changing norms and expectations of members.

Norms and Change

Norms come in two types: general benefit norms, such as institutional loyalty, expertise, and hard work; and limited benefit norms, such as seniority, apprenticeship, and specialization, which reward primarily a small subset of powerful senators (Rohde, Ornstein, and Peabody 1985). In the 1960s every new member heard the advice a thousand times that the route to success in Congress was hard work and keeping quiet. Members were expected to serve an apprenticeship of a number of years before beginning to climb into leadership. The norms of behavior were as well known, and as closely followed as the Boy Scout's oath. Matthews (1960) called them "folkways" and described them for the Senate: apprenticeship, legislative work, specialization, courtesy, reciprocity, and institutional patriotism. Newly elected senators were expected to be workhorses, not show horses, and to do the highly detailed, dull, and politically unrewarding tasks that make up the Senate's work (Sinclair 1989).

By the 1980s the norms had changed. Apprenticeship was first to go as newcomers refused to find mentors and stand in their shadow. Subcommittee chairs or membership on a power committee could be expected quickly, especially in the Senate. Even first-year representatives started arriving with seasoned press agents to help make names for themselves and their committees through hearings, public appearances, and television interviews. The limited-benefit norms, seniority and specialization, also began to decline in importance. Junior senators now participate freely in Senate discussion both on the floor and in committee. Researchers in 1963 could classify only twelve senators in the Eighty-eighth Congress as generalists who offered amendments to bills from four or more committees. By the Ninety-sixth Congress, in 1980, that number had tripled to thirty-five (Sinclair 1989).

Expertise and hard work remain important, but the source of expertise has changed. Sitting through committee hearings is too inefficient for a generation raised on sound bites. Many now seek an infusion of knowledge from specialized staff and briefing visits from experts. Loomis (1988, 55) called this learning outside the "committee classroom." It appears to reflect the evolution of a new norm, which might be called participation or "playing the game." As Henry Waxman put it, "If you don't try, you've lost already" (Loomis 1988,

63). Evidently following this new norm, more than one-third of the members elected in 1974 managed a bill on the floor during their first session of Congress.

Does this mean the norms have vanished? Probably not, because loners still have a hard time. Cooperation and responsible behavior remain the way to make friends who can lend support when it is needed. Bernie Sanders, Vermont's only House member and the 103rd Congress's only independent member, found that he had to make common cause with Democrats: "The way this institution works is that you have to have friends" (Grover 1993, 17).

Expertise is still valued. Members who really know their topic and manage staff who are real experts can dominate their area of legislative interest. Senator Ted Kennedy of Massachusetts has shaped health legislation for decades. In 1991 his Labor and Human Resources Committee pushed fifty-four of its bills into legislation—the most for any committee since the heady Great Society days of the mid-1960s (Priest 1994).

ENTREPRENEURIAL MEMBERS OF CONGRESS

New norms, more staff support, opportunities for rapid advancement, press coverage, and diminished power of committee chairs have made it easier for what Loomis called "a new breed" of national politicians to be elected. They are issue oriented, independent, impatient, and savvy in the use of staff resources and the media (Loomis 1988). The new breed can be characterized as individual policy entrepreneurs, promoting policy issues unilaterally (Parker 1989). As Loomis put it, "More than any other single metaphor, the politician as entrepreneur captures the essence of how most top-level officials operate today, in or out of Congress" (Loomis 1988, 13). Shepsle and Weingast (1984, 349) said that "each house of Congress, more than at any time in history, now consists of members free to pursue their own electoral ambition, through service to constituencies, geographic or otherwise."

Congressional Staff

One of the reasons that members can follow the entrepreneurial path is that they are well staffed. No one would expect Congress to operate without an efficient and capable staff. As Congress began to take on more and more tasks and responsibilities through more committees and subcommittees, it began to hire more staff. Recent tallies exceed 30,000 employees who work for the legislative branch. Canada, with the next best-staffed legislative branch in the world, has about one-eighth of that total, fewer than 3,500.

Figure 1.3 shows the increase since 1965. The biggest growth has been in personal staffs, much of them in the member's home district where constituent services are performed. Two-fifths of the personal staffs of representatives and one-third of those of senators work in district offices (Ornstein, Mann, and Malbin 1994). Committee staffs have grown too, but at a lower rate. Support agency staff, a third type of staff important to the functioning of Congress, also has grown. Interestingly, when the Republicans initiated cuts in staff in 1995, it was the committee—not personal—staffs that were targeted. House committee staff was slashed by one-third, while the members' personal staffs were largely spared.

Personal Staff

Personal staffs link the member and the district. They keep the member in touch and, when the opportunity arises, make the pitch that the member is working hard on constituents' behalf. Personal staffs become expert on issues that the member may find boring but that concern constituents. They also offer expert advice on issues in which the member wants to "specialize." Personal staffs work with committee staffs on issues of concern to their bosses in roughly two stages. The first is a monitoring mode, in which the personal staff spends relatively little time keeping up with major issues likely to come before the committee. The second is a more active "cramming" mode, gathering information and getting help from committee staff and others to help their member prepare for deliberations.

As demands on members have grown, the personal staff has had to assume a greater role in policymaking. Staff members consult and engage in initial negotiations with one another, then with their bosses, to resolve conflicts. Staff members are expected to come up with new ideas; provide support for desired positions, draft language for proposed laws and press releases, and give advice on political issues. They are also the surveillance crew, on the lookout for issues that will garner media and public attention, whether or not a solution is viable. Not atypical was the experience of one personal staffer who was given the dates on which the member planned trips home. She was told to come up with a major policy proposal and draft a bill for him to unveil in a press conference on each return visit. She did, he did, and one

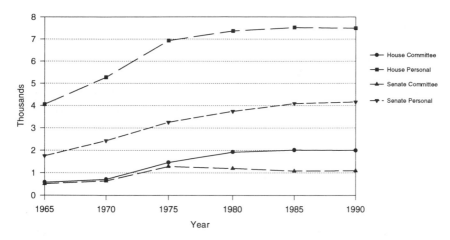

Figure 1.3 Growth in Congressional Staff, 1965–1990

Source: Data from Ornstein, Mann, and Malbin (1994).

Note: For personal staffs, the years reflected are 1967, 1972, and 1976.

of her ideas—a proposal to remove the requirement for a three-day hospital stay before Medicare home health care eligibility—became law.

Some people worry about these developments. Perhaps congressional staff members play too important a role in policymaking, particularly since they tend to be young, smart, and eager, yet generally inexperienced. "If people only knew how important decisions are really made, with exhausted staffers in their 20s sitting around a table at 2 in the morning, they would be very upset," confided one health staffer of a U.S. senator, referring to negotiations in the budget reconciliation packages. The comment is heard again and again.

A second concern relates to turnover. A study of congressional legislative assistants (LAs) found that in one five-year period (1977–1982), 95 percent of the LAs changed in the House and 91 percent in the Senate. Even these figures mask the extent of change, since the positions turned over more than once during that period in several offices. The 435 House offices had 888 changes of legislative assistants between 1977 and 1982 (Grupenhoff 1983). Women staffers came and went slightly more frequently than men; from 1977 to 1987, the average length of service for women was 2.63 years, while for men it was 3.05 (Friedman and Nakamura 1991).

Committee Staff

The expert staff work for committees. Their colleagues described them to political scientist David Whiteman (1987, 223) as "the people who really know what's going on." Whiteman found that on health committees a small inner core of one committee staffer and perhaps two or three personal staff were knowledgeable on dominant issues. Staff outside the core were better informed in the Senate than in the House.

House committee staff doubled between 1972 and 1976 as a result of the expansion of the number and importance of subcommittees. The Senate staff grew by about two-thirds. These differences in growth rate also reflect differences in the way the two houses use staff. Until 1995, House staff was decentralized, hired by and under control of the subcommittee chair and ranking minority member. Some Senate committees allow subcommittee chairs to hire their own staffs but others do not, preferring to use committee staff to assist the subcommittees. Several Senate committees do not have subcommittees or subcommittee staffs. Despite improvements, women still hold relatively few top positions on committees staffs. In a 1987 tally, they held fewer than one-fifth of the top staff positions in Senate committees (Friedman and Nakamura 1991). Parkinson's law applies to Congress just as it does to the bureaucracy: more work for Congress has led to more staff, which takes on more work. Committees hold widely publicized hearings and conduct in-depth investigations. Even confirmation hearings can lead to enormous staff involvement scrutinizing past actions, writings, and opinions as well as interviewing friends, associates, and relevant interest groups.

Staffs, of course, tend to reflect the personalities, styles, and political desires of their bosses, although Price (1971, 325) identified some staff as policy entrepreneurs that served as independent sources of policy initiation, reflecting "an interest more lively in some cases, than that of their bosses."

Though staff must trade in the currency of politics—loyalty—their degree of commitment to the cult of personality varies considerably. Typical is the staff of the Senate Commerce Committee. When chair Warren Magnuson (D–Wash.) was nearly defeated for reelection in the 1970s, the staff set out to remake him in the image of a consumer advocate. Consumerism, they figured, would sell well back in Washington state. That the topic also fit well with the staff's own interests was, of course, nice too. On the other hand, highly trained professionals are likely to be more blatant in pressing their own view of the public good, feeling that their primary commitment should be to the norms of their profession: economics, law, or social work. Salisbury and Shepsle (1981) added a third staff type: a politico, whose major concern is the career of the member for whom he or she works. Salisbury and Shepsle felt that the ranks of politico staff have swelled in the past two decades at the expense of the other two types.

Some worry that the staff are running the place. "There are many senators who felt that all they were doing is running around and responding to the staff. . . . It has gotten to the point where the senators never actually sit down and exchange ideas and learn from the experience of others and listen," said Senator Ernest Hollings, from South Carolina (Smith 1988, 282). "Sometimes when the members do talk, they find that they agree; it was the staff who disagreed." Staff are key in translating general congressional desires into legislative mandates. In the hours before the July Fourth weekend of 1994, both the Senate Finance Committee and the House Ways and Means Committee passed bills that contained sections with vague directions. Members fled to their districts or to the beach, leaving it to the staff to fill in the details and produce a coherent legislative product by their return to Washington (Broder 1994c). While the 1995 curbs in committee staffs may help counter this trend toward staff dominance, it is noteworthy that the cuts were not extended to personal staff—the source of major growth. Cynics might point out that it is personal, not committee, staff, that is most closely associated with the reelection of members, clearly an important concern for members of both parties.

Congressional Staff Agencies

Congressional staff agencies, what Martha Derthick (1990) called the congressional generalist staff, have also grown. In 1965 the Congressional Research Service (CRS), which researches and provides analyses of issues or problems, had 231 employees; by 1990 it had 864 employees. The CRS is not very visible to the public or even most policymakers, but it serves an important policy role in congressional decision making. Part of the Library of Congress, the CRS answers questions, provides information, and synthesizes research that is later used in a variety of congressional committee reports and members' speeches.

The massive General Accounting Office is much better known and has a much clearer impact upon congressional action and policy decisions. It has not grown as much as congressional staff and other staff agencies, partly because it is so well established and so big. It had roughly 4,300 employees in 1965 and had grown to only about 4,600 by the mid-1990s. Its fiscal year 1995 budget was $443 million. As competition from new policy analysis agencies made it look stodgy, it changed from a "green eye shade" agency dominated by accountants to an aggressive policy analysis shop staffed by lawyers, social scientists, and policy analysts. More than 80 percent of GAO's work is commissioned by Congress, usually in the form of a request from an individual member. It is required to do work requested by a committee chair and ranking minority member, and responds to requests from other members as resources allow (Pear 1990). It typically issues well over 1,000 reports and more than 4,000 legal rulings each year, claiming to save more than $20 billion a year in its advice to Congress (Pear 1994b).

Reports on flaws in long-term care insurance oversight by state insurance commissioners, problems with the quality of home health care, and the impact of Medicaid mandates on states are typical of the early, succinct, and provocative reports it issues. Between June 1990 and June 1992, it sent 182 reports on health to the Hill, on issues ranging from a survey of state policies on access to health care to recommendations on the distribution of maternal and child health block grants, from a description of worksite programs and committees on occupational safety and health to recommendations on federal action against health maintenance organizations (HMOs) violating federal standards. In that two-year period, reports on Medicare and Medicaid made up more than 20 percent of the total. Health financing and access accounted for 15 percent, and military and veterans health care for 12 percent of the GAO report total. A study in the early 1990s highlighting the small number of women in clinical trials sponsored by the National Institutes of Health (NIH) put the spotlight on the problem and resulted in a rapid increase in the funding of women's health issues, such as breast cancer (Miller 1994). But its primary mission is evaluation. It evaluates every major program enacted by Congress at least once, assessing the effectiveness of the program and making recommendations for improvement. When GAO talks, Congress listens; some two-thirds of its recommendations are adopted (Pear 1990).

Nonetheless it has critics. A nonprofit research group's study of its performance found that members of Congress increasingly felt it had been giving too many opinions along with its facts. "Some in Congress have expressed concerns . . . that GAO has on occasion moved too far in advocating policy, pushing into policy formulation more appropriate to elected officials," the National Academy of Public Administration study said (Pear 1994b). But the panel said Congress was as much at fault as the agency for encouraging findings tailored to the views of the requester. In 1995 a Senate Republican task force recommended cutting GAO by 25 percent.

In the 1970s two new and important congressional research arms were created: the Congressional Budget Office and the Office of Technology Assessment (OTA). Each is small, with approximately 225 employees at CBO by 1990, and fewer than 150 at OTA. CBO's mission and burgeoning importance make it seem certain to grow much larger. It provides Congress with cost estimates of every bill reported by a congressional committee, as well as estimates of the costs to state and local governments of federal mandates and laws, and forecasts of economic trends and spending levels. The CBO "mark," or how much money the agency thinks a proposed law will cost, is essential in determining the feasibility of a provision. Controversies between the OMB and the CBO frequently arise over whose estimates are correct. Congress tends to believe the CBO. The Clinton administration estimated its health care reform package would *save* nearly $60 billion over then-current spending. CBO said it would *add* nearly $75 billion to current outlays. CBO also settled an argument over whether employer-mandated premiums were taxes or private spending. To the administration's great consternation, CBO said they were taxes.

CBO cost estimates were pivotal in the subsequent hearings and debates over the health reform proposal. David Broder (1994c, A9) described the scene in the Ways and Means Committee markup in which every proposal made by a member would lead to a telephone call to a CBO analyst for a quick cost estimate. Most resulted in the proposal's elimination from consideration (or subsequent defeat) despite the member's plaintive protest, analogous to baseball hitters questioning a strike.

CBO cost estimates may also have contributed to one of the health care reform bill's most politically unattractive features: its level of detail (1,342 pages as it came from the president). A top White House official said CBO was at least partly to blame because it needed such details to improve the accuracy of its cost estimates. Many elements that might better have been left for regulation were part of the draft proposal, the official said, increasing its bulk and offering more targets for interest group opposition.

Technology, very broadly defined, is the business of the OTA. It works only for committees, not individual members. Its studies in health include a 1986 policy analysis of nurse practitioners, physician assistants, and certified nurse-midwives, and a 1990 study on health care in rural America. At times, looking at OTA reports, sorting technology from more-or-less routine procedures or standards does not seem all that easy. In 1995, as part of an effort to reduce spending, OTA was dismantled.

In the mid-1980s Congress set up two important research and advisory commissions in health care policy: the Prospective Payment Assessment Commission (ProPAC) in 1983 and the Physician Payment Review Commission (PPRC) in 1985. These agencies are small and nearly invisible to even the informed public eye, yet they can deliver a powerful punch. ProPAC is a seventeen-member expert panel of health economists, hospital reimbursement specialists, hospital financial management analysts, and related experts. Originally, ProPAC had the limited job of giving advice on implementation of the Medicare prospective payment system for hospitals. Like many other agencies, ProPAC's charge has broadened over the past few years. It now analyzes and drafts prospective payment policies for all Medicare facilities and services. It looks broadly at the effects of Medicaid hospital payment rates and, like many others, proposes changes that it hopes will stop the spiral of health care costs. A mid-1990s recommendation that Medicare graduate medical education payments go directly to training programs rather than through hospitals created a major controversy in the congressional debate over how to fund medical education.

PPRC is newer, established to give advice on Medicare physician payment reform. Its thirteen members, also experts in health economics and finance, were directed by Congress in 1988 to recommend policies to put the brakes on spending for physician services. Congress had grown tired of waiting for the executive branch to come up with answers (Oliver 1993).

Congress requests advice from PPRC on issues including medical malpractice reform, graduate medical education, physician supply issues, and the application of the resource-based relative value scale (RBRVS) to Medicaid, to name only a few. PPRC's "success" rate is high. RBRVS was one of its biggest successes. Early reforms to make RBRVS more acceptable to specialists and the decision to include volume performance standards were clearly traceable to PPRC's recommendations. The panel also oversees the implementation of federal law, reviewing experience with the Medicare fee schedule and volume performance standards, and recommending refinements. It was called on frequently for advice in the Clinton health reform debate and was asked to develop a national data system and to make recommendations to reform graduate medical education.

At a more practical level, both agencies give Congress political cover for some of the tough choices it must make to control health care costs. Members simply point to the commissions' recommendations and say they had no choice. Drawing outside experts into the inner circle as they do, these agencies serve that uniquely Washingtonian function of creating informal links among experts from various agencies and institutions of government. Despite the fact that the two commissions serve a congressional master, members rather frequently leave the panel to become high-level administration officials.

THE CONGRESSIONAL ENTERPRISE

Current and former congressional staff and congressional campaign workers who help develop and operate a political policy organization headed by the member have been called the "congressional enterprise" (Salisbury and Shepsle 1981). The turnover of congressional staff is so high that an alumni network can be the largest element of the enterprise. One indicator is that four years after the passage of the tax reform act of 1986, a *Wall Street Journal* reporter found that half of the staff involved in the passage of that act had become lobbyists. *The Washington Monthly* found that, of 170 former key congressional staffers, only five remained as staff; 115 had moved to the administration and fifty to lobbying or consulting jobs (Meacham 1993). Campaign staffs exist—unnoticed—as ongoing organizations, funded by PAC money and other campaign contributions (Loomis 1988). Yet they may play an important role in defining the policy persona of the member and especially for members of the House, provide ongoing political advice. At the center of it all sits the member of Congress, ready to respond to fax machine, phone call, angry letter, or delegation visit, passing on the request to an army of staff and supporters, tossing a bill in the hopper, or making a speech denouncing an agency ruling or promoting a new program.

How Members of Congress Make Decisions

Congressional decision-making is not easily dissected. The system is complex, including district preferences, interest groups' impact assessments, demands from party leadership, individual members' preferences, the characteristics of the issue on the table, and the distractions of other issues and demands for attention. Some have suggested that how members vote is not as important as where they put their resources and focus their energy. Back in the (what now seem to be) lazy days of the mid-1970s, a political scientist decided that time was "a House member's scarcest and most precious political resource" (Fenno 1978). Today's member is even more stretched—sandwiching committee introductions, votes, and responses to constituents in the few minutes when the member is not feeding the persistently yawning jaws of the campaign coffer or questing for thirty more seconds of media coverage. Grier and Munger (1993) concluded that reelection tops the list of activities that occupy their time.

Reelection also takes top billing in deciding how to vote. Only those in moderately safe seats enjoy the privilege of frequently pursuing other goals, such as enhancing their influence in Congress or producing good public policy (Arnold 1990). Members do a type of personal impact assessment to answer two questions: How will this decision enhance the chances for reelection? How might it be used against me by opponents?

Sometimes the answer may be to vote yes and no: No to add a provision to a bill, yes to report the bill to committee. No to a rule permitting no amendments, yes to crippling amendments if the member wants to kill the bill. Yes to recommit the bill to committee, yes to substitute another bill, no to a motion to cut off a filibuster. Yes on a vote to postpone the final vote, no on a voice vote to pass the bill, but yes on a final roll call vote that may be reported back home.

Arnold (1990) argued that members vote in ways that reflect both current and "potential" preferences of constituents. They anticipate what the voters will think and how voters will interpret an issue and an action, then respond accordingly. Constituents are not equally informed. Only a few can be called "attentives," those who have opinions about a policy, know what Congress is doing, and communicate those opinions to their legislator. Interest groups affected by the policy are part of this attentive public. "Inattentives" have no preferences and no knowledge of congressional activity. To make a decision, Arnold (1990, 84) said, a legislator needs to

—identify all the attentive and inattentive publics that might care about a policy issue;
—estimate the direction and intensity of their preferences;
—estimate the probability that potential preferences will be transformed into real preferences;
—weigh all these preferences according to the size of the attentive and inattentive publics;
—give special weight to the preferences of the legislators' consistent supporters.

Conflict can lead to different decision-making strategies. Kingdon (1977) believed that a member will implicitly ask whether there is any controversy in the issue. No controversy means vote with the consensus in the member's "environment" of party members, ideological companions, predispositions, and constituency. In the face of controversy, Kingdon believed the member subsets the environment into the most critical factors: constituency, party leadership, and fellow members. When these three conflict, the member will most likely vote with the constituency. The reality is that on many issues, the constituency is uninterested or uninformed. This leaves the choice between party and policy goals. From that set, the member will most likely choose the policy goal.

The saliency or visibility of the issue in the press and with the public also plays a key role. On highly salient issues, the constituent role is the dominant decision-making criterion. For low-saliency, complex issues of little broad public concern, policy or party considerations are more important.

Policy content is also important. Clausen (1973) described it in terms of a dimension, such as more or less government or saving money. The member's other decisions flow from this initial view of the policy content. Health issues tend to be viewed in an ideological manner, affected by the framing of the problem. Mueller (1986) examined nine health policy votes in the House of Representatives between 1973 and 1980 and found that ideology (measured as conservative coalition support) was the most important explanation of health policy voting behavior.

Finally, personalization is important to congressional decision making—what Browne (1993, 22) called the "I Know a Man Theory." Browne's example is a former Senate Budget Committee staffer who said when the time to make a decision came, a member of the committee would say something like, "On the contrary, I know a man from Illinois . . .," and language would be drafted to avoid that man's problems.

Though legislators prize their own decision-making prowess, they are also affected by the positions of respected colleagues, and to get their own bills passed, they need to be owed some favors, bargaining and exchanging votes with them. Bargaining includes more than just vote trading, which also goes on. It can include compromising on a $1.5 billion appropriation rather than the $2 billion the member might have preferred. With the severe budgetary restraints now in effect in Congress, "logrolling," or exchanging support for another's bills, tends to be in the form of equalizing sacrifices rather than distributing rewards (Davidson and Oleszek 1994). Bargaining is also constrained by the size principle: the bargainer will bargain only as much as necessary to produce a minimum winning coalition, and no more (Riker 1962).

Congress at its worst may also be Congress as a collective body. Clearly it seems to suffer from the classic "tragedy of the commons" problem. Individual decision making puts district interests first, as in "that's what I'm here for." Collectively, that may break the budget and hurt the country. Davidson and Oleszek (1994) referred to this situation as the conflict between the two congresses: the Congress of individual wills or guardian of constituents' interests, and the Congress of collective decisions. Several institutional mechanisms exist to mitigate this problem, including the newest one, the president's enhanced rescission authority, a type of line item veto. If working as planned, individual members of Congress are discouraged from adding items to the legislation that the president is likely to veto because few particularized benefits will hold up to a two-thirds vote requirement for veto override. Of course, chief executives can and do make promises not to veto certain items in exchange for cooperation on things important to his own agenda. Since the president represents a larger constituency, these items are more likely to be of a general benefit nature. But when such horse trading is involved, they are probably not everybody's idea of a broad benefit.

Several other mechanisms remain important motivators. First, budgetary restrictions force Congress to look at overall totals and hold down spending. Arnold (1990, 142) argued that legislators will rise above their district's concerns and vote for general benefits over particularized ones under certain circumstances:

—the general costs or benefits are salient to a large number of citizens;
—these general effects can be easily traced to the member's vote, permitting credit taking;
—the costs to the district are small.

Second, in tough, targeted decisions that can adversely affect a member's district, mechanisms can be adopted essentially to release Congress from the decisions through delegating authority to a commission named by the Congress but with independent decision-making authority. One of the more successful is the base-closing commission, a bipartisan commission with the authority to close military bases. The list produced by this commission is given to the Secretary of Defense, who has the authority to close the bases. The only formal way Congress can intervene is to pass a joint resolution blocking the entire package, but pressure on the Secretary of Defense to delete some bases from the list continues to be an informal way that Congress tries to protect its own. Recent congressional commissions on Social Security, the budget, and entitlements were told to make tough choices in the public interest, but they were weaker in the sense that their recommendations were not as automatic as those of the base-closing commission. In at least one instance, the PPRC has remained to oversee the implementation of the policies it proposed and Congress enacted.

Finally, Congress can pass the decision on to the bureaucracy, forcing it to make the tough choices Congress cannot. When Congress could not decide whether to include atomizers and nebulizers in a list of equipment to be rented (rather than purchased) under Medicare, it asked HHS to make the choice (Brinkley 1993).

Congress and the Press

The press plays a key role in the packaging of the modern member of Congress. The number of reporters covering the Congress has soared in recent years to more than 4,000 (Loomis 1988). These media representatives are extremely responsive to the actions and reactions of the member and provide almost universally positive coverage. Reporters representing local newspapers, particularly those in small or medium-sized cities, are generally uncritical and unwilling to examine issues in depth; whatever the member says must be true. Local television stations are similarly happy to have video feeds from their members, even those produced by the party's own camera crew, often featuring the member's press secretary asking the "probing" questions. For members primarily concerned with reelection, local coverage is more important than national exposure. Kansas Representative Dan Glickman said, "I can be on Tom Brokaw but it is not as important to my reelection as being on the NBC affiliate in Wichita" (Benenson 1987, 1552). Cokie Roberts, a longtime congressional correspondent for public radio, felt that the emergence of local television "has made some members of Congress media stars in their hometowns and has done more to protect incumbency than any franking privilege or newsletter ever could" (1990, 94). Especially for House members, who control the local media to a far greater extent than senators, the president, or governors, there is an apparent symbiotic relationship with the local press: the press gets the story and the members, positive exposure. According to Loomis (1988, 81), "In a fragmented Congress where information is often at a premium, media representatives and legislators regularly help each other perform their jobs."

The national press, a harder "sell" for many members of Congress, can also be useful if the member is more concerned about influence in the Congress or national public policy (or running for national office at a later date).

"Visibility leads to credibility," said California Representative George Miller (Loomis 1988, 77). The plethora of talk shows and the advent of C-Span have brought the names and faces of once-unknown members into living rooms across the country and into those of their colleagues. Members can use the media to enhance the importance and improve public knowledge of favored issues and perhaps persuade viewers to support their position. National media coverage can also serve to help build winning coalitions and inform colleagues, the White House, and top-level bureaucrats. It can enhance the legislator's career, as Speaker of the House Newt Gingrich and Texas Senator Phil Gramm discovered. Both have made themselves available to the media with snappy quotes and a willingness to speak on a range of issues. While known primarily for his deficit-reduction efforts, Senator Gramm has also appeared on national television on issues ranging from family values to health care, unemployment to international affairs (Georges and Boo 1992).

This media-oriented environment not only has affected the behavior of members already elected but also has perhaps its greatest effect in attracting a new kind of member—one who is photogenic and fast on his or her feet. Television personalities, movie stars, and sports heroes have successfully used the media and their experience with it to win primaries and seats in the Congress.

Jacobson (1987) concluded that the media, taken together, have not done much to damage the members of Congress but have damaged the institution of Congress, at least a little. When an announced Senate candidate appearing on a Sunday television talk show calls the chair of a Senate subcommittee "misinformed" on the president's health care proposal, which his staff helped draft, both attacker and attackee are diminished in the process. Kansas Senator Nancy Kassebaum noted that news media coverage "can make the outlandish claim and the fervent war cry seem to be the most effective tools for a successful campaign for or against an issue. The frequent victim of such tactics is effective government, the ability and the willingness to accommodate and shape a consensus" (Cohodas 1987). The confrontational style encouraged by the media may stir the fires of a cynical and dissatisfied public viewing audience.

Finally, the broadcasting of congressional hearings and floor action by C-Span has provided the public with access to congressional decision making and offered the member another way to get name recognition and attention. It has also helped improve the feeling of efficacy, at least of some avid viewers. It is not unusual for viewers to call up the staff of members, advising them on what arguments their bosses should make or providing corrections for misinterpretations or misstatements on the House floor.

THE MODERN CONGRESS AND
HEALTH POLICYMAKING

In 1965 the executive branch was the primary source of legislation, the few congressional staff were largely long-time friends of the member, there were several hundred lobbyists, and a few committee chairs were the dominant players. Today the Congress has no need to wait on the executive branch for ideas or expertise. In a town where power is everything, Congress has the most. "The Imperial Congress" or "King Kong of Washington's political jungle" was how long-time political player and former health advisor Joseph Califano Jr. put it in 1994 (40). Yet clouds hover over the congressional parade.

Despite the tendency to send incumbents back to the House and Senate (with the glaring exception of *Democratic* incumbents in 1994), Americans were also willing to express their dissatisfaction with their officials and their government. In 1993 less than one-fourth of the public said they could trust Washington to do what is right all or most of the time—a drop from three-quarters in the year Medicare passed (1965). Only 30 percent of the public approve of the job Congress is doing (Abramson and Pearl 1993).

Some feel the congressional process has debilitating weaknesses, particularly the decentralization and the shared power that it entails, which limit the role of Congress as key policymaker. Ippolito (1981) believed that Congress's capabilities are modest because it has its greatest difficulty in providing comprehensive policy leadership, something the liberal policy agenda of the 1970s assumed, incorrectly, it could provide. Indeed, in health, in the spring of 1994, it was easy to discount key votes in the Ways and Means Health Subcommittee, since they were only the beginning of the process that would include hundreds of votes by more than a dozen committees and subcommittees. The answer to the question "Who's in charge?" was not clear.

Ideology has also played a role in congressional action in health (see Chapter 7). In 1994 the 90 staunch members supporting a single-payer system, led by Washington Representative Jim McDermott, were at one end of the Democratic ideological spectrum. At the other end were Tennessee Representative Jim Cooper and Louisiana Senator John Breaux, whose more incremental, go-slow approach fit well with a bipartisan appeal. The unenviable task of the House and Senate leadership was to "hold" the Democrats, a task made more difficult by ideological issues, such as abortion. Democratic House leaders were promised by 35 Democrats that they would never support any health reform bill that included abortion. Some 70 Democrats promised to vote against any health reform bill that omitted abortion. As McDermott put it, "Peeling off 40 votes in here is not very hard" (Toner 1994b, A7)—or conducive to reform.

Finally, the issue of comprehensive health care reform is difficult for a relatively decentralized, independent body of 535 members to tackle. It is salient, complex, and affects nearly everyone. There are few places to hide from constituents or concerned interests. While there stand to be some winners in most proposals, the likelihood is that more groups, and constituents, will lose. Interests resist delegating too many details of such important policy to the bureaucracy. The comprehensiveness of health policy, however, allows the Congress many venues to claim credit and declare victory. In other unlikely areas, such as tax reform in 1986 and welfare reform in 1988, the Congress bucked the notion that nothing could be done and made major policy change. The tax reform case, in which public discontent and bipartisan support were key, may be particularly instructive in strengthening the congressional backbone. In cases where it feels it must, Congress does act.

2

The Presidency

A LOOK BACK

1965

ON 27 JULY 1965 President Johnson and his cabinet assembled for their twentieth cabinet meeting and congratulated themselves heartily. Medicare had just come out of the House-Senate conference, and final passage was hours away. The voting rights bill was right behind it in conference, with agreement expected within the week. The landmark Elementary and Secondary Education Act had become law in April, and the War on Poverty was a year old. In all, thirty-six major pieces of legislation had been signed into law by the time of that twentieth cabinet meeting; twenty-six others were moving through the House or Senate.

Tom Wicker, writing in August 1965, said, "They are rolling the bills out of Congress these days the way Detroit turns super-sleek, souped-up autos off the assembly line" (Johnson 1971, 323). There was an activist president, elected with 61 percent of the popular vote, and a heavily Democratic Congress (68 percent in both the House and the Senate). There was also strong public support. Although in the fall of 1965 Johnson sensed "a shift in the winds" or a fading of public support for change (reflected in some congressional calls for a slowing down of legislative action), he pushed forward, largely through the work of ten task forces, each on a critical area of need.

By the end of the year, major laws had been enacted dealing with issues ranging from higher education to the formation of the Department of Housing and Urban Development (HUD), from law-enforcement assistance to manpower training. Of these laws, seven were in health (Medicare; heart, cancer, and stroke program; mental health; health professions; medical libraries; child health; and community health services) and four dealt with the environment (clean air, water pollution control, water resources council, and water desalting). But at the top of the list, and the one Johnson and others considered the premier issue of that year, perhaps of his term, was Medicare.

In 1964 President Johnson had been very disappointed that Medicare had failed to pass the House, after its success in the Senate, and he was determined that the Ways and Means Committee should not bottle up the measure again. He worked closely with House leaders, encouraging them to change the ratio of the Ways and Means Committee to reflect the Democratic majority in the House, thus adding two crucial seats. He asked the leadership to designate Medicare HR 1 and S 1, indicating they were the first bills introduced in both houses, symbolizing its importance. He highlighted Medicare in his State of the Union message on 4 January and in a special message on health. When consulted on a compromise proposed by the Ways and Means chair, Johnson enthusiastically supported any reasonable move "to get this bill now" (Johnson 1971, 216). He met personally with House and Senate leaders following the favorable recommendation of the bill by the House Ways and Means Committee. When the bill passed the Senate, Johnson called it a "great day for America."

1981

The situation facing Republican President Ronald Reagan in his first year after election was not as rosy as that enjoyed by Lyndon Johnson sixteen years earlier. While Reagan's winning margin was substantial (by nearly 10 points over incumbent Jimmy Carter), he faced a Democratic majority in the House and a slim (53–46) Republican majority in the Senate. Nevertheless, Reagan, like Johnson, moved quickly. In his first nine months in office, he helped push through major domestic budget and tax cuts, and a massive defense buildup. One of his greatest achievements was the passage of much of the administration budget and program reform package in the OBRA of 1981, which consolidated twenty-one health programs into four block grants: primary care, maternal and child health, preventive health and health services, and alcohol, drug abuse, and mental health. The consolidation included a reduction in federal dollars of 21 percent for the programs over the previous year's funding (Feder et al. 1982).

By the fall of 1981, the congressional tide had turned. The Congress was less enthusiastic about the administration's cuts and approved only half of those proposed. By February 1982, even the Republican-dominated Senate Budget Committee rejected the administration's budget, which was defeated 21–0 two months later (Salamon and Abramson 1984). Yet in those early months, some argue that the long-standing principles governing social welfare policy in this country were questioned, if not revised. The administration felt that public welfare should focus on only those who were unquestionably unable to care for themselves. For those who were marginally disabled or less needy, the approach was to reduce or eliminate benefits, and encourage them to work or seek help in the private, not the public, sector. In health, President Reagan's philosophy encouraged less government and had the effect of promoting the idea of market competition and the provision of services by the private sector.

1993

The political climate surrounding newly elected President Bill Clinton was inauspicious. He was the governor of a small state, with limited Washington experience. Elected with only 43 percent of the vote, he clearly lacked any "mandate." He had what one writer called the "worst first week of any President since William Henry Harrison who caught pneumonia while delivering a long Inaugural speech and died a month later" (Blumenthal 1994, 36). There were problems with nominees for attorney general and enormous opposition to changes in policy on homosexuals in the military. Yet the Congress he faced was seemingly sympathetic—with Democratic majorities of 60 percent in the House and 57 percent in the Senate. This president was enthusiastic and diligent in his efforts to court the Democratic members of Congress in his first year of office, making trips to Capitol Hill and inviting members individually and in groups to accompany him jogging, ride on Air Force One, attend meals or a movie screening, to the point that "few on the

Hill . . . managed to escape a talk with Clinton" (Blumenthal 1994; 38). Early successes were a difficult budget vote (by two in the House, one in the Senate), ratification of the North American Free Trade Agreement (NAFTA), legislation on family and medical leave, earned income tax credit, and national service. In his first year, his presidential success rating as measured by the *Congressional Quarterly* was 86.4 percent—the highest for a president in his first year since Lyndon Johnson's 88 percent in 1964. (The score reflects presidential victories on votes on which the president took a position. It combines major and insignificant bills and reflects the position of the president at the time of the vote.)

Like Lyndon Johnson, Bill Clinton worked the Congress to promote his health care agenda, but unlike Johnson, he also used television in what has become known as the town meeting format, in which citizens ask questions of the president in an informal setting. After a highly publicized appearance before a joint session of Congress in September 1993, the real "selling" of the program began. Hillary Rodham Clinton made five televised congressional appearances and had interviews with five network reporters. The president answered questions about his health care proposal for two and a half hours on a popular network news show, conducted a town meeting in California, invited two dozen newspaper reporters to lunch, and allowed fifty-five radio talk-show hosts to broadcast live from the White House lawn (Kelly 1993).

But Clinton faced many more obstacles and had fewer resources than did Johnson. Both were Democratic presidents dealing with Democratic Congresses, but the nature of the relationship was starkly different. Members of Congress in 1994 were a largely independent enterprise and could raise their own money and strike their own deals. Another "plum" from the Johnson era and before—presidential support and appearances in congressional campaigns—was of little use when the president's public support reached a low of 37 percent (as Clinton's did before the midterm elections), and there were relatively few calls for campaign appearances. The party leaders, while Democrats, had less power than those of the 1960s, and were unable to deliver votes or coerce many votes from party members. With the advent of the Congressional Budget Office, the president's own numbers—on the cost of health care reform, for example—were questioned and discounted in favor of those of the less partisan CBO.

The interest group world into which President Clinton's health agenda was thrust also varied enormously from that of the mid-1960s. In 1993 interest groups used strategies to mobilize their members and sway public opinion in ways that only one or two powerful groups could have mustered in

Johnson's time. President Clinton's "bully pulpit" was shared, at least in part, by fictional characters, Harry and Louise, developed by the Hospital Association of America and wildly successful in framing the public debate on health care reform. Interestingly, Harry and Louise apparently made their biggest initial impact on Washington rather than on the people back home. When the Clintons began to refute and parody the ads, they gained more legitimacy and standing (Clymer, Pear, and Toner 1994).

Finally, President Clinton faced budgetary constraints unlike those confronting any other modern president. In the summer of his first year in office, the Congress imposed strict spending limits, freezing discretionary spending at the previous year's levels with no allowance for inflation. Under the agreement, any new spending must be offset by spending cuts and/or revenue increases. To make up for inflation and add money for priority initiatives, such as health care, Clinton was forced to cut back hundreds of programs. It was a far cry from the days of earlier presidential power. Bill Clinton, the president with an activist agenda topped by health care reform as the defining element, was relegated to near-observer status in the spring and summer of 1994 when the legislative drafting set about in earnest.

OVERVIEW OF PRESIDENTIAL DECISION MAKING

The presidency is the institution of executive power in the United States; the president is the person who exercises that power for a limited period of time. While many young boys and girls (and their parents) may aspire to be president, few achieve it, and those few are closely watched, examined, and analyzed, especially in recent years. Yet, as Jones (1994, 281) pointed out, the American presidency "carries a burden of lofty expectations that are simply not warranted by the political or constitutional basis of the office." As Jones and others indicated, the president is one institutional player among many in the crafting of national public policy.

The president's primary policy-making role is putting items on the agenda. When a measure is introduced in Congress, his role shifts to one of monitoring and encouragement. The president's margin of victory, popularity with the public, and dominance of his party in the Congress make up what is known as political capital, which is an important factor in his ability to persuade Congress to adopt his desired programs. Presidents like to "go public," or take their case to the American public in the hope that the public will then pressure their congressional members to support the president's policy. In 1994 going public was not a successful route for President Clinton; strong interest groups invested in advertising to inform the public on issues not to the president's liking. The press coverage of presidents is massive and can be helpful, but it can also prove problematic. The president is responsible for overseeing the executive branch, a task that many presidents do not like, but some try to use to their advantage. The president's most significant role in health policy has traditionally been in putting health issues on the national agenda and urging public support for adoption by Congress.

Presidential Power

The founding fathers were leery of giving presidents too much control—their experience with kings and their henchmen convinced them that control vested in one individual was not to their liking. Yet they were also fearful of the "impetuous vortex" of the legislative branch and wanted to prevent "legislative usurpations" as well (Hamilton, Madison, and Jay 1961, 309). So they set up a system of balanced powers with three branches of government, each providing a check to any overzealousness of the others. Since the ratification of the Constitution, the struggle between the Congress and the president over control has been waged almost continually, with some presidents exercising strong leadership, and others acquiescing to a more dominant Congress.

The president personally embodies most of the power of the executive branch (compared with Congress and with the judiciary, which is highly decentralized and dispersed). This gives the president power because he can act more quickly than other branches and can be the focus of press attention, thereby focusing the attention of the entire nation on a particular problem.

The president is the only person (except for the vice president) elected to represent the nation as a whole, thus having a national constituency. The president represents all of the people and is the personification of the national interest. In the development of policy, the president's concerns for the broad national interest can conflict with the more specialized congressional concerns focused on the costs and benefits of policies to their local constituencies. Department of Health, Education, and Welfare (HEW) Secretary Caspar Weinberger in 1973 referred to this difference when he defended the administration's call for cuts in health programs, saying that while the administration's proposals to scale down the federal health establishment might hurt special interest groups, the presidential proposals reflected the interests of the American people, implying that Congress was responsive only to interest groups (Iglehart 1973). President Nixon himself was equally pointed when he said in his 1973 inaugural address, "I am going to stand for the general interest" (Marini 1992, 116).

Another way to look at the president is a bit more narrowly—that he represents the 200 million or so Americans who are not directly represented by lobbies of some sort. Representing these Americans was the role President Truman ascribed to himself in a television interview with Edward R. Murrow in 1958 (Bolling 1964, 132). President Clinton seemed to be appealing to these Americans as well when he said in August 1994 that his White House was really "the home office of the American Association for Ordinary Citizens" (Wines 1994, A9).

Presidents are a symbol for the country as a whole, and people sleep better when a president they trust is watching over the country (Kernell, Sperlich, and Wildavsky 1975). Journalists focus Washington coverage on the White House, and even scholars highlight the power and leadership in the office of the president. Presidents themselves encourage their identification with the nation and the national interest in their speeches and addresses (Hinckley 1990). In his emotional speech upon resigning the presidency, Richard Nixon drew on this bond, which he called "a personal sense of kinship with each and every American" (Price 1977, 348).

Yet the president soon learns that promoting unity in the face of the basic pluralism of the American political system is extremely difficult. Much is expected—often too much. Louis Brownlow (1949) noted that to whatever else a president new to the White House may look forward, he will, if he is wise, realize from the first moment that he is certain to disappoint the hopes of many of the members of his constituency who collectively compose the nation.

The public-presidential relationship can be tenuous: useful when presidential popularity is high, more problematic when it is not. Further, as President Clinton found in 1994, other groups also have access to the public and can use television and newspaper advertisements to raise questions about key presidential proposals and goals.

Presidential Roles

The president is clearly the most visible governmental official in the land. Television appears to cover nearly every move he makes—even jogging stops at fast-food restaurants, helicopter trips to a forest getaway, and attendance at church worship, parental funerals, and Parent-Teacher Association meetings. The formal speeches, press conferences, and state dinners are well covered by the press and closely followed by many others. Yet the presidency is more than a photo opportunity or dress-up dinner. The president must lead. But how? And in what direction?

Cronin (1970) described three overriding functions of the presidency: to recast the nation's policy agenda in line with contemporary needs, to provide symbolic affirmation of the nation's basic values, and to galvanize the vast machinery of the government to carry out his programs and those he has inherited. In so doing, the president has to deal with two distinct policy domains: domestic affairs, and defense and foreign policy (Wildavsky 1966). Of the two, the president has more control over (and perhaps more success in) the second. He must deal extensively with the Congress on domestic issues, and convincing Congress can be tough indeed. The president's time and attention are often devoted to mustering congressional support rather than determining the desired policy. In defense and foreign policy, the reverse is often true. "Selling" the plan is not the hard part; coming up with the best policy choice seems to be much tougher. The public knows little about defense or foreign policy, and tends to trust the president on his proposals. People often like a decisive president in foreign affairs; presidential support as measured by polls often rises after the president takes action to deal with a difficult foreign issue. And relatively weak interest groups oppose presidential actions in this area. In domestic policy, especially economic issues, the public is more informed and more likely to object to the president's preferences when interest groups are active. Finally, the preferences of the president and Congress may differ more markedly on domestic rather than foreign policy issues (Rohde 1990).

This chapter focuses on the domestic presidency—the one in which the president has major roles in setting the policy agenda, persuading the Congress and the public to support the proposed policies, and overseeing the implementation of the policies once enacted.

Setting the Agenda

Unlike members of Congress, reelection is not viewed as the raison d'être of presidential decision making. Presidents want their policies to be adopted, they want the policies they put in place to last, and they want to feel they helped solve the problems facing the country (Ceaser 1988). However, for the first-term president, reelection is an ever-present concern. In *The Agenda* (Woodward 1994), reelection concerns came up in the first year of the Clinton presidency over such issues as freezing Social Security cost-of-living increases and NAFTA, and their effects on key states like Florida and California in 1996. The closer to an election, the more likely the president is to be concerned with reelection.

Light (1991) said presidents choose issues to minimize political costs and maximize political benefits. One way to do this is to alternate the promotion of broad policy redirection and noncontroversial incremental changes. Indeed, not all of the president's agenda items are bold steps. Peterson (1990) found that of the presidential initiatives he examined, only 12 percent involved large, new programs. Most of the proposals (58 percent) were best categorized as small changes to existing programs.

Presidents can choose certain issues for strategic, political gain. For example, Torres-Gil (1989) argued that part of the rationale behind President Reagan's decision to put catastrophic health care on the agenda was a careful determination that the Republicans needed an issue that would illustrate their compassion and family orientation. Torres-Gil noted that the "compassion agenda" came on the heels of Iran-Contra hearings and a loss of party control in the Senate, at a time when the president needed to regain public support.

There is a tendency for the modern president to focus on short-term, rather than long-term, issues. However, values are important to the modern presidency. According to Reagan pollster Richard Wirthlin, values "must be linked to policies and both must be contrasted with the values and policies being rejected" (Broder 1993a, 4). Yet in so doing, the president faces a number of limitations or constraints. As Kennedy advisor Theodore Sorenson put it, the president is free to choose "within the limits of permissibility, within the limits of available resources, within the limits of available time, within the limits of previous commitments, and within the limits of available information" (Cater 1964, 87).

When the president decides an issue is a national concern, whether it is health reform, drug abuse, energy conservation, or the alleviation of poverty, that issue is propelled to the top of the nation's policy agenda. Typically, presidents use the prestige and prominence of their office to focus national attention on the desired policies. Davidson said that "framing agendas is what the presidency is all about" (1984, 371). Presidents communicate their agendas through State of the Union addresses and other major speeches, television addresses and televised news conferences, and the release of special reports and analyses. They use highly visible cabinet members to spread the word and highlight key issues across the country. To effect policy, presidents must convince the Congress, and the president has little trouble getting members' attention. Kingdon (1984, 25) quoted a lobbyist as saying, "when a president sends up a bill [to Congress], it takes first place in the queue. All other bills take second place."

Kingdon (1984) offered an example in health policy of the strength of the president's agenda prowess. In interviews he conducted in 1976, only 18 percent of the congressional respondents mentioned hospital cost containment as a current agenda item. In 1977 interviews, some 81 percent cited the issue. Costs had not jumped comparably, and no other major event had occurred— save President Carter's emphasis on the issue.

While the president cannot introduce legislation, he can and does provide draft legislation or legislative guidance for translating his agenda into legislative language. A leader of the president's party or another key party member usually introduces the president's proposal. The president is also responsible for the presidential budget proposal, submitted to Congress in January before the fiscal year begins, which often sets the baseline for further discussions. Congressional budget reforms adopted in the mid-1970s dramatically affected the president's budget-making power, providing Congress with the staff and procedures to formulate its own budgets and allowing it to declare (as it did with Presidents Reagan and Bush) that their proposed budgets were DOA—dead on arrival.

The trend in the 1970s and 1980s to enact entitlement programs, which are not appropriated but are automatically part of federal spending, limited the president's power to reduce spending, a desire of both Republican and Democratic presidents since Richard Nixon. More recent budget changes have shifted the power back a little in the president's direction. In 1991 the White House and congressional leaders put in place budgetary procedures likely to increase the power of one key executive branch player, the Office of Management and Budget. Under the new pay-as-you-go system, any new entitlement spending programs or tax reductions that are not "revenue neutral" have to be accompanied by a plan to cut current spending, or OMB could sequester or automatically cut the necessary funds from other entitlement programs (Spitzer 1993, 115).

The president must make three decisions concerning the agenda: what problems should be addressed, what solutions seem most appropriate, and what the relative priorities are (Light 1991). The decision calculus for the three differs markedly. Light argued that the evaluation of problems is made on what problems are most likely to be politically beneficial to the president. These are likely to be chosen from problems that have been around for a long time, rather than newly identified problems. The evaluation of solution options relies on costs; solutions that involve high costs—either budgetary or political—are not likely to be proposed. The search for alternatives is important yet very difficult, particularly with budget and political constraints of recent years. Clearly, the Clinton White House's careful (and time-consuming) choice of solutions was a case in point. Light (1991) advised presidents to adopt a "satisficing" approach, whereby the first alternative that meets the policy needs is chosen rather than continuing the search for a "better" solution. (He also argued against innovation, at least in the first term.) The Clinton administration sought to dramatically change the health care system in this country—after extensive study by some 500 experts for nearly six months. A year later, the task force process and product were roundly criticized and credited, at least in part, with the failure of the Clinton health care plan. Clearly, Clinton would have been better advised to follow the recommendation of Light (1991) and others to adopt and amend proposals already before Congress rather than launching on a new policy path.

Presidential priorities are also key. The president will often choose to put his prestige behind one or two issues prominent in the campaign and those ideologically important to him. As Sullivan (1991) put it, the lesson is one of "concentrate or lose." The targeting of priorities is necessary, because resources, especially time and energy for both the president and the Congress, are scarce and need to be directed to those programs of highest support. President Carter discovered the value of prioritized issues in 1978 when he began sending up a variety of programs with little guidance on the relative standing of each, with little success. President Reagan learned from the Carter experience and was clear about his priorities: cutting government spending, reducing taxes, and increasing defense spending. Similarly, President Clinton focused on several key issues, but only after he suffered an embarrassing defeat on improving the treatment of homosexuals in the military—not a defining issue of his presidency but one on which he expended much political energy and time. President Reagan's health agenda was focused on two goals: the reduction of federal responsibilities and expenditures, and the reform of public or private insurance mechanisms that promote rapid increase in health care costs (Feder et al. 1982).

Putting items on the agenda and getting them passed are very different; the second is much harder. Once the president has put the item on the agenda and offered a preferred solution, it is then up to the Congress to act. At that point, presidents operate "at the margin" of coalition building in the Congress—they must rely on congressional party leadership for support, and their legislative skills are essentially limited to exploiting rather than creating opportunities for leadership (Bond and Fleisher 1990; Edwards 1989). Presidential skills have less to do with changing votes than with getting the right issues on the floor (Schull 1989), and presidents prefer to influence the design of legislation rather than the votes on it.

The president's proposals can be dismissed, ignored, substituted for those more acceptable to Congress, compromised, or (sometimes) adopted in full. Most presidents recognize that the probability of success is improved with their active monitoring and encouragement. Presidents can help mobilize public support and assist in the coalition formation necessary to successfully guide the bill through both houses of Congress. They can use their office to encourage legislators "leaning" in their direction and to provide encouragement to friends. They can use their prestige and visibility to counter strong interest groups by alerting the public to their tactics. A long-time member of Congress and chair of the House Energy and Commerce Committee argued that the president's role was pivotal in the consideration of 1994 health care reform. According to Representative John Dingell, of Michigan, the resistance of "vested interests" was too powerful for congressional leaders to overcome without a sustained focus by the president (Weisskopf 1994, 14).

Personal appeals, on the telephone or in person, can be persuasive, although not conclusive. Harry Truman summed up his role as sitting all day "trying to persuade people to do things they ought to have sense enough to do without my persuading them. . . . That's all the powers of the president amount to" (Neustadt 1960, 10). Such persuasion includes inducing them "to believe that what he wants of them is what their own appraisal of their own responsibilities requires them to do in their own self interest, not his" (Neustadt 1960, 10).

Presidential influence is often wielded through cabinet secretaries who work closely with the Congress and interest groups to forge legislation. For example, HHS Secretary Otis Bowen was an active participant during congressional consideration of the 1988 catastrophic health insurance bill, informally participating in the conference committee deliberations. The White House had argued throughout the process that respite care, where the government paid for homemakers or aides while a family caregiver took a break, was not germane to this proposal dealing with acute, not chronic, care. When the secretary agreed to an amendment limiting the eligibility to receive respite care, the conferees quickly concurred, and the deal was done.

In the 1994 congressional consideration of health care reform, President Clinton was asked by congressional leaders to stay out of the first round of decisions and refrain from public comment on what was going on. The White House activity directed at Congress in the spring and summer of 1994 was confined largely to providing expertise as asked and inviting members identified as pivotal to the White House for special attention and persuasion (Kosterlitz 1994). Yet by summer, the president was visibly concerned about the slow congressional pace and began meeting with key congressional leaders. Public appearances of the president, the first lady, and key cabinet members were stepped up.

THE PRESIDENT'S RELATIONSHIP WITH CONGRESS

According to Lyndon Johnson, "There is only one way to deal with Congress, and that is continuously, incessantly, and without interruption" (Kearns 1976, 226). Indeed, Johnson understood the workings of Congress and was able to work with it very successfully. His successors had a more difficult time. Bob Woodward's chronicle of the first year of Clinton's presidency, *The Agenda*, frequently illustrated the president's preoccupation and frustration with Congress. On the budget deficit–economic stimulus package of 1993, the president was involved daily, counting votes, making calls to key members, sitting in on strategy sessions with congressional leaders. At one point, Hillary Rodham Clinton claimed her husband had become "mechanic-in-chief"—put in a position of "tinkering" with policy rather than leading the charge to a higher vision (255). Yet President Clinton managed to squeeze out success with only the closest of votes on the economic plan, NAFTA, and, later, in 1994, the crime bill. Clinton expressed his frustration by using the analogy of the nation as a ship: "I can steer it but a storm can still come up and sink it. And the people that are supposed to be rowing can refuse to row" (330).

Some researchers believe there are swings in dominance between the White House and the Congress such that in some years the president is more powerful and in other years the Congress is. Other researchers see the system as much more stable and cooperative, what Peterson (1990) called tandem institutions both contributing to national decision making. Indeed, as Davidson noted (1984), cooperation between the Congress and the president is at least as common as conflict, although we hear more about the latter. The president's relationship with the Congress is far from static, varying with the president's political capital, outside influences, and the nature of the policy proposed.

Political Capital

Political capital is the strength of the president's popularity and the president's party in the Congress. Political capital is important because it affects the receptivity of the president's proposals in Congress. The president's popularity, reflected in public approval polls, is a key component of political capital, because presidents who can arouse and mobilize the public are apt to "greatly lessen" their problems in Congress (Sullivan 1987, 300). Rivers and Rose (1985) estimated that a 1-percent increase in the president's popularity leads to a 1-percent increase in the president's legislative approval rate. Even legislative sponsors can be persuaded by public opinion influenced by the president (MacKuen and Mouw 1992); similarly, potential opponents may think twice about voting against a measure supported by a particularly popular president. The president's popularity is especially important when the president is from the party of the congressional majority.

The first measure of the president's popularity in a new term, the size of the electoral victory, is also a factor in political capital. John Kennedy squeaked by in 1960, with a change of one state, or even a large city like Chicago, potentially changing the election. Bill Clinton was elected by a scant 43 percent in 1992 (table 2.1). Lyndon Johnson, Richard Nixon in 1972, and Ronald Reagan in 1980 could (and did) claim a mandate for change that the Congress recognized. Members are sometimes reluctant to face the wrath of an electorate by opposing the implementation of such a mandate.

Another factor important in political capital is the strength of the president's party in the Congress. Thomas Jefferson is purported to have said, "great innovations should not be forced on slender majorities" (Light 1991, 106). Indeed, Lyndon Johnson's successes of 1965, including the passage of Medicare, must be attributed in large part to the election of a large number of liberal Northern Democrats in the November 1964 election. The amount by which presidents lead or trail congressional candidates from their party can be important as well. If the individual members drew more votes in their districts than the president, the perceived political value of the president to that member is reduced. Peterson (1990) found that the proposals of presidents with smaller winning margins than the party's House candidates when the opposition controlled the Congress faced difficulty in reaching a con-

Table 2.1. Presidential Political Capital, 1965–93

President	Year	Senate Seats Held by President's Party	House Seats Held by President's Party	Public Approval	Percentage of Popular Vote
Johnson	1965	68	295	80	61.1
	1967	64	248	46	—
Nixon	1969	42	192	59	43.4
	1971	44	180	51	—
	1973	42	192	65	60.7
Ford	1975	37	144	39	—
Carter	1977	61	292	66	50.1
	1979	58	277	43	—
Reagan	1981	53	192	60	50.7
	1983	54	167	38	—
	1985	53	182	62	58.8
	1987	45	177	48	—
Bush	1989	45	175	51	53.4
	1991	44	167	58	—
Clinton	1993	57	258	58	43

Source: Adapted from Light, table 1, (1991): 32; updated using Ornstein, Mann, and Malbin (1994) and first approval rating of the year according to the *Gallup Opinion Index.*

sensus and that public fights over the proposals were common. Although Bill Clinton did not face a house controlled by the opposition party in his first two years, he was in the unenviable position of having trailed every member of the House and one-third of the Senate in voting in November 1992. In the fight over health care, consensus was slow in coming, and public fights, even among members of his own party, were frequent.

Unfortunately for the president, political capital tends to decline over time (largely due to lower popularity with the citizens and loss of seats in the midterm election). Indeed, presidents tend to think of themselves as being strongest politically in the earliest months of their tenure and act accordingly. Lyndon Johnson was especially concerned in the early days following his election that he "use his strength while it still existed," pointing out that the popularity of other presidents had diminished, and their problems with Congress increased very quickly (Johnson 1971, 323). Edwin Meese, a key Reagan aide, told a reporter that the White House knew that if it wanted to get the radical changes proposed through the Congress, it had to do it in the early months of the administration. "We're fighting the clock," he said. "We think about that all the time" (Kernell 1984, 256). Indeed, by the fall of the first year of the Reagan administration, presidential victories declined abruptly, and the following spring even the Senate Republicans on the Budget Committee voted against the president's budget (Salamon and Abramson 1984). However, some political scientists feel the value of "hitting the ground running" has been overestimated. Sullivan (1991), for example, thought quick action is secondary to the value of a focused presidential agenda.

Of course, events can occur to bolster the president's popularity, such as an international crisis handled well, like the Gulf War, or a domestic victory, such as the passage of NAFTA for President Clinton in 1993. Generally, the pattern is one of declining popularity. Ironically, as Light (1991) noted, the cycle of decreasing presidential influence coincides with a cycle of increasing effectiveness as the president learns about the office, makes mistakes, and learns from those mistakes.

The president's influence is greatest when some event has occurred that shows the current policy is no longer acceptable and presidential leadership can help forge the new alliances necessary to come up with a new solution (Miller 1993). He plays a much less important role in issues that are not salient and on which the Congress has already reached agreement.

The midterm elections, the end of the president's second year when one-third of the Senate and all of the House members are up for election, are an important outside influence affecting the relations between the president and Congress. As the election nears, members may shy away from controversial issues and may prefer to provide visible programs to their districts. After the election, the president may be worse off, because midterm elections generally go against the incumbent's party, regardless of the occupant's efforts or popularity. In the 1994 health care reform debates in Congress, the approach of midterm elections was a crucial outside influence. The Republicans wanted to delay a vote until the new Congress was seated in January 1995—hoping they would have greater numbers, perhaps even a majority in one or both houses. (They were right: they took over both houses in 1995.) The Democrats wanted to make health care a campaign issue, ideally taking credit for the passage of a laudatory bill or alternatively, taking the opportunity to blame the Republicans for any failure to do so. Yet health was markedly absent from most campaign debates, and Pennsylvania Senator Harris Wofford lost in November 1994. The loss was significant, because Wofford's election to an abbreviated term in 1991 was credited with alerting politicians to the public's concern over health care and catapulting health care to the top of the national agenda. Some felt that his subsequent loss symbolized the coming dormancy of comprehensive health care reform in Washington.

Presidential Persuasion

Kernell (1991, 90) called the president "doubtless the Washington community's most prominent and active dealmaker" who can provide the "much-needed coordination in assembling coalitions across a broad institutional landscape."

Consultation with Congress is important. The likelihood of meaningful consultation between the president and the Congress is greatly enhanced when the issues involved are salient and the president wants a solution; the White House cannot solve the problem alone and prominent figures on the Hill want to reach an agreement; or the president desires to work with the Congress on a solution (Peterson 1990).

Bargaining, whereby the member agrees to vote with the president in exchange for the president's support for a pet issue, is extremely common and an important weapon in the presidential arsenal. The president must bargain even with those who agree with him, because most members have interests of their own beyond policy objectives, and their votes cannot be ensured (Edwards 1980). Bill Clinton was accused of "giving away the store" for key votes on the 1993 budget bill and NAFTA. Other presidents have been similarly accused. Ronald Reagan, for example, angered party leaders when he offered not to campaign personally against Southern Democrats supporting him and gave them policy concessions beneficial to their constituents (Salamon and Abramson 1984). Coercion, or "arm-twisting," is generally relied on as the last resort and then only on particularly important votes (Edwards 1980).

Compromise is obviously an important factor in the relations between the president and Congress, but compromise can be difficult for a president whose every move makes national news. In the spring of 1994, for example, Bill Clinton was criticized for compromising too much to make his health reform plan pleasing to a variety of people. When he seemed to be wavering in his support for universal coverage—or at least its definition—he was criticized as retreating or backsliding, and was forced to reiterate his full support for coverage of all Americans. Interestingly, Ronald Reagan was criticized for the opposite behavior—for not compromising enough, for what Salamon and Abramson (1984, 59) called "ideological intransigence." George Mitchell, Senate majority leader, described the situation in 1994 as one in which Clinton would be criticized for whatever he did. If he took an inflexible position or refused to compromise, he would be attacked for not knowing the ways of Capitol Hill or not having the experience to win. If, on the other hand, Clinton participated and made the necessary compromises to get the plan approved, he would be attacked for being willing to give in. "You can't escape criticism in the process," Mitchell said (Woodward 1994, 183).

The personality component of the presidency can be key on some issues but may be overstated. Some presidents (Clinton and Johnson) seem to enjoy meeting with and attempting to persuade members of Congress; others (Nixon and Carter) prefer a hands-off approach, with minimal personal interaction. President Reagan was widely viewed as an excellent communicator whose informal, friendly style was disarming and charming to members of both parties. Barber (1985) characterized presidential personalities into four types based on the level of energy and enthusiasm the president brings to the job, and his positive or negative views about himself in relation to that activity. Reagan would be classified as passive positive, Clinton as active positive, Eisenhower as passive negative, and Nixon as active negative.

Another presidential "tool" is the veto—a disapproval that requires a two-thirds vote in both houses to overturn. Unlike forty-three state governors, the president of the United States does not have a line-item veto but is forced to veto the entire law rather than offensive parts of it.

Typically, the veto has served more as a threat than a reality, although presidents facing a Congress controlled by the opposite party and those with declining public popularity are particularly likely to use them (Rohde and Simon 1985). Gerald Ford, the only unelected president who assumed office without serving as an elected vice president, had no electoral margin of any kind and faced a heavily Democratic Congress. He used the veto more than any other modern president; vetoing thirty-seven bills in the Ninety-fourth Congress (1975–76), compared to Reagan's fifteen vetoes in the Ninety-seventh Congress (1981–82) and Carter's twelve vetoes in the Ninety-sixth Congress (1979–80). A veto override is relatively difficult to achieve. For example, Bush vetoed a total of forty-six bills in four years and was overridden only once (Ornstein, Mann, and Malbin 1994). When the president prefers less spending than Congress, the veto can be an effective potential constraint. However, when the president supports more spending, the veto can offer little political leverage (Kiewiet and McCubbins 1991).

The president's threat of a veto—particularly one issued early in the policy process—greatly increases his stake in the policy outcome and clearly articulates his priorities. Such a threat means the president has thrown down the gauntlet (especially to the opposition party) that certain policies must be enacted or he is willing to sacrifice the entire policy package. It also provides "comfort and cover" to members inclined to follow the president but who want assurances that he will back them up (Priest and Broder 1994). President Reagan "drew the line in the dirt" on tax cuts in 1981; President Bush uttered a "no new taxes" pledge. President Clinton, in his speech to a joint session of Congress introducing his health care reform proposal, used the threat of a veto to attempt to prove his intractability over universal coverage. Although he offered to compromise on other aspects of the proposal—managed competition, health care networks, and global budgets, to name a few—he continued to demand that universal coverage be in the legislative package or it would be vetoed.

The position is risky, however, since the president may lose credibility if he must compromise in some way (as Bush did in 1990 and Clinton did in 1994). Yet, as Henry Waxman put it, "It holds out the prospect for Republicans and some nervous Democrats that they will be held responsible if health care fails and that's a tough label for those people to have when they go back home to face the voters in November" (Priest and Broder 1994).

The use of the veto reminds the Congress that the president can be a powerful constraint, especially since successful override votes are difficult to muster. Franklin Roosevelt was known to ask his supporters for something he could veto as a reminder to the Congress that this form of policy enforcement could and would be applied (Spitzer 1983).

Institutional Constraints

Key among the institutional constraints are the decentralized nature of congressional policymaking, the expansion of interest groups and policy networks, and the reduced importance of political parties in the past thirty years. A modern president cannot work with a few key committee chairs and party leaders and a few dominant interest groups; rather, the president must deal with a spate of individuals and groups, all of whom have their own particular interests in the forefront. As Jimmy Carter (1982, 80) put it, "Each member had to be wooed and won individually. It was every member for himself, and the devil take the hindmost!" Further, the underlying consensus that animate the national majority politically and philosophically is different from that which animates the majority party of the legislature (Marini 1992). In a time of weak party discipline, ideology, not partisanship, is key. The modern president has little to offer individual members, who are largely independent in their fund-raising and campaign organization. These changes mean that coalition build-ing is more complicated, said Peterson (1990), and the president becomes only one more player among many in congressional policy choices.

Light (1984) believed that presidents must now "pay more for domestic programs." And the cost is high. Joseph Califano, former White House staffer and HEW secretary, noted that President Clinton's willingness to compro-mise on most things in his health care package reflected the dominance of Congress and the recognition that he would have to sign whatever it sends to him and "declare victory" (1994, 41). In fact, as Light noted, the president often does not get "star billing" for his domestic agenda. Light concluded that the presidential aura has lessened because of increased competition among the other policy initiators, more resources for such initiation, and less reverence for the wisdom of presidential planning (1984, 207).

Recent presidents are also constrained by the fiscal realities of the federal budget deficit. Even though presidents are often expected to be activists, federal spending constraints can stymie the president's policy plans. For ex-ample, President Clinton, facing a Democratic House in 1994, was able to get only one-third of the increase he sought in Head Start and one-half the ad-ditional money he wanted for his national service program.

Presidential Successes

The president generally has an easier time when the Congress is controlled by members of his own party. When one party controls both branches, the president's success scores do not drop below 75 percent (Ornstein, Mann, and Malbin 1994, 189). Since 1947, however, this has occurred less than one-half the time—only ten of the past twenty-four Congresses have been controlled by the sitting president's party. Ronald Reagan was successful an average of 62 percent of the time over his eight years in office (table 2.2). Richard Nixon's average in office was 67 percent; Gerald Ford's, 58 percent. Lyndon Johnson, in contrast, had an average success rate of 83 percent.

The success rates shown in table 2.2, compiled by the *Congressional Quar-terly,* are used frequently by presidential researchers and the press. These rat-ings probably overstate the president's successes for several reasons. First, the scores are based on votes on which the president took clear-cut positions, and

Table 2.2. Presidential Victories in Votes in Congress

President	Year Elected (or Assumed Office)	Percentage of Bills Supported by the President That Were Enacted		
		Highest	Lowest	Mean
Johnson	1963	93.1 (1965)	74.5 (1968)	82.6
Nixon	1968	76.9 (1970)	50.6 (1973)	67.2
Ford	1974	61.0 (1975)	53.8 (1976)	57.6
Carter	1976	78.3 (1978)	75.1 (1980)	76.4
Reagan	1980	82.3 (1981)	43.5 (1987)	61.9
Bush	1988	62.6 (1989)	43.0 (1992)	51.6

Source: Data from Ornstein, Mann, and Malbin (1994) based on success rates compiled by the *Congressional Quarterly*.

treat seminal legislation and more trivial pursuits equally. Further, the *Congressional Quarterly* score considers the president's position at the time of the vote, not his position much earlier when the item was first placed on the agenda. Finally, roll-call measures, such as this, understate the complexity of the policy process where the president is only one of many actors, making "victories" attributable to the efforts of one player somewhat suspect.

In a more in-depth look at a sample of some 300 presidential proposals of five presidents (Eisenhower through Reagan), Peterson (1990) found that some 54 percent of presidential proposals between 1953 and 1984 were passed, with more than one-third passed exactly as introduced. However, presidential success varied with the nature and scope of the proposal. For example, Peterson found that for new and costly comprehensive policy initiatives, presidents "won" some measure of what they proposed only 29 percent of the time and had some of their proposals accepted in less than 40 percent of the proposals. Presidential proposals were rarely ignored (only 20 percent were not acted on), but they did tend to engender strong opposition (40 percent). An analysis of twenty health policies in the final two years of the Carter administration and first two years of the Reagan administration (Heinz et al. 1993) found that while 50 percent were initiated by the White House, only 12.5 percent of those administrative proposals were enacted.

Divided Government

A president facing at least one house controlled by the opposite party has to use a different strategy from one blessed with a Congress led by his own party. Traditionally, presidents facing a unified Congress often rely on informal party mechanisms to achieve their goals. When facing a divided Congress or one controlled by members of the other party, the president must resort to the veto (or threat of the veto) and support from the public. Yet both are somewhat risky. Clearly the president cannot veto every bill he does not like but must pick those in which there is public interest or strong public opinion. Similarly, the president cannot take every issue to the public.

Presidents facing a Congress of the other party tend to avoid congressional interactions wherever possible. For example, Nixon and Reagan both relied heavily on an administrative strategy composed of reorganization, careful appointments, and (in the case of Nixon) budget impoundments. While presidents have long been able to withhold money appropriated by the Congress if the spending was unnecessary or could not be done usefully, Nixon in his second term greatly expanded the concept, withholding (or impounding) money for programs he did not wish to continue. As Allen Schick (1980, 48) described it: "When Nixon impounded for policy reasons, he in effect told Congress, 'I don't care what you appropriate, I will decide what will be spent.'" Reagan also used threats of reduction in force (RIF) to push out civil servants he did not trust and used the senior executive service to bring in people whom he did (Marini 1992).

One reason that relations between the president and Congress are especially dicey when there is divided government is that opposition politicians will often gain electoral advantage in frustrating the president. Kernell (1991) said that the main business of an opposition Congress is to prepare for the next election. The minority party will tend not to bargain in good faith—it is not in their best interest. As Republican Representative Richard Cheney, from Wyoming, explained it in 1985, "If there are no real issues dividing us from the Democrats, why should the country change and make us the majority?" (Barnes 1985, 9). For electoral reasons, minority members might take positions inconsistent with the policies that members might prefer if given other circumstances.

Interestingly, President Clinton had a Democratic Congress in his first year, yet encountered difficulties not unlike those of a president in divided government. The Republican leadership talked about "sitting at the table" but spent more time carping at the Democrats' plan and forming coalitions with conservative Democrats to defeat key portions of the proposal. In the second two years of his first term, Clinton faced an opposition Congress, and his tactics changed as expected. He had fewer meetings with members, was less visible to the public, and offered little in the way of legislative initiatives.

DEALING WITH OTHERS

Going Public

Closely tied to presidential success in Congress is the desire of the public at large. Presidents often make direct appeals to the public to urge that pressure be placed on their elected officials. Ronald Reagan often tried "to go over the heads" of the Congress to mobilize public opinion behind a desired policy. While this tactic is not new—Woodrow Wilson used it in an attempt to engender public support for the League of Nations—it has been used increasingly in the past two decades, thanks to advances in technology that allow interactive communications from a variety of sources and direct, targeted satellite feeds to television stations across the country. From Franklin Roosevelt's "fireside chats" to Bill Clinton's "town meetings," the purpose is the same: to mobilize public support and build coalitions. As Miller (1993, 314) put it, "The president's most powerful weapon . . . is a public aroused on a specific issue."

Presidents and their advisors fully understand the role of strong public support. Kernell (1984) recounted the desires of President Reagan and his staff to take advantage of his popularity after the assassination attempt in 1981. They decided to push the president's desired budget cuts in a televised joint session of the Congress and the first major appearance of Reagan since the shooting. The broad public support helped; the budget passed, nearly intact. The problem with such an appeal is that the public is typically fickle and can often provide only fleeting support. It is also susceptible to messages from other interested parties and can easily grow bored with a subject. Policy dependent on the public may be quite volatile indeed. As Tip O'Neill, then Speaker of the House, said in 1981, "The opinions of the man in the street change faster than anything in the world. Today, he does not know what is in this program and he is influenced by a President with charisma and class. . . . But a year from now he will be saying 'You shouldn't have voted that way'" (Kernell 1986, 117).

President Nixon also fully understood the importance of developing a message and making certain it got out. According to speechwriter David Gergen, he would say over and over, "about the time you are writing a line that you have written so often that you want to throw up, that is the first time the American people will hear it" (Kelly 1993, 68).

A president's access to the media and strong allegiance to the national interest make the public approach appealing. A key challenge to the president comes in seeking to shape opinion. The Clinton administration recognized the importance of public opinion and established a "war room" that served to put the best "spin" on information, such as the Congressional Budget Office's estimates of the cost of the Clinton health care plan, and congressional pronouncements, such as New York Senator Daniel Patrick Moynihan's questioning of the seriousness of the health care "crisis." Nevertheless, public support for the plan began to drop in the spring of 1994, when, for the first time, most Americans opposed Clinton's plan—although, ironically, they continued to like many aspects of it (Kosterlitz 1994). As the vote on health care reform neared, the White House stepped up its efforts, scheduling a Health Security Express bus tour and offering nightly short addresses on cable television in which the president highlighted health issues of public concern. But the public's support continued to dwindle.

In its "selling of the health care reform plan," the Clinton administration tried to promote broad principles and goals, such as health security, and to avoid details regarding health alliances and employer mandates. This policy backfired when commercials by interest groups took the opportunity to inform and persuade the public that such aspects of the plan were harmful and unwise. President Carter, too, found the public difficult to persuade concerning rising health costs, because most people were insulated from the problem by insurance and could not get worked up over the need for change (Peterson 1990).

Probably the best example of public misunderstanding involved the passage, then repeal, of catastrophic health insurance for the elderly in 1988. Passed by substantial margins in both the House and the Senate and strongly supported by the president, the law was not well explained by elected officials, and the public was easily led astray by scare tactics of opponents. Although the bill adversely affected primarily the well-to-do and helped the poor, many of the elderly poor thought they would have to pay high premiums for services they valued little. The final blow came when initial cost estimates of the program turned out to be extremely low—the new figures estimated costs at six times the first estimates (Broder 1994b).

Sometimes the president uses the public as a sounding board for possible solutions, solutions quickly forgotten if the cues are wrong. For example, the

Clinton administration abandoned consideration of a new value-added tax (VAT) to finance its health program because a poll conducted by the White House pollster indicated no support for it (Peters 1994, 5).

The President and the Press

The days when a close-knit and small press corps crowded around Franklin Roosevelt's desk to hear the latest presidential pronouncements are long gone. Today's press corps covering the White House numbers in the hundreds, and it covers every move, and failure to move, in seemingly excruciating detail. The first modern media president was John Kennedy, who used television to project the image of an energetic, talented, and handsome leader. Richard Nixon, "burned" by television in his campaign against Kennedy in 1960, learned to use it in his effort to remake his political career in the mid-1960s. Nixon institutionalized the process of communications and put in place a series of innovations designed to control the news and put the best spin on it.

Nixon established an Office of Communications and an Office of Public Liaison, which worked to "orchestrate" the news and organize grass-roots efforts supportive of the president. The Office of Communications focused in large part on local media—using them to reach the people without filtering through the larger, more cynical (and perhaps unsupportive) Washington and East Coast media. This communications office understood the importance of symbols to presidential activities and worked to provide short, meaningful messages that could be captured in sound bites. The Nixon staff developed the notion of a "line of the day," which was highlighted on a given day by the president and other spokespersons. The communications staff tried to control the media's agenda and access, rewarding reporters who wrote good stories and attacking those who were critical. The Office of Communications staff met weekly with the public relations staffs from federal agencies to make certain that the message was clear and unified.

President Reagan, using some of the staff trained in the Nixon White House, followed the same highly coordinated, well-developed plan to control the media and reach the public. James Baker, while he was chief of staff, spent thirty-five hours a week talking to journalists. He gave an hour a day to three networks and four major newspapers (Kelly 1993). The Reagan team was also good at "leaking" information to reporters in exchange for valuable information from the press, such as what members of the White House press corps were working on and what they were hearing from other people.

President Clinton had a tough time getting his message across in the first two years of his term. Missteps, such as troublesome nominees for attorney general, expensive haircuts, and aides using helicopters to play golf, were emblazoned across newspapers with such headlines as the *New York Daily News'* "Bumblin' Bill" or *Time* magazine's "Incredible Shrinking President." More serious issues involving allegations of influence peddling and sexual harassment from his gubernatorial tenure followed him into his second year. President Clinton appeared to suffer from what Larry Sabato called a "boom-and-bust cycle—where things are either perfect and beautiful and wonderful or they're terrible and awful," with little in between (Kurtz 1994, 10). While Sabato believed that the press tends to follow public opinion rather than help shape it, others feel that media coverage helps define the presidency and form the perceptions key to public opinion (Kurtz 1994).

The press coverage and congressional oversight combined in the summer of 1994 to rivet much of the nation's attention on hearings on an Arkansas development called Whitewater. The spectacle of White House aides and a treasury secretary being grilled on their knowledge of attempts to "cover up" or influence federal agencies in decisions related to the treatment of persons and entities associated with Whitewater diverted attention from health care— just at the time that the House and Senate leadership were preparing their proposals for consideration on the floor.

Policy Implementation

While the president may spend enormous amounts of time setting the policy agenda and trying to get desired policies put into place, the office also brings with it another important policy function: carrying out or executing those laws. The president is charged with overseeing the executive branch of government—some 3 million strong, with approximately 300,000 of those working in the Washington, D.C., metropolitan area.

One important way the president exercises such oversight is through appointing cabinet positions, commissions, and subcabinet posts, offices with leadership responsibility for federal programmatic functions. There are thirteen cabinet posts and about 190 key subcabinet posts, all subject to Senate confirmation. The "inner cabinet" is made up of the secretaries of defense, state, justice, and treasury. "Outer cabinet" members (interior, agriculture, commerce, labor, education, HUD, transportation, and HHS) do not generally have the access and influence of inner cabinet members. They deal both with groups whose political resources are few (welfare recipients, Native Americans) and with groups whose well-established influence presidents could not change substantially even if they wanted (large manufacturers, corporate farmers, organized labor) (Dolbeare and Edelman 1985). However, some outer cabinet members can exercise more power if they are particularly close to the president, such as Robert Reich, President Clinton's labor secretary.

Cabinet members are appointed by the president and serve at his pleasure. The popular Joseph Califano, HEW secretary in the Carter years, found out the tenuous nature of his position when he was rather ignominiously fired for reasons quite apart from his role as cabinet secretary. (He got too cozy with potential presidential primary challenger Senator Ted Kennedy.) Or as Light (1984) quoted Abraham Lincoln following a cabinet vote over a heated issue, "One aye, seven nays. The Ayes have it" (436). The presidentially appointed positions serve important functions linking the president and his plan for government with a huge body of civil servants who do the day-to-day work of implementing federal programs.

The Bureaucracy

Presidents are important to federal agency employees (Moe 1985). In addition to appointing the agency leadership, presidents and the Office of Management and Budget recommend agencies' budgets to the Congress and oversee the promulgation of agency recommendations.

The bureaucracy is important to the president; it can provide useful expertise and an institutional and policy memory that can mean the difference between success and failure of a treasured policy or program. Ironically, while the president often understands the importance of "getting the bureaucracy under control," he is usually relatively uninterested in administration, and presidents of both parties tend to distrust the federal bureaucracy. Some presidents try to control federal agencies with careful selection of agency heads who share the president's ideological and policy vision. Others prefer to "work around" agencies by having policy expertise and control located in the White House, rather than relying on the agencies. President Nixon tried both. He carefully selected cabinet officials and other high officials to ensure that the bureaucracy would be helpful, not harmful, in his policy goals, and he also centralized control of policymaking in the White House, using agencies as little as possible.

Presidents can also reorganize the executive branch to best fit their goals and to improve overall efficiency—to some extent. For example, President Nixon sent a reorganization plan to Congress in 1971 that would have abolished the Departments of Agriculture, Labor, Commerce, HUD, Interior, HEW, and Transportation, and consolidated their functions into four new departments: Human Resources, Natural Resources, Community Development, and Economic Affairs. His plan went nowhere in a Congress lobbied by groups that wanted to keep the existing agencies and where such a shakeup would make changes in congressional committee responsibilities—changes that could mean some committee chairs and members would lose authority and standing. Nixon later accomplished some of his changes with a functional reorganization corresponding roughly to the proposed superagencies with staffers responsible for coordinating policy in those areas.

The trend is toward a more "politicized" bureaucracy—presidential appointments further and further down the ladder, more careful choices of ideologically compatible appointees, and less reliance on career bureaucrats in making policy. Some feel this is a good idea (Moe 1985); others believe it is detrimental to the system (Rourke 1991). Many believe that Congress controls or dominates the bureaucracy (Weingast and Moran 1983; Calvert, Moran, and Weingast 1987; Marini 1992).

The White House Staff

The White House staff typically consists of about a thousand people. Like the congressional staff, the White House staff is an important source of expertise and political guidance—often more of the latter than the former. While most presidents fill these positions with trusted and loyal assistants and aides, sometimes persons who are most trusted are not the best staffers. Bill Clinton's first chief of staff, long-time friend Thomas McLarty, was loyal but not best suited to the tough job as gatekeeper and left after eighteen months. Many of the Clinton White House aides were young (in their twenties) and inexperienced in Washington norms. Not a few "old hands" were offended by what they felt was brusk or inappropriate treatment by the "youngsters." Having such young and inexperienced staffs has been a recurring problem for presidents. Jimmy Carter's staff managed to enrage Speaker of the House Tip O'Neill by denying his personal request for extra inauguration tickets. Even before the president was in office, the congressional-presidential relationship was off to a rocky start. Other problems can arise if aides isolate the president and tell him only what he wants to hear (Presidents Nixon and Johnson are possible examples) or are not well informed on political relationships and mores in Washington (President Carter comes to mind here). President Clinton was criticized for having "government by inner circle" and for relying on "adhocracy" or ad hoc groups, rather than established experts in the bureaucracy and elsewhere, for advice (Haass 1994). Traditionally, Democratic presidents have preferred what is known as spokes-of-the-wheel organization, whereby the president works with a few cabinet-level persons who report directly to him. Republicans tend to use a chief-of-staff model, where one person serves as the gatekeeper to the presidential office. In reality, however, these organizational forms simplify the differences in presidential interaction with staffs (Jones 1994).

In recent years the White House staff has grown considerably as the president desires to have more of his "own people" in key policy-making roles. For example, the Domestic Council often serves as the president's window on domestic policy and the mechanism for presidential coordination of agencies. The Office of Communications in the White House is a very important vehicle for presidential links with people—especially key since Nixon. The Council of Economic Advisors is responsible for the annual economic report and provides advice to the president on economic issues. The National Security Council provides advice on defense issues. The staffs of these agencies are usually small. As Light (1991, 55) said, "The number of [White House] staff directly involved in policy choice is quite restricted. The bulk of the staff is usually engaged in firefighting while the rest are forced to tackle one or two problems at a time."

The Office of Management and Budget

Of the eight agencies within the Executive Office of the President, the Office of Management and Budget is pivotal to domestic policymaking. Established in 1921 as the Bureau of the Budget, its formation is viewed by some as the beginning of the institutional presidency (Moe 1985). In 1970, it added management to its name and function and became the "eyes and ears" of the president (Benda and Levine 1986). It has increasingly taken on broad domestic policy coordination issues, in addition to its traditional budgetary one. Its primary function is the preparation of the president's budget; it reviews agency requests and coordinates them with the president's priorities

and desires. For example, President Nixon asked department heads to identify their chief presidential objective so OMB could monitor the agency's
performance.

OMB has long played the role of budgetary "heavy"—arguing for reductions in spending, or the elimination or a scaling back of programs. Behn and
Sperduto (1979, 56) dubbed the agency "the terminator." During the Nixon
and Reagan administrations, OMB played a key role in targeting health programs for reduction. In 1973, for example, the president's budget proposed
the termination of Hill-Burton, the regional medical program, allied health
training, public health training, and public health school grants. When HEW
department heads were called before Congress to justify the elimination of
these programs, they were "short of solid explanations . . . because the decisions were made at the Office of Management and Budget, largely on budgetary grounds" (Iglehart 1973, 647). Light (1991, 169) quoted a newspaper account of the development of an urban assistance package in the Clinton years
in which "the influential and penny-pinching Office of Management and
Budget broke out a fresh supply of wet blankets for the occasion."

In the Reagan years, the agency's role was to coordinate the political priorities "top down" from the White House with the more "bottom up" preferences of the agencies. Also in the Reagan years, OMB took on a stronger
regulatory role. Agencies were required to submit "major rules" (involving
an estimated economic impact of more than $100 million a year) to OMB
sixty days before publication of notice in the *Federal Register* and again thirty
days before publication. OMB could delay or recommend the withdrawal of
regulations. The agency promulgating (or writing) the regulations was also
required to submit a cost-benefit analysis of the regulation's expected impact. While most rules were approved (81 percent between 1981 and 1985),
nearly 500 a year were withdrawn or approved after the agency made changes.
This number probably understates the informal interactions and changes made
to garner OMB support (Cooper and West 1988).

THE PRESIDENCY AND HEALTH

Since Harry Truman, every president, Democrat or Republican, has proposed major health legislation, many involving national health insurance.
Most presidents wanted to expand the federal role in health; the Reagan and
Bush administrations proposed the addition of protection against catastrophic
losses under Medicare and a number of additional Medicare benefits, in an

attempt to make public coverage more efficient and better targeted. Presidents have varied in their efforts to inform the public and to influence the Congress and their success. President Ford offered a major plan and (due largely to economic considerations) never pursued it with the Congress. President Clinton pulled out all the stops in drafting a comprehensive plan and encouraging its adoption. Yet no comprehensive national health insurance reform plan has been enacted, although some cost controls and efforts to revamp the delivery system supported by presidents have been put in place.

One reason for the notable lack of success of presidential proposals in health reform may be the different constituencies discussed earlier. For the president, concerned with a national and broad constituency, national health insurance can be easily understood and explained, making broad policy changes that will improve the efficiency and effectiveness of health care for all Americans. For a member of Congress, national health reform comes down to the effect on that member's local hospital, medical school, or small business. The member will see the issue in terms of pharmacists and optometrists and nurses and drug companies and dry cleaners—many of the issue's components rather than the entire issue. By deconstructing the national program for the public good into its 535 components, problems arise that have, to date, stymied the enactment of a comprehensive, universal health policy for the country.

Other major "sticking" points for presidents have concerned the cost of a broad, comprehensive health care program—and how to pay for it. Increased taxation is something no president relishes, yet major change must be accompanied by resources to pay for it. Issues of unemployment also arise at the presidential level, although not with the personal possibilities that they do in congressional districts. Finally, all modern presidents have promoted cost controls. Going back to Richard Nixon, there was a great deal of concern about rising health care costs and how to get a handle on them. So far, many answers have been elusive to presidents and congresses alike.

The Clinton Health Care Proposal

Although many earlier modern presidents had proposed major health reforms, none did so with the fervor and dedication of President Bill Clinton. With the first lady as the point person, a major effort involving more than 500 experts in more than a dozen task forces was launched to write a health reform plan in 100 days. The effort was largely conducted in secret, without the involvement of key interest groups that would be directly affected by the reforms, and was highly decentralized, with task forces working independently and generally without concern for potential costs and likely political support (or opposition). In a speech before Congress in the fall of 1993, the president challenged the members to ignore "scare tactics by those who are motivated by self interest . . . in the waste the system now generates" and produce a program providing universal, comprehensive health care for American citizens. But it was too late. The plethora of interest groups waiting to attack parts of the proposal that they did not like (and largely silent on those parts they did approve) were lying in wait with millions of dollars at their disposal. Several weeks later, some 280 days after the process began, a 1,342-page bill, entitled the Health Security Act, was unveiled to the Congress, the public, and the affected interests. The timing, the process, and the product were problematic. Criticism was rampant and shrill, and questions designed to shake public support were being asked in television commercials and emblazoned across full-page newspaper ads.

The timing—nine months into the presidency—meant that the proposal was well past the halcyon "honeymoon" period, when Presidents Reagan and Johnson had been most successful with their sweeping new proposals. The process enraged those who were not a part of it (court cases were pending long after the Clinton plan had been put on the shelf). The press railed against the secrecy and complained about the waste of money. It was a "policy wonk's" dream—months of high-level policy deliberation. But the political realities appeared to have been sorely missed. The product, a reflection of the rarified air of a protected policy analytical discussion, was simply too complex and too academic, containing something to offend everyone and without a simple theme understandable to the public. Finally, as Light (1984) noted, the president can often succeed by adopting and amending proposals already before the Congress. The Clintons chose not to take this path, but rather forged an ambitious, comprehensive proposal making massive changes in the current system, with limited congressional involvement. The path they chose—what Skocpol (1995) called "competition within a budget" (69)—was also not endorsed by health policy elites who could have helped shape, alter, and direct public opinion (Jacobs and Shapiro 1995).

The public, which seemed initially supportive of the proposal, began to question the need for and complexity of national health care reform. In public polls conducted in February 1994, those against the plan and those supportive of the plan garnered the same percentages. After that time, the "nays" began to pull ahead. Even those in favor of reforms may have had a rather modest adjustment in mind. Focus groups and some polls found that many people were interested mainly in insurance forms, not the problems of the uninsured, and about whether they could obtain insurance if they left their jobs, an issue of portability rather than whether the entire system needed a major overhaul (Clymer, Pear, and Toner 1994). As Skocpol (1995, 79) put it, there were "not enough payoffs to organized groups and middle-class citizens pleasantly ensconced in the existing U.S. health care system."

President Clinton, given an opportunity to choose early in his term between a more targeted program to cover only large, catastrophic costs and the more comprehensive, universal approach, chose the latter (Woodward 1994). He was simply unwilling to compromise his vision of major reform. To do so, he felt, would be to violate the trust of the people and his office. As he said later, when the future of any plan was bleak (August 1994), "We didn't say, 'vote for me, in a representative form of government and I will make all the necessary decisions to solve the problems of the country, except those that are difficult, controversial and make the people mad.' That was not the deal" (Wines 1994, A9). But it was a deal—at least in health care—that was not to be. President Clinton joined his predecessors in his inability to fashion a successful health reform package.

CONCLUSION

Some argue that the domestic policy-making powers of the modern president are weaker than they were in the days of the Roosevelts or Lyndon Johnson. Light (1991) called the modern presidency a "no-win" situation, noting that the cost of presidential policy has grown while the president's ability to influence outcomes has declined. A powerful and decentralized Congress, a slew of well-financed interest groups, weakened political parties, a fickle public, and budgetary constraints on new policies limit the success of a president's policy initiatives.

The president can still command the public's attention and garner massive press attention, but the public is also hearing contrary messages from other interests, and the press attention is often critical and downright negative. In health the presidential role has long been an initiator of change in health care access and delivery. But the president is stymied at many points and has been generally unsuccessful in achieving major health legislation since the passage of Medicare in 1965. Republican and Democratic presidents have offered surprisingly similar proposals for national health insurance, which met similar, unsuccessful fates in the Congress (Chapter 7 goes into more detail).

The president clearly has the trappings of power, but that power is shared and must be negotiated carefully, not wielded at will. The inability in recent years of Democratic presidents with a Democratic Congress to enact their top policy proposals, including health, can be explained by the small amounts of presidential political capital; the strengthened, independent congressional entrepreneur; the complexity of the issues; budgetary constraints; and the inherent differences in constituencies. The public too is part of the explanation. In health and other areas, the public's attention span is short and susceptibility to counterargument high. Without a public clamor of support, the presidential voice is weakened, and the likelihood of success greatly reduced.

3

Interest Groups

A LOOK BACK

1965

CHARLS WALKER, a top Washington lobbyist, described lobbying Congress in the days of Speaker of the House Sam Rayburn as highly personal, direct, and easy. In a fifty-minute meeting with the Speaker, "for forty-eight minutes we would talk about Texas, family and friends. In the remaining two, we would settle what I had come to talk about. He always knew what I was there for, and would say, 'It's taken care of, Charlie,' or 'I just can't do that for you'" (Colamosca 1979, 16).

In 1965 the American Medical Association was the strongest health lobby and probably the most powerful lobby of any kind in the country. A spokesperson could say that "medicine" opposed a bill and be correct. The *New York Times* had not long before claimed the AMA was the "only organization in the country that could marshal 140 votes in Congress between sundown Friday night and noon on Monday" (Morone 1990). Yet in 1965 the powerful

AMA met its first major defeat with the passage of Medicare, after spending $1.2 million to fight it.

The 1965 Medicare fight was unusual, a blip on the otherwise relatively blank screen of national health insurance. In 1966 things had settled down, and the physicians' group spent $49,000 lobbying in Washington. That same year the American Dental Association (ADA) spent $18,000; the American Hospital Association (AHA), $41,000; and the American Nurses Association (ANA), $45,000.

1981

The pace of politics and interest group competition had picked up by the early 1980s. A plethora of health interest groups had opened offices along K Street, N. W., and more and more of the lunches consumed at the Rotunda, the Monocle, and other long-time power-lunch eateries huddled at the foot of Capitol Hill were being bought by professional lobbyists whose clients wore white coats or worked closely with those who did. President Jimmy Carter's demand for spending controls on hospitals had aroused the powerful Chicago-based AHA, which stepped up its lobbying and built up its campaign contribution base. Business lobbyists too had health care on their own menus. Costs had caught business executives' eyes as the fringe benefit lines in their annual reports began to show a higher rate of growth than wages, sales, or profits.

Chatty lunches were only a small part of the health care policy influence story. Reelection campaign costs had mushroomed as expensive television ads became the weapon of choice in the battle for votes. Campaign costs had risen tenfold in less than two decades. With so many digits in their reelection budgets, those elected might not even notice the generosity of moderately sized individual contributions. Enter the political action committee, which packages campaign contributions of interest groups, corporations, labor unions, and others to represent a single set of interests (Sabato 1985). In 1981 PACs had become a major factor to help fund (and speed the growth of) the campaign vortex.

While a handful of PACs had been around for years, the PAC movement became a feature of the political landscape only in the 1980s, thanks in part to the reformers of the 1970s. Trying to shrink the influence of a few well-heeled givers, those who wanted more citizen-financed campaigns had pressed the Congress to cap individual contributions and those of interest groups as well as setting up a public financing mechanism for major party candidates for president. The authorization of PACs in the 1974 law led to an extraordinary increase in their number and influence.

Health care associations took notice. Clearly there were many whose interests were not being represented by the AMA, AHA, or the insurance companies. With their own PACs, optometrists, osteopaths, dentists, nurses, nursing homes, group practice associations, family doctors, pharmacists, chiropractors, drug companies, occupational therapists, and others could mount lobbying efforts or make campaign contributions that would ensure that when the body politic wrote national health insurance, it did not neglect the part of the body in which they had a particular interest. Well-placed contributions could ensure that a group's services were included in insurance coverage proposals and that the givers' scope of practice was protected from would-be poachers.

Cash became a p.r.n. (as needed) prescription for the whole health care industry. The 1978 spending totals for federal elections alone reached major proportions for a wide range of groups: for the AMA nearly $2 million; for the dental PAC $573,000; nurses, $100,000; for-profit hospitals, $144,000; and optometrists, $112,000.

PACs seemed to be taking on a life of their own. Groups without them needed them; those with them needed bigger ones; and those in a PAC representing interests that might be a bit too broad for their particular concerns could splinter off, form their own PAC. But there never seemed to be enough. More money chasing the same number of candidates inflated the cost of campaigns, intensifying the need for larger and larger PAC contributions, and more and more fundraising efforts by the candidates. More PACs would have to raise more money.

1993

Washington seemed to be overrun with lobbyists, many with health care reform on their minds. Groups had proliferated, mutated, multiplied, spread, bred, and fed on one another: specialized physician groups, specialty hospitals, insurers, businesses, labor, corporate interests, pharmaceutical firms, home care companies, prepaid health plans, walk-in clinics, and groups representing poor people, elderly people, disabled people, and children. Nursing homes in one southern state could not afford their own lobbyist, so they put on retainer a Washington professional who lobbied for a variety of health care groups. Enterprising, he contacted the nursing home association in a contiguous state and picked up another client. The story was being repeated all over town. When the White House began to count noses as it sized up the potential opposition to its reform plan, the numbers stunned everybody. Staffers identified more than 1,100 interest groups with substantial stakes in the health care battle (Broder 1994a). No one wanted to be left out. Every interest group in the land seemed "to have something to say on health care restructuring—from dentists to the Christian Coalition. It has created a daily, unrelenting round of Health Care Events" (Toner 1994a, 1).

"This is the biggest-scale lobbying effort that has ever been mounted on any single piece of legislation—both in terms of dollars spent and people engaged," said Ellen Miller of the Center for Responsive Politics (Seelye 1994, A10).

The *New York Times* described a "typical day" in the capital—March 8, 1994—in the "Year of Health Care Events":

> [Eight hundred] doctors were massed at the American Medical Association conference; 210 restauranteurs were tromping to Capitol Hill, ventilating their opposition to the idea of requiring businesses to pay for health insurance; President Clinton was making the case for health care overhaul to the American Society of Association Executives (a kind of trade group for trade groups); Ralph Nader was denouncing the AMA at a news conference; former First Ladies Rosalyn Carter and Betty Ford were arguing for mental health coverage before the Senate Labor and Human Resources Committee, and the line of interested parties stretched down a very long hall when the House Ways and Means Subcommittee on Health began considering a health care bill. And this was all before noon. (Toner 1994a, 1)

Health care lobbying had become a team sport. The AMA was just a player. No longer could its president boldly declare that "medicine is opposed to this measure as a total package" (Campion 1984, 275). There was no "genuine peak association" in the health domain, concluded researchers Salisbury, Heinz, Laumann, and Nelson (1987), who found that the AMA was best described as only one among several sets of interest group participants, though a highly significant set.

Changes in the world of health interest groups were similar to those in other issue areas: more groups, many formed from specialized membership of traditional groups, and more citizen or public interest groups than in the days of Lyndon Johnson. And there was more money, much more. In the first eight months of 1993 (not an election year), the AMA PAC spent more than

Table 3.1. Key Health-Related Interest Group Players in 1993–94 Reform

Group	Membership	Annual Budget (in Millions)	PAC Spending in First Six or Eight Months of 1993
American Medical Association	300,000 physicians	$205	$747,250 (8)
Blue Cross and Blue Shield Association	69 Blue Cross and Blue Shield plans	131	72,610 (6)
American Hospital Association	5,000 hospitals; 50,000 personnel	70	264,140 (8)
American Dental Association	140,000 dentists	50	205,400 (8)
American College of Physicians	80,000 internists	41	—
Pharmaceutical Manufacturers Association	More than 100 research-oriented drug companies	32	7,500 (6)
American Nurses Association	200,000 nurses	21	25,024 (6)
Health Insurance Association of America	250 insurance companies	21	50,900 (6)
Group Health Association	350 HMOs	10	5,500 (8)
Health Industry Manufacturers Association	More than 300 producers of medical technology	9	2,000 (6)
American Health Care Association	11,000 nursing homes and other providers of long-term care	8	187,620 (8)

Source: Data from Bendavid, Goldman, and Kaplan (1993).

Note: Parentheses in column 4 indicate whether spending reflects six or eight months.

$747,000. Other big health contributors were the AHA ($264,140) and the ADA ($205,400) (see table 3.1).

Style changed too: "It's not about going up and tugging on Rosty's sleeve (Dan Rostenkowski of Illinois, the then-chair of the House Ways and Means Committee) and saying 'I need something,'" a former Clinton administration functionary told the *Washington Post*. "That gets you absolutely nowhere. It's knowing how to mobilize, having access to information, making the right moves at the right time" (Boodman 1994a, 6).

AN OVERVIEW OF INTEREST GROUPS AND POLITICAL LIFE IN AMERICA

The body of theory that describes interest groups and helps us understand their actions reflects the changes the groups themselves have undergone. Key elements of this theory include how and why they form and why they persist. Interest groups have evolved from closely knit alliances through rapid proliferation to their current position as diverse, large, and powerful players in federal (and state) policymaking. While many groups occupy somewhat narrow niches in policy, they also participate in coalitions that allow them to pool their efforts to affect or deflect broad policy change.

Interest groups provide information and campaign support to elected officials and tend to utilize three strategies to influence policy: lobbying, grassroots organizing, and campaign giving through PACs. While interest groups spend most of their time attempting to influence Congress, they also recognize the importance of lobbying the executive branch. Interest groups use the courts, often as a final avenue for action when other means fall short. In sum, the role of interest groups in defining and shaping health care policy is pivotal. Next to Congress, interest groups may well be the most important actors in health policy.

Interest groups are individuals who have organized themselves around some common interest and who seek to influence public policy. Interest groups include organizations as diverse as the Federation of Behavioral, Psychological, and Cognitive Sciences and the Association of State and Territorial Health Officials, as broad as the American Public Health Association, and as narrow as the American Society for Gastrointestinal Endoscopy. They also include corporations and institutional interests, such as hospitals, medical schools, HMOs, and schools of public health.

Some scholars have called their role in policymaking indispensable. They clarify and articulate citizens' preferences, warn policymakers of problems with their proposals, and suggest ways to make them more palatable or point out why what is being proposed will damage and enrage their groups' members. Simply put, groups represent the interests of their members. Those may be abortion rights or medical colleges or the nation's Catholic hospitals.

Whether interest groups are good guys or bad depends on who is making the decision. To the National Citizens' Coalition for Nursing Home Reform, the American Health Care Association, which represents for-profit nursing homes, is a money-hungry bunch who care nothing about patients. But to the nursing homes that make up the association's membership, the coalition is a bunch of "crazies" who know nothing about managing a business and demand that resources be wasted on silly, unnecessary rules and regulations.

Interest groups also serve to educate their members and others on issues and help form a feasible public agenda. They monitor activity, public and private, and can "blow the whistle" on a bad idea when it is proposed. Their job is to make the case for their constituents before government, plying the halls of Congress, the executive branch, the courts, and other interest groups' offices to provide a linkage between citizens and government. For many decades in this country, political parties provided this linkage. But in recent years, surveys show that people prefer to have more kindred spirits minding the store for them. The more well-heeled the group, the more likely it will make its own way rather than turn the job over to a broader group like a political party.

Interest groups are as American as talk shows and much older. James Madison, in Number 10 of the collection of political tracts arguing for support of the U.S. Constitution, the *Federalist Papers,* bemoaned the mischief of "factions," which he defined as "a number of citizens . . . who are united and actuated by some common impulse of passion or of interest" (Hamilton, Madison, and Jay 1961, 78). Though Madison put a negative "spin" on the factions by suggesting their interests might be adverse to the rights of other citizens and interests of the community, the right to associate is one of the first defended in the Bill of Rights.

A century later, Alexis de Tocqueville, the French visitor whose uncannily accurate observations still resonate today, observed that "in no country in the world has the principle of association been more successfully used or applied to a greater multitude of objects than in America" (1956, 95). He continued, "Wherever, at the head of some new undertaking, you see the government in France, or a man of rank in England, in the United States you will be sure to find an association" (198).

Interest group representation has long been a fact of life in Washington—much to the chagrin of many in government. Woodrow Wilson in 1913 said, "Washington was so full of lobbyists that 'a brick couldn't be thrown without hitting one'" (Brinkley 1993, A14). Eighty years later, President Bill Clinton, outlining his economic plan to Congress, noted that "within minutes of the time I conclude my address to Congress . . . the special interests will be out in force. . . . Many have already lined the corridors of power with high-priced lobbyists" (Brinkley 1993, A14).

Interest groups are essential to the American notion of pluralism—groups competing to put items on the agenda and to achieve their members' goals in public policies. Ideally, as Madison speculated, groups check each other and come to agree only on the common interest. James Madison's ideal has not, in fact, emerged. Groups are not equally endowed and fail to provide representation for all. As Schattschneider (1960, 35) put it, the pluralists' "heavenly chorus sings with a strong upper class accent." Poor people, immigrants, and ethnic minorities frequently are not as well represented as middle-class business interests. Even middle-class interests are not equal. The National Rifle Association is a very strong national lobby whose success is only partially checked by antihandgun groups and police associations. Such powerful interests as the AMA have the potential to be heard more strongly than organizations of nurse midwives or health consumers.

Groups do not always act in the public interest either. Frequently their contribution to public policymaking is to exercise a veto power over policy changes and innovation. Kingdon (1984) found that interest groups' power lies less in moving subjects onto the agenda than in keeping other subjects off. If they are well organized and well supported, things must be going well for them, suggesting that they are unlikely to welcome change. Often their goal is to block new initiatives from gaining widespread support, and they tend to be very good at this. A minority represented by a strong interest group can stop or delay legislation or a proposed rule. The system is set up that way, to make it hard to change policy. Lose one round, live to fight another: subcommittee, full committee, house floor, repeat the process in the second house, move to the more informal setting of the conference committee, and if you still have not succeeded, seek a presidential veto, try to influence the agency writing the regulations, or sue them in federal court for violating the due process clause of the Constitution.

The AMA reflects this penchant for maintaining the status quo, preserving existing benefits provided by government, and avoiding additional regulation. Since the 1920s, it has opposed national health insurance, restrictions on physicians' behavior, the development of alternative forms of health delivery, such as HMOs, and anything that encourages competition, such as advanced nurse practice. Interestingly, one exception to the AMA's opposition to expansion of the governmental role in health was its 1916 support of compulsory state health insurance, a proposal supported by the American Association of Labor Legislation. Four years later, the AMA withdrew its support for the proposal (Weeks and Berman 1985).

One term for this ability of a strong interest group minority to ride roughshod over majority interests is "interest group liberalism." President Jimmy Carter tried to sound the alarm that it was not good for the republic.

Making the growth of special interest organizations the topic of his farewell address, he said that "the national interest is not always the sum of all our single or special interests" (Carter 1981, 196). He called their growth a "disturbing factor in American political life."

How Interest Groups Are Formed

Analogies help scholars make sense out of complexities. Madison wrote the *Federalist Papers,* Number 10, at a time when educated people thought of the universe as a collection of forces pressing against one another. The point at which they equaled the other's force was called equilibrium and seemed somehow natural or right. Applied to politics, they concluded that this point of equilibrium was the public interest. Political scientist David B. Truman (1951) used the term equilibrium in one of the first efforts to describe why groups formed. Some disruption or disturbance upsets the equilibrium. People would then band together to restore the equilibrium by exerting countervailing force. Sometimes the formation of one group might lead to a disturbance that upset another group, which might in turn cause another to form, until a new social equilibrium was reached. Group formation might stabilize for a while, only to start again with another disturbance.

While this explanation goes a long way toward explaining the formation of most groups, it does not explain why groups stay together once the threat or event that caused the group to form has disappeared or attenuated. It also assumes that anyone can easily organize those who share their interests into a group during disturbances.

A second explanation for group formation highlights selective benefits. Olson (1968) offered what can be viewed as a "rational choice" argument: people join groups because they will directly benefit from membership through material rewards, such as the ability to serve on the staff of a hospital, to bid on certain construction jobs, or even just to receive discounted travel services or an informative magazine. Selective benefits also help overcome another problem with groups seeking public policy change: the free rider. Why join the Sierra Club when anybody can enjoy the clean water and unspoiled wilderness the club's policy advocacy has produced? The answer is selective benefits: to receive maps, camping tips, and other benefits of membership.

No group does this better than the American Association of Retired Persons (AARP), which has 33 million members, roughly one-fourth of the registered voters in the United States. With a low membership fee, anyone fifty years of age or older qualifies for rental car and hotel discounts, cut-rate prices on drugs, group health insurance, investment programs, or car and mobile home insurance.

Clark and Wilson (1961) built on the selective benefits notion, labeling three types of benefits that attract group membership: material benefits (magazines, discounts, tips, etc.); purposive benefits (those associated with ideological or issue-oriented goals without tangible benefits to members); and solidary or social benefits, which can also include the benefits from achieving worthwhile policy goals.

Salisbury (1969) offered a market-oriented view. He believed that interest groups are formed by entrepreneurs who invest capital to create benefits, which they offer to a market of potential customers at a price. In effect, an "exchange" takes place between the leaders who offer the incentives and the members who provide support. Exchange theory is useful because it explains not only how groups begin but also how they retain their membership and survive.

Walker (1991) said that 80 percent of American interest groups have emerged from preexisting occupational or professional communities. He could have been looking at health groups. There the link to jobs is clear: groups representing health professionals, health providers, and the health industry dominate the field.

Finally, interest groups can be launched directly or indirectly by governmental action. More government equals more groups. Walker (1991) said that groups are created more as a consequence of legislation than as an impetus for it. Governmental policies are adopted that provide new benefits or jobs to people who form groups to protect (and expand) those benefits and rights. The National Association of Retired Federal Employees was created after the passage of the first federal pensions for employees in the 1920s. When hospitals serving many Medicare patients experienced problems under a new financing scheme, they joined together to form the Association of High Medicare Hospitals, a group lobbying for the interests of these hospitals. Almost every time the federal Health Care Financing Administration (HCFA) funds a series of demonstration projects to study a new policy approach, it creates the core of a new interest group, which immediately starts lobbying for legislation to make the policy permanent before the research results are available.

There are many examples of interest groups launched directly by governmental agencies, in part to provide support in Congress for the continuation (and expansion) of programs for which they are responsible. The American Farm Bureau Federation and the U.S. Chamber of Commerce are the two best-known examples of groups started by governmental agencies. A health example is the genesis of the National Association of Community Health Centers. Federal grant dollars helped establish neighborhood health centers across the country, which then formed an association to lobby Congress for more funding. The federal funding agency facilitated the survival of the fledgling group by giving it additional grant money. Federal agencies often financially support citizen groups to participate in agency proceedings. Governmental sponsorship appears to be most successful in areas of low controversy. When groups oppose one another, policy professionals and bureaucrats cannot count on support from political leadership to protect their agencies against hostile critics (Walker 1991).

Groups are also formed in anticipation of federal action. Hospitals that wanted reclassification from rural to urban (to qualify for higher reimbursement) started a lobby-oriented association (Kosterlitz 1992). Other groups organize to prevent federal action. The Tobacco Institute was formed to fight the regulation of cigarettes (Walker 1991). The American Association of Blood Banks organized to fight a proposal for a national blood system (Tierney 1987). The National Council of Senior Citizens was created in the early 1960s to help fight for Medicare (Harris 1966).

Knowing why groups form and how they stick together is important for understanding their goals. Feldstein (1977) noted that health associations pursue policies that will allow a monopoly position for their members. This applies whether the group comprises professional members or nonprofit organizations. Feldstein argued that health interest groups are likely to support policies that will

—increase the demand for their services,
—enable them to be reimbursed as price-discriminating monopolists,
—lower the price of complementary inputs,
—increase the price of substitutes,
—restrict additions to their supply.

Simply put, health interest groups support policies to get them more patients, set their own prices, reduce their costs, make their product the best deal, and freeze out the competition. While pursuing these policies of self-interest, the groups will say they are acting in the best interests of the public. Health groups often "frame" the issue so their support is seemingly in the public interest.

In a typical example, the AHA opposed the Carter cost-containment proposal, noting that a "limitation on inpatient revenues related to the cost of living will reduce hospitals' ability to expand services to meet the medical needs of patients and will, in some institutions, reduce those services" (Iglehart 1977, 1530). The AMA, trying to curb nurses' efforts to increase their autonomy and range of care, resorted to the quality-of-care rationale as well, saying that expanding nurses' roles would "raise questions of patient safety" (Priest 1993). Interestingly, the same AMA board of trustees report discounted the public's preferences, saying that "patient satisfaction is not useful to differentiate between or prove the congruity of 'quality of care' between doctors and nurses" (Priest 1993, A3).

For many years the world of interest groups was dominated by "peak associations" or umbrella organizations representing large groups of farmers, businesses, or labor unions. In the 1990s the landscape became much more varied, with the larger organizations still in existence but sharing space with smaller, more focused groups, often formed from the peak associations. For example, complementing the AMA at the time of the Clinton administration's health proposal efforts were at least eighty medical specialty groups representing surgeons, pediatricians, emergency room physicians, ophthalmologists, plastic surgeons, and others. Similar diversification occurred in the hospital industry, where the interests of small community hospitals, large nonprofit hospitals, teaching hospitals, and inner-city hospitals differed so substantially that one organization (the AHA) could not fully represent them all. What frequently happens is that the larger umbrella organization must take general positions that minimize conflict, while the specialized, smaller groups are free to adopt more specific positions targeted at their members.

Interest Groups Working Together

The fragmentation of interest groups and the fragmentation of power in the Congress has made the formation of coalitions especially important. In these coalitions, interest groups can maximize their resources and their lobby strength. They can work to influence a wider array of policies and to a degree that was not possible by going it alone.

Some coalitions are of long standing, with long-term relationships of support over many years and numerous policy battles. Such groups can be called policy communities or networks of interest groups active in a particular domain or representing similar constituencies. Sometimes these coalitions are well funded and staffed. An example is the 113-member National Health Council, founded in 1920 to improve the health of the nation. With a budget of about $1 million, the National Health Council encompasses voluntary and professional health societies, federal agencies, national organizations, and business groups with strong health interests.

More typical are temporary coalitions, formed to work together on one issue or policy, only to disband when the issue dies or becomes law. The 1994 health care debate launched a number of coalitions formed expressly to present a certain view or opinion. One of the most visible coalitions during the debate was the Coalition for Health Insurance Choices, made up of independent insurers and businesses that dealt with them. The National Leadership Coalition for Health Care Reform, whose members included larger employers, and the Health Care Reform Project, whose members included the American Association of Retired Persons, Citizen Action, and American Airlines, were often more positive to the Clinton proposals. A usual pattern is for these temporary coalitions to be funded by special member assessments. For example, the Health Care Reform Project was funded with $5,000 contributions from each of its seventeen members ("Coalition Starts" 1993). In some coalitions, such as the more than fifty-member Mental Health Liaison Group, member organizations fund their own activities.

Groups are free to join multiple coalitions, and many do. The ANA joined no fewer than forty coalitions in 1993, including the Health Care Reform Project, the National Leadership Coalition for Health Care Reform, the Campaign for Women's Health, and the Long-Term Care Campaign (Bendavid, Goldman, and Kaplan 1993). Sometimes coalitions are useful for highly visible groups to get support for their preferences from other, more "legitimate" groups. For example, a coalition of citizen groups and public health advocates opposing limits on Medicaid spending for prescription drugs was formed in 1993 by the Pharmaceutical Manufacturers Association (PMA). A PMA spokesperson acknowledged that the coalition was formed to give more credibility to Congress than if the PMA made the apparently self-serving arguments (Pear 1993a).

Interest groups see coalitions as a way to maximize their likelihood of success with a minimum of staff effort by devising joint strategies with like-minded groups. Most coalitions have no staff or formal organizational structure, and their membership is fluid, with groups joining or leaving at will. Coalitions often best serve the needs of smaller resource-poor groups, which can improve their probability of success by joining with larger, more powerful groups and can often use materials and information from the larger members of the coalition for their own purposes. The larger groups benefit from coalitions by having their positions endorsed by a number of other groups and broadening their base of support. Their positions often prevail in these coalitions, since staff members from larger groups often lead and provide resources to the coalition.

Salisbury, Heinz, Laumann, and Nelson (1987) looked at the stability of coalitions or alliances in four different policy domains—energy, health, agriculture, and labor—and found that the interests varied considerably in how groups worked together from issue to issue. They found that interest groups involved in agriculture tend to be nonpartisan and work quietly together; those involved in labor issues were noisy, conflictive, and partisan. Health interest groups were highly visible but less rancorous than others.

Respondents were asked by the researchers to name three "adversarial" and three "allied" groups in their policy domain. Some clear differences emerged among the health groups. For example, hospital groups were much more closely allied than medical associations. Hospital groups named forty-one other hospital groups as allies and only one as an adversary. But medical associations named forty-one medical associations as allies and nineteen as adversaries. When the focus shifted to intergroup perceptions, medical associations felt much more embattled by those outside the fold. They named twenty-seven adversarial groups. Academic groups named only one adversary; hospitals named twenty-two. Although adversaries tended to be citizen and labor groups (eleven for hospitals, for example), citizen and labor groups were also chosen as allies to hospitals, more often than in other policy domains studied. Yet compared to respondents in the other domains the researchers examined, health representatives were fairly collegial. According to Salisbury et al., they "perceived their issues to be less conflict ridden and less partisan" than did other participants in the study (1987, 1226).

Niche Theory

Unlike the pluralistic notion of interest groups competing against one another to reach some type of accommodation, in some interest areas, the groups tend to stake out policy domains that are recognized as theirs and accommodated by other groups. A group does this by finding a recognizable identity, defining a highly specific issue niche for itself, and fixing its political assets (i.e., recognition and other resources) within that niche. Often groups with special expertise can establish a niche and are not threatened by other interests. Clearly, such a staking out of territory has a practical appeal, since one interest group cannot influence everything.

Another key component of finding a niche is the instability of the policy world. Without the security of friends in the Congress and bureaucracy, and with such forces as the decentralization of Congress, citizen groups, the president, and the press exerting influence, interest groups can attain some sense of security by staking out a policy niche and devoting resources there (Browne 1991). For example, the Association of American Medical Colleges (AAMC) focuses on policies affecting the nation's 125 medical schools. AAMC has not often ventured into broader health care issues, but it has been perceived as the dominant force in issues related to medical education.

Niche politics prevail when the issues are narrow and involve few interests. Cigler and Loomis felt that the "bulk of group politics" takes place within these policy niches or policy communities (1991, 392). As long as discrete policies do not cross niche boundaries, these accommodations can continue, even as more and more groups are added.

Comprehensive proposals for change can disrupt the niches. When reforms touch financing, education, quality, cost, and a host of details, the scope of the conflict is widened. Choices have to be made about what to fight for and against. Old alliances and dominance of an issue can break down, opening opportunities for new patterns of dominance (Baumgartner and Jones 1993). Often niche groups participate in coalitions when comprehensive change is proposed as a way to ensure that the major change will encompass issues of concern to the niche group or that damage to the status quo of major concern to them will be minimal.

Health policy has long been characterized as niche politics with highly specialized groups dealing with focused, even arcane, issues. The issues are often resolved without much outside attention.

From Iron Triangles to Issue Networks

The dominant political model of interest group influence for many years was the iron triangle, where decisions were made by congressional committees, interest groups, and bureaucrats as the three vertices of the triangle. This triumvirate was so strong that it tended to prevail over all others, including the president. Sometimes called subgovernments, or policy subsystems, or policy monopolies, these relationships were viewed as impermeable and lasting. Major decisions were said to be made by a few experts who benefited from working closely together. The interest group benefited from close access to decision makers and implementors. The bureaucracy benefited by ensuring adequate appropriations and public support. Congressional staffs benefited by garnering the substantive and political resources of these key actors—making members look good to other members and constituents. To understand policymaking on an issue, one had only to look at the interest groups affected by it, the congressional committee making the policy, and the bureaucracy implementing the law. In the health area these iron triangles were dominated by experts, often health professionals, and were buttressed by a lofty goal so well acknowledged by the citizenry that few questions were asked (Baumgartner and Jones 1993).

While intuitively persuasive, the notion of iron triangles proved to be simplistic and wrong as American policymaking moved into a world of competing interests, complexity, and tough choices. Instead, a view popularized as "issue networks" developed to describe the more free-floating, varied groupings of many individuals, including specialists outside government, journalists, academics, and policy entrepreneurs.

Issue networks are fairly open collections of people who help shape governmental policymaking. The term, coined by Heclo (1978), describes loosely connected interest groups, experts within and outside of government, and others with expertise, working together on some aspect of public policy. The definition is somewhat nebulous because members of issue networks can have varying degrees of expertise and commitment to the policy, and can move in and out of the policy domain. Issue networks are sloppy, unpredictable, and very difficult to describe, much less predict or explain.

Another aspect of the shift to networks relates to the complexity of issues like health care policy. Since jurisdiction is widely shared among many committees, rather than focusing on one or two committees, most interest groups now tend to work with four or five separate committees or agencies and, on some issues, with committees not generally in their purview. Even an issue as specific as prospective Medicare reimbursements caught the attention of the Gray Panthers, the National Council of Senior Citizens, and a host of others as well as traditional physician and hospital interests.

Recent empirical studies of interest groups have increased our understanding by charting the acquaintance networks of groups identified as influential in several key policy domains, including health (Heinz et al. 1990; Salisbury et al. 1987). The researchers looked for interest groups that were influential in more than one of several different fields: health, labor, agriculture, and energy. They found none. Had the research been done thirty years earlier, some feel they would have found that the American Federation of Labor and Congress of Industrial Organizations (AFL-CIO) was influential in multiple issue areas, such as health, income and poverty policy, aging policy, housing, and labor relations.

Likewise, the researchers found that for each of these issues (health, labor, agriculture and energy) few mediators or facilitators worked closely with their colleagues concerned with the same issues. Instead, influential people talked with others who agreed with them, based largely on their organization's or clients' interests. This the researchers dubbed a network of interest groups with a hollow core or empty center, sans actors who bridge various aspects of policy. Again, thirty years earlier they might have found such mediators or coordinators in the form of the Farm Bureau in agriculture and the AMA in health care policy.

In short, the interest group world appears to have come full circle: from tightly knit, closely coordinated, closed, and impervious to atomistic, uncoordinated, and highly permeable.

The Invasion of the Externality Groups

"Externality groups," so dubbed by Salisbury (1992), are primarily citizen groups, "good government" or issue organizations, formed around specific causes or proposed changes. Though still small in both numbers and resources, their growth curve is impressive, and their potential for influencing policy is substantial in both Washington, D.C., and the states. They have helped to displace the iron triangle because they force legislators to consider a broader electoral base on many policy questions. They can also destabilize the policy process because they often use dramatic, headline-grabbing strategies that can arouse the public and force elected officials to take public positions instead of working behind the scenes for consensus (Heinz et al. 1993).

These groups have grown for the same reasons that other groups have grown, namely, the expanding scope and size of the government. Citizen groups are now a larger proportion of national lobbying associations than ever before, and they are growing at a faster pace than other groups. Walker (1991) found that citizen groups (which he defines as those whose membership is not based on occupational or professional status) made up nearly one-fourth of the total groups he identified in 1985. Over one-half of the citizen groups he surveyed had been created within the preceding twenty-five years.

Oddly, the growth in the importance of citizen groups is not reflected in health. While some have found relatively large numbers of citizen groups, there is little evidence that these groups have had much effect on health policy. A few well-known citizen groups target health issues, such as Planned Parenthood, the Public Citizen Health Research Group, the National Women's Health Network, and the National Citizens' Coalition for Nursing Home Reform. However, these and other smaller groups seem to lack both the membership and the resources to be significant players in national health policy formation. As evidence of their lack of visibility, citizen or consumer group was not listed as one of the 146 categories of health group in a prominent directory (National Health Council 1993). The group with many members and resources that is very concerned about health issues is the American Association of Retired Persons. When asked to name the citizen groups active in the 1994 health care discussions, one well-placed participant named only the AARP. Cigler and Loomis (1995) note AARP as the exception to their point that consumers of medical care are not well represented. While AARP fits Walker's definition of a citizen group, its role of protecting current and expanding future health care benefits under Medicare seems to fit the spirit of an occupational or professional group protecting its concentrated interest in regulation (or in this case reimbursement) and imposing costs on a broad population base (Feldstein 1977). More successful are groups of citizens whom Foreman (1995) calls grass-roots victims organizations—persons who are directly and often suddenly and tragically affected by a health hazard or disease. Such groups, the Love Canal Homeowners Association and the AIDS Coalition to Unleash Power (ACT-UP), for example, can achieve limited, targeted policy success.

Citizen groups often have little grass-roots support in the districts of members. Browne (1993) concluded that environmental public interest groups were often disadvantaged in their interactions with Congress because members rarely heard from constituent-members of these groups when they went home to their districts. Often the local activists were more concerned with local issues than national ones, and other constituents had only general views about better national environmental conditions.

Why Iron Triangles Are Out

Salisbury believed that iron triangles are outdated because they cannot survive in a "destabilized world of fragmented interests and multidimensional challenges from externality groups" (1992, 347). No longer do interest groups direct politicians, said Salisbury, but rather politicians now very often exploit the interest groups. Policy instability is key, according to Cigler (1991, 121), who added less hegemonic interests, more openness in the decision-making process, intergroup competitiveness, and a willingness among partisan officials to intervene even in narrow policy arenas as reasons for the demise of iron triangles. The sheer number of interests and the increase in citizen groups also contributed to the demise of iron triangles (Walker 1991).

Iron triangles were further weakened by changes in regulatory patterns. Rather than having one administrative agency writing regulations and overseeing programs of concern, businesses and others today must deal with "cross-industry" regulation. Rules governing environmental protection, occupational safety, and health and energy conservation apply across industries, making participation much more difficult and involving several different federal agencies. As Heinz et al. (1993, 385) put it, "Policy making had become more significant for more groups, but less controlled by the groups it affected."

Finally, the congressional actors have changed. The decentralization of congressional power means that interest groups cannot simply work with leaders or a few committee chairs. Rather, they must inform and attempt to persuade several committee chairs and probably dozens of members to maximize the likelihood that their positions will prevail. The party leadership changes in 1995 also made it tough for interest groups accustomed to working with Democratic chairs and their staffs.

Nevertheless, it would be misleading to say that the iron triangle is completely gone from the scene. On some complex, nonsalient issues or those with little opposition, the iron triangles may still prevail. For example, on policy for the disabled, Scotch (1984) found a tightly unified subgovernment with no effective opposition. Veterans policy is heavily dominated by the influence of the disabled veterans organization and a few other veterans groups, a small number of House and Senate committees, and the Department of Veterans Affairs. Few others concern themselves with policy decisions affecting veterans. At the state level, groups representing mentally retarded and developmentally disabled persons often work closely with legislative supporters and agency staff to achieve policy goals, rarely questioned by other policymakers.

Influencing Decision Making

Many interest groups use a three-pronged strategy to influence policy-making: direct lobbying, grass-roots lobbying, and campaign contributions (through PACs). Direct lobbying may be viewed as an "inside" strategy in which groups use their financial resources and expertise to work directly with political and administrative leaders (Walker 1991). This strategy works especially well in Congress. Grass-roots lobbying is an "outside" strategy involving the mobilization of members and appeals to the broad public. It is more indirect but can be powerfully effective and has grown enormously in popularity over the past few years. Campaign contributions are provided through PACs in a type of outside strategy but are often dispensed in coordination with the desires of the group's lobbyists, who may include the allocation of monetary resources as part of their broad lobbying strategy.

WHAT LOBBYISTS DO

Defining lobbying might seem easy to most people, but not so to the U.S. Treasury Department. Its 1994 proposed rules to implement a 1993 law repealing the tax deductibility for lobbying took thirty pages. Boiled down, all those words seemed to define lobbying as activities that seek to influence legislation (Hershey 1994).

Salisbury (1992) found that lobbyists report spending most of their time monitoring issues and providing information, much of it to other groups. This makes sense, they say, because of the rapid expansion of new groups and the burgeoning growth of the list of activities into which government now injects itself. More and more interest groups are commissioning research to support their positions. As one lobbyist put it, "commissioning studies gives us more persuasive position to argue from" (Stone 1994, 2842).

Information is most useful in the early stages of bill consideration—when members must get up to speed on the issue and its impact on their districts. Later in the process things change. "We've long passed informational lobbying; now we're at the break-your-arm lobbying," said Senator John Breaux of Louisiana late in the 1994 health reform debate (Seelye 1994, A10).

To make use of what they see and learn, lobbyists must meet the most important proximate goal of their profession: gaining access. A chance to tell their story is key to most lobbying strategies. To the interest group, access may mean having telephone calls answered and meetings arranged regularly with members and their staffs. Sabato (1985, 127) quoted one PAC official as saying, "frequently all it takes is the opportunity to talk to a legislator 10 or 15 minutes to make your case. He may not have 10 or 1 minute to hear the other side." Wright (1990) found that the number of lobbying contacts was a better predictor of legislators' votes than the amount of campaign contributions.

Access alone is not always enough, of course. Lobbyists must be able to present a case so persuasive that the member will support their position. They do this in part with good, timely information on complex issues. More than 90 percent of interest group respondents to a 1981–82 survey indicated that their organizations provide research results and technical information (Schlozman and Tierney 1986). The form and content of this information are key. Smith (1984) argued that lobbyists must show how the position that the lobbyists favor is also the one most consistent with the goals of the members. Baumgartner and Jones (1993) refer to it as the "policy image" or definition of an issue.

Successful lobbyists understand they must do more than simply convince the member of the value of the desired position. They must also provide them with acceptable explanations of their position, explanations that can be used to justify their position to constituents and others. Ellen Merlo, a Philip Morris executive, described how this is done (Rosenblatt 1994, 55):

> Once you have the access, you have to be able to deliver a message that makes sense. If it's a tax that we're against, then we have to be able to prove that there are going to be job losses, that it's not going to produce the revenue that is being projected, that if a state raises its taxes so high and it's next to another state with low taxes, there are going to be cross-border sales and those sales will not only be a loss in tobacco revenue, but once someone goes over a border to buy their tobacco or their liquor or something else, they're probably making a lot of other purchases.

Yet in grass-roots lobbying, groups sometimes rely on emotion, even misinformation, rather than facts, in calling the public to action. One example was the 1993 effort by the makers of nebulizers and aspirators to enlist the elderly users of their products to help persuade the Congress that their devices should be rented rather than purchased under Medicare. The manufacturers apparently persuaded the public that their lives were in danger if the Congress made a change in the current rental provisions, and the Congress faced a barrage of mail from senior citizens pleading to retain the current system. Unable to make the tough decision, Congress asked the Department of Health and Human Services to decide whether nebulizers and aspirators should be rented or bought (Brinkley 1993).

Lobbyists are often most successful in the seemingly small, highly technical issues. Partly this is just the experience of the lobbyist who is likely to be expert at noticing small differences within broad legislative categories. When a tax-staff-expert-turned-lobbyist looked over a new tax bill, she saw important distinctions missed by the bill's drafters and wrote to the tax committee's staff with an argument that hotel and airline club membership were distinctly different from the kinds of executive club membership that the committee sought to tax. These kinds of clubs should be excluded from the definition of those newly subject to taxation, she argued. One of her letters reached a congressional staffer who agreed and wrote the exception into the law even though he never met or spoke with the lobbyist (Rosenbaum 1993). Her alert eye helped the committee avoid unintended consequences and the cumbersome task of repealing an amendment, should the provision have become law and then proved unworkable.

Lobbyists also earn their money by keeping issues off the public policy agenda. Kingdon (1984) calls these negative blocking activities to preserve what the group has and to maintain the status quo. He believes interest groups spend more time blocking agenda items or proposing amendments to or substitutes for proposals on the agenda than they do creating new policies.

With budget declines and pressures to shrink the size of government, nowadays it is at least as important to maintain existing successes or minimize cuts as to get more. The efforts of the National Citizens' Coalition for Nursing Home Reform led to the modification of rules they supported instead of to their cancellation, as the administration had initially proposed—an effort the group counted as a lobbying success (Tierney 1987).

Lobbying Congress

While good lobbyists will work with key officials in the executive branch as well as the Congress, they will focus more attention—and often rack up more successes—on Capitol Hill than elsewhere in the city. Former AHA president John McMahon said it this way: "Congress has a greater understanding and more sympathy with our problems" (Iglehart 1977, 1527). The understanding stems, in no small measure, from the important role hospitals play in the economies of local communities; the standing of hospital administrators, boards, and staffs in the district; and the likely campaign support derived from them and their employees.

The old adage "It's who you know" has traditionally been very important in the lobbying business. Lobbyists rely heavily on legislative "friends" or advocates and spend much of their time trying to retain or increase the intensity of members' commitment to an established, favored position. As Matthews put it in 1960, "the principal effect of lobbying is not conversion but reinforcement" (191). Seeking to curb the growing legislative zeal to promote HMOs in the early 1970s, the AMA devoted most of its time to the House Commerce Committee rather than the more liberal Senate counterpart chaired by HMO advocate Senator Edward Kennedy of Massachusetts. The American Association of Foundations of Medical Care, a group representing individual practice associations (IPAs), used a different tactic. It convinced a key member of the Senate Labor and Public Welfare Committee to support the inclusion of IPAs in the bill with adequate funding. In the same legislative debate, the Group Health Association asked a top labor leader to talk with West Virginia Representative Harley Staggers, chair of the House Interstate and Foreign Commerce Committee, about the importance of HMOs, and Staggers became "an ardent supporter" (Falkson 1980, 161).

Today lobbyists must often cast their legislative nets wider than the already converted. Lobbyists spend much of their time on uncommitted members. Neither side can ignore them, because in a close vote, the uncommitted members can make the difference. Both supporters and opponents of the Clinton plan targeted the same 100 House members and fifteen to twenty Senators, mostly moderate Democrats, for special attention during the 1994 health reform debate (Boodman 1994).

Finally, some political scientists argue that interest group lobbyists must target unfriendly legislators with the idea that the group can persuade them to change their minds. Austin-Smith and Wright (1994) found that many interest groups lobbied senators who were disposed to vote against the group's position on the 1987 Senate confirmation of Robert Bork to the Supreme Court. They argue that groups' lobbying of senators who agreed with their positions was not to reinforce their support but to counter the influence of opposition groups lobbying the same senators.

Lobbyists also buttonhole staff. It gives them someone to work on when the member is too busy, but they also recognize the reality that the staff make many of the decisions on specific issues of concern to the interest groups. Groups often sponsor staff seminars in exclusive resorts, giving lobbyists a chance to fully discuss issues of common interest (Noah 1993, A16).

Lobbyists provide valuable information to members about the policy consequences of a proposal and about how policy will affect the member's reelection chances. In the words of political science, lobbyists help reduce the member's uncertainty about the proposed policy and in so doing affect the voting decision (Smith 1995, 99).

While a 1993 law eliminating the tax deductibility of lobbying expenses affects some lobbying efforts, especially by smaller groups, it does not reduce the influence of lobbyists by much. Why? Because in the final analysis, Congress appreciates lobbyists. They tell members what will not work and how things will play back home, warn of unwanted consequences, and help at election time.

The decentralization of Congress in the 1980s and early 1990s made lobbying a much tougher job. Some 57 percent of interest group respondents in a Schlozman and Tierney (1986) survey said increasing the number of subcommittees in Congress made it harder for their organizations to operate effectively. The growth in the number of committee staffs has made the job harder for 48 percent of the respondents. While the role of committee chairs has diminished somewhat as the entrepreneurship of individual members of Congress has increased, the likelihood that committee chairs will be key members of conference committees makes them an important target of lobbying efforts.

The change of political control of the House and Senate in 1995 jolted the interest group world made up of lobbyists accustomed to working with Democratic committee leadership. Groups scurried to hire former Republican staffs and to acquaint themselves with Republican House members and seek common interests. Firms that "bagged" Republican staff bragged in press releases about their "understanding of the dynamics surrounding the Republican control of New Congress" (Moore 1994, 2768). While the Republicans' efforts to reduce the House staff and cut the number of committees made it somewhat easier to reduce lobbying staffs, most of the impact was in a shift in political connections, not a reduction in size. With massive federal cuts as a top federal priority, lobbyists were needed to protect current favorable policies and to prevent cutbacks and reductions that adversely affect the interest group.

Lobbying the President

Good lobbyists target both the president and the agency responsible for implementing a law. In the 1972–73 efforts to pass HMO legislation, lobbyists from groups both supporting and opposing the effort met with Department of Health, Education, and Welfare staff and with White House officials to make their case. In opposing key provisions of the bill, the AMA put pressure on the White House, often reminding key officials of the importance of the Physicians Committee to Reelect the President. AMA lobbyists met almost daily with the White House staff at one point and succeeded in getting the president to reverse his policy on the preemption of existing state laws (Iglehart 1972).

Although the Office of Management and Budget and the Executive Office of the President are important policy actors, they are often difficult for lobbyists to reach. Their staffs are smaller (compared to the entire federal bureaucracy and Congress) and are less likely to be swayed by particularistic concerns for one region or state, since they work for the president, the only elected official (other than the vice president) who represents the nation as a whole. This may not be quite so true in an election year, of course, when electoral votes and key primaries begin to be considered. It is also true that interest groups' concerns are often specific and most relevant to legislative or regulatory language—not in the scope of presidential activity.

The Bureaucracy and Interest Groups

Some argue that bureaucracies are acting like interest groups and compete with them for congressional influence. "Surely the single most cogent explanation for the decreased ability of the traditionally dominant interest to dictate health policy is that the federal government itself is now the major protagonist in health interest politics" (Tierney 1987, 102–3). Government is paying a large part of the health care bill for Medicare, Medicaid, and other services (well over $250 billion in federal spending in 1994). It operates a huge system of hospitals and clinics for veterans, and it administers grants to states and localities for home health care, maternal and child health care, family planning, and health centers for migrants. To deal with its interests, the federal government has a large bureaucracy, staffed with experts in day-to-day activities of health financing and the provision of health care. Because bureaucrats oversee federal health programs, they have more at stake than many players. Should the federal government sit by idly and wait for Congress to write bad policy or fail to make important policy improvements, or should it protect its interests by sending its experts to the Hill to meet with staffs, brief members, help with bill drafting, and testify at hearings? Both Congress and the agencies appear to have answered that question with a resounding "yes." The range of opportunities expands when bureaucrats are detailed to key subcommittees to pitch in on such major issues as the Medicare prospective payment system (PPS), RBRVS, and health reform. "I was probably the only guy on the Hill who really understood what was in the RBRVS bill, because I wrote so much of it," said one agency staffer detailed to the Congress.

The increasing size and complexity of governmental health services has led to a subsequent increase in the power given to the federal bureaucracy (Morone and Dunham 1985; Tierney 1987). Congress often delegates the power to make key decisions to the bureaucracy regarding how programs will work and provides inconsistent oversight of implementation (see Chapter 4). The dominating concern for controlling health care costs has focused attention on the executive branch in its role as the implementor and source of expertise about the details of major health care programs, such as Medicare and Medicaid.

Interest groups understand this transfer of power and focus some portion of their efforts on executive agencies. In the Schlozman and Tierney (1986) survey, some two-thirds of interest group respondents said executive agencies were an important focus for their activity; 78 percent said their organization helped agencies draft regulations. The AHA and the AMA were key actors in formulating the regulations associated with Medicare. Both succeeded in achieving many of their desired changes because the success of the program depended on the participation of the nation's hospitals and physicians (Campion 1984; Feder 1977; Weeks and Berman 1985).

Lobbyists must change their tactics when they hail a cab for the short trip from Capitol Hill down to HHS headquarters at 200 Independence Avenue. PAC dollars are not an option. Bureaucrats also tend to be less easily persuaded by local physicians or hospital board members. But there are other avenues available to these groups. Sometimes interest groups attempt to influence the selection of agency heads. In his memoir, *The Vantage Point*, former President Lyndon Johnson noted that he received more than a thousand telegrams asking him not to appoint Wilbur Cohen Secretary of Health, Education, and Welfare because he was "an enemy of American medicine" (1971, 218). But information—the stock in trade of the lobbyist—can still be useful to bureaucrats. Lobbyists develop contacts with midlevel experts, tell them what is going on with their industry, what they have heard on the Hill, what other agencies with overlapping jurisdiction are doing, and in the usual ways gain entrée. This can result in them gaining opportunities to comment informally on possible changes and run up a red flag if a provision is likely to cause a major flap (Tierney 1987, 111).

Interest groups often form coalitions to fight regulations, much as they do to fight legislation. When the Occupational Safety and Health Administration (OSHA) was drafting proposed indoor air-quality standards to ban smoking in most workforce arenas, the National Federation of Independent Businesses, American Dental Association, and National Restaurant Association formed a coalition to fight ventilation system requirements (Stone 1994, 2842).

In one sense, lobbying these midlevel personnel is easier than lobbying Congress: the staff tends to be much more stable, and long-term relationships can be developed more easily with them than with the much more highly mobile congressional staff. It is also easier to get an appointment. When they are not able to sway the agency involved, lobbyists often go back to Congress. A good example was the experience of the Federal Trade Commission (FTC) with cigarette labeling in 1965, when the cigarette lobbyists were able to stall FTC regulations by including a four-year moratorium on the FTC's rule-making power over cigarette advertising in federal law (Fritschler 1989). Similarly, a concerted effort by the diet food and soft drink producers in 1977 led to legislation postponing a proposed Food and Drug Administration (FDA) ban on saccharine (Schlozman and Tierney 1986).

Lobbyists can also sometimes gain access to the agency head more easily than can a midlevel bureaucrat working on a policy draft. Bureau staffs know that lobbyists possess these access-to-power weapons and are loathe to simply ignore lobbyists' requests. They may choose to resist and carry the fight forward, but they are likely to make a careful job of it when they know that their administrative and political bosses are going to hear the other side from the lobbyists. As one example, one HHS department head was lobbied hard by the nursing home industry concerning soon-to-be-issued regulations of quality. The word filtered down that the regulations were not to be stringent and must be acceptable to the industry.

Lobbyists are also likely to have to answer to the Office of Management and Budget. Probably responding to fierce lobbying efforts on the Hill, OMB vetoed efforts by HHS to merge capital into the prospective payment system and to establish national fee schedules for physician payments under Medicare in the 1980s. On the other hand, OMB also refused a plan favored by the HHS secretary to provide Medicare coverage for heart transplant surgery (Tierney 1987, 113).

If lobbyists fail to get the desired outcome in the regulation, the fight is likely to continue in the courts. Of the thirty health standards issued by OSHA since the early 1970s, twenty-seven have led to lawsuits. The courts have blocked only two (Stone 1994, 2842).

Outside Strategy

Interest groups recognize the importance of using their own members as constituent-lobbyists. Members of Congress value their constituents' views and weigh them heavily in their decisions. How better to influence a member's vote than by sending your message through constituents? Though it seems only recently to have hit the big time, the grass-roots strategy has been employed for decades. Skocpol (1992) told of the successful effort of the National Congress of Mothers in 1920 to write letters, visit members, and get publicity in local papers in support of a federal program to promote maternal health education (the Sheppard-Towner bill). To assist the women in their effort, the official National Committee of Mothers magazine included blank petitions as its last page.

Interest groups motivate their members to correspond with their senators and representatives by writing letters, sending faxes, or meeting personally with them in their districts or in Washington. Their scope can be impressive. In a 1990 effort the AMA initiated 100,000 letters to Medicare officials to protest budget cuts affecting physicians (Kosterlitz 1992). Four years later the AHA launched a $1-million grass-roots effort to get its 4,900 member hospitals and their workers to advocate community-based networks, employer mandates, and universal access ("AHA Launches" 1994). In 1994 groups representing drug manufacturers, insurers, and a myriad of health care providers blanketed Capitol Hill offices with postcards, letters, and telephone calls. Advocates of more funding for breast cancer research were more proactive: in the early 1990s they held candlelight vigils on the Capitol steps and crowded congressional offices with breast cancer survivors.

Probably most effective is hometown folks directly lobbying their representatives in person. Some 80 percent of the Schlozman and Tierney (1986) respondents reported using this technique, dubbed "the Utah plant manager theory of lobbying." The idea is that a senator from Utah may not make time to meet with a lobbyist from a large conglomerate or interest group but will agree to see the manager of a local branch plant or a delegation of local physicians. As frequent AMA critic California Representative Pete Stark noted, "My colleagues listen to folks from home and that's the AMA's strength" (Feder 1993).

In the 1993–94 health reform debate, the National Federation of Independent Business (NFIB), representing thousands of small business owners, was very successful in mobilizing its members to write and call their representatives and tell them the potential harm employer mandates could wreak on them. The NFIB bombarded its members with taxes and mailings, targeted telephone campaigns just prior to key votes, and scheduled hundreds of meetings during members' visits to the dentist. "What the NFIB did in the local community was to give the issues a larger meaning," said one member of the House Energy and Commerce Committee who was heavily lobbied by NFIB members in his district. "Their information was literally corroborated by first-hand stories," he said (Lewis 1994, A9).

The grass-roots movement was initiated by citizen groups, especially Ralph Nader–sponsored groups, and labor unions. By the mid-1980s other groups recognized the movement's importance and were able to expand the grass-roots scope with resources and technology. Satellite networks can instantly connect Washington offices with affiliates in the states. Fax machines can send messages quickly all over the country. Local callers are assisted in reaching their own representatives and provided with a script of what to say and ask (Brinkley 1993). A variant on the grass-roots strategy was employed by Health USA, a citizens' health group that sent staffers to live in the states of key members of Congress in 1994 to build up support and highlight the need for health care reform.

While popular, there is some sentiment that grass-roots efforts have been overused. If the effort is clearly programmed, with every postcard and phone call providing identical pleas, the recipient may discount it. Former Texas Senator Lloyd Bentsen once derogatorily called an effort more "Astroturf" than grass roots when, as chair of the Senate Finance Committee, he received reams of programmed responses (Toner 1994a).

Persuading the Public

A related "outside" strategy is targeted at the broader public—getting people to "buy in" to policies or positions advocated by interest groups. Some use their grass-roots members to inform others in their communities. Dentists and physicians can use their waiting rooms to distribute information and encourage the political voice of patients. A 1993 AMA campaign urged physicians to lobby their patients and mailed out questions patients might ask and answers the physicians should give them. AMA leadership said the organization would "activate an unprecedented national network of physicians" to achieve AMA objectives that reflect "their patients' interests, not just their own economic interests" (Pear 1993b, A1). In their own way, brewers used their resources, outfitting beer trucks with huge placards urging beer drinkers to call an 800 number to fight potential taxes on beer.

Sometimes the groups go directly to the public. Often a concerned group's first step in developing a strategy to blunt the effect of reform on its interests is hiring a pollster who can help the group "shape" its message to "resonate" with the public. The Consumers Union, questioning the appropriateness of forcing citizens into HMOs, commissioned a poll that found that nearly one-half of Americans would be willing to pay more money to choose their own doctor, and 91 percent said it was important to choose a specialist (Rubin 1993a). Community-based primary-care training consortia funded surveys revealing that the public highly valued primary care and supported more federal dollars going to the training of generalist physicians and nurses.

The next step in a public-oriented campaign is usually bringing on an advertising consultant to help design a television and print ad campaign aimed at consumers (Toner 1994a). In the 1980s the AMA was highly successful in its print campaign designed to inform the nation's elderly citizens of the harmful effects of restrictions on Medicare payments to physicians (Kosterlitz 1992). One ad showed a sad elderly woman under a headline asking "How do you tell someone on Medicare she's an expenditure target?" The timing of the ad—run during a period when elderly people were revolting over an unpopular (and later revoked) catastrophic health bill—was key. The AMA called the ad, its first directed at Congress, "a bold step." Many in Congress were furious (Alston 1989).

In the 1993–94 health care battle for the public's support, television was the weapon of choice. An estimated $60 million was spent on television alone—$10 million more than the total spending for advertising in the 1992 presidential campaign (Seelye 1994, A10). The most highly visible advertising campaigns launched in 1993 were those of the insurance industry, featuring a fictitious Harry and Louise questioning the Clinton health care plan over the kitchen table. While several coalitions and the Clintons themselves tried to counter, and later parody, the ads, they were widely cited by media and members, and set a questioning or dubious tone for the public debate. The ad's sponsors, the Health Insurance Association of America (HIAA), the 300-member association of insurance companies, spent more than $12 million on advertising on Harry and Louise and related health reform ads. One evidence of the success of Harry and Louise was the ad's role in HIAA negotiations with a key health committee. The HIAA agreed to muzzle Harry and Louise while the House Ways and Means Committee considered health reform legislation. In return, the committee made some concessions sought by the insurance industry in insurance reform. The deal was off when another committee chair took over and a new set of ads hit the television across the country.

Again, the public strategy is not a new development for health interest groups. The AMA raised more than $3 million in 1949 to educate the public against public health insurance. Lobbyists of the 1960s, described by Douglass Cater, understood what he called "building a climate of public opinion" as important to a major lobbying strategy (1964, 209). According to Berry

(1984), interest groups recognize the simple truth that ideas are powerful. If they can change the public's view or image, significant changes may follow.

There was some evidence of overkill in the 1993–94 health reform debate, however. So many groups used the public-directed strategy that members of Congress reported they did not have time to schedule all the "face-to-face meetings that have been requested from dance therapists, masseurs, chiropractors and podiatrists, armed with scripted palm cards provided by one trade association or another" (Krauss 1993, A1, A12). One long-time Washington hand and former White House official told the *New York Times* that the 1993 effort to reach the public on health care was "the largest mobilization since the establishment of Social Security" (Krauss 1993, A1).

PACS

For interest groups, contributions to political action committees are the price of admission. PACs are campaign funding arms of an organization or group. PACs exist only to give money to candidates. They come in several varieties. Connected PACs are affiliated or coexist with some parent organization. More than 80 percent of PACs fit this description (Wright 1985). Unconnected PACs have no sponsoring organization and tend to be ideological in nature, often promoting a single issue. Some PACs are associated with one business. Candidates and elected officials often have their own PACs. Representative Henry Waxman raised more than $1 million between 1980 and 1990, which he funneled to influential Democrats in the House and the Senate (Morgan 1994). PACs can be permanent or temporary, devised to support or oppose a policy on the institutional agenda.

PACs guarantee access and a chance to present their case. PACs are relatively new players in the election scene. Until the mid-1970s members of Congress got about two-thirds of their campaign money from individual donors. PACs had only "bit" roles, providing less than 20 percent of House and Senate spending in the 1974 campaigns (Matlack, Barnes, and Cohen 1990). By 1992 PAC contributions made up 36 percent of House spending and 21 percent of Senate spending (Ornstein, Mann, and Malbin 1994). As campaigns became increasingly expensive and public concern grew over large quantities of unreported contributions during the Nixon election, Congress passed a series of statutes in the 1970s defining and institutionalizing PACs.

AMPAC, the AMA's PAC, is the third oldest PAC in the country, established in 1961 (Campion 1984). It is big, well funded, expert in election

Table 3.2. Registered Political Action Committees, 1974–92

Type of Committee	1974	1976	1978	1980	1984	1988	1990	1992
Corporate	89	433	784	1204	1682	1816	1795	1735
Labor	201	224	217	297	394	354	346	347
Trade/membership/health	318	489	451	574	698	786	774	770
Unconnected			165	378	1053	1115	1062	1145
Cooperative			12	42	52	59	59	56
Corporation without stock			24	56	130	138	136	142
Total	608	1146	1653	2551	4009	4268	4172	4195

Source: Data from Ornstein, Mann, and Malbin (1994).
Note: Data as of December 31 for every year. The trade/membership/health category includes all noncorporate and nonlabor PACs through December 31, 1976.

laws, and not afraid to innovate ways to spend money to produce the most payoff. Looking for things it could do to make itself more useful to candidates, it hit upon running polls for them. Under federal law, AMPAC can depreciate the cost of the poll by 50 percent by waiting for sixteen days to share the results with candidates. The depreciation goes to 95 percent if the wait is more than sixty days. By delaying the presentation of results, AMPAC provides a valuable service to members at a very low cost—allowing it to give more dollars to that candidate before reaching the spending limit. AMPAC gets "more" for its money by requiring that the member of Congress (rather than a staff member) help design the poll and receive the results from the AMPAC staff.

AMPAC provides favored candidates with opposition research on the public record of their opponents. This kind of help qualifies as an "in-kind" contribution and slips outside spending ceilings (Pressman 1984). PACs also lend staff to officials to help organize schedules and events and to pitch in on fundraising. It will pay for television ads or pick up the travel costs of congressional staff who visit the member's district.

Growth

PACs grew rapidly following the 1974 revision of the Federal Election Campaign Act. Before then, 608 PACs were registered with the Federal Election Commission. Two years later the number had nearly doubled. By the early 1990s there were more than 4,000, most of them (1,735) associated with corporations (table 3.2). The money changing hands grew too, though not quite so impressively: from donations of $34 million in 1978 to more than $178 million in 1992 (Ornstein, Mann, and Malbin 1994).

Talk about health reform spawns new PACs and fills the coffers of old ones. Between 1989 and 1992 the number of health PACs grew by 28 percent. Groups representing pathologists, anesthesiologists, and plastic surgeons formed their own PACs. In the same time period the chiropractors' PAC increased its contributions by 270 percent, emergency physicians by 154 percent, and a drug company, Snytex, Inc., by 439 percent. Explaining the growth, a pathologist told the *Washington Post* he was afraid pathology "might get lost" on the AMA agenda (Babcock 1993, 14).

Democrats rely on PAC contributions more heavily than do Republicans: 43 percent of 1992 House Democratic campaign spending was paid for by PACs, compared with 26 percent for Republican candidates. Party differences were only about 3 percent in the Senate. Many PACs prefer to donate to House campaigns because the total cost of the races is lower, and PAC dollars are more valued. The limitations of $5,000 (per race) for multimember PACs apply whether the candidate is running for the Senate or the House. House races cost less than $500,000 in the early 1990s, compared with nearly $3 million for Senate races (Ornstein, Mann, and Malbin 1994). Though the PAC contribution limit is $5,000 for the primary and another $5,000 for the general election, few come close to the limit. The mean contribution to a candidate in the 1992 election was $1,600; the median donation was $1,000, and the mode was $500 (Babcock 1994).

More than 200 PACs are associated with health issues. Besides the AMA, ADA, ANA, and AHA—probably the most visible interest groups in health—there are PACs for Philippine Physicians in America, Society for the Advancement of Ambulatory Care, Hospital Corporation of America, and Kentucky Physical Therapy. Businesses in health are represented by PACs for Miles Laboratories, Mutual Benefit Life Insurance, Upjohn, and Pfizer.

The health PACs generally contributing the most money to congressional campaigns are the big ones—the AMA, ADA, and AHA—although contributions from smaller, more specialized groups are not unsubstantial. In the 1993–94 health care reform debate, contributions from health PACs increased dramatically. Contributions to congressional candidates from health and insurance PACs swelled by nearly 25 percent between the first fifteen months of 1991–92 and 1993–94 (*Health Care Policy Report* 1994). According to the Washington-based, non-profit Center for Public Integrity, health-related interests contributed more than $25 million to Congress between January 1993 and March 1994. "Money follows hot issues," said Ellen Miller, the Center for Re-

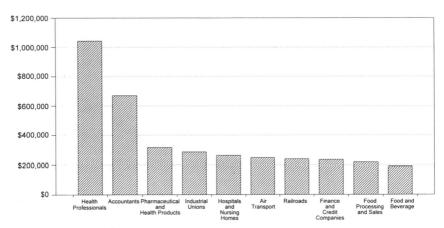

Figure 3.1 The Biggest Increase in PAC Giving (1994 Compared with 1992)

Source: Data from the Center for Responsive Politics (1994).

sponsive Politics' executive director (1994). While health spending increased in 1993–94 over the previous election cycle, PAC dollars for energy and natural resources, labor, and communications declined. Figure 3.1 shows the increase in PAC giving by interest group category. Among the health interests, those representing health professionals upped their giving ante the most.

The increasing importance of PAC contributions may have worked against interest groups, which often are expected to contribute to many candidates and sometimes feel that they are not rewarded for their contributions, but rather are punished for noncompliance. What used to be a system of incentives for access may now be a baseline for playing in the game—and the price of admission has increased substantially. Particularly irksome for many PAC staff members are the ubiquitous fundraisers, which they are expected to attend and often to help organize. Clawson, Neustadtl, and Scott (1992) found in a series of interviews with corporate PAC managers that politicians press PAC managers for contributions as much as lobbyists press politicians for favors. A survey by the National Association of Business found that in 70 percent of the cases, the PACs were responding to, rather than initiating, a request for money (Rubin 1993b).

Strategies

PACs can employ one of several strategies for distributing their dollars. They can seek to change the composition of Congress to make it more ideo-

logically pleasing, or they can maximize their access to members. The former strategy leads more often to funding of challengers; the latter to favor
ing incumbents, particularly party leaders and committee or subcommittee
chairs. Since challengers are usually cash-starved compared with well-placed
incumbents, PACs have the potential to be better appreciated for their contributions to these upstarts. Politicians tend to be aware of who gives "early
money," especially when they are desperate to fund media campaigns and
mailings to increase their name recognition.

Nonetheless, the largest share of PAC money goes to incumbents (Berry
1984). As Sabato (1985, 78) put it, incumbents have an "irresistible charm" for
PACs. In the 1990 House elections, the AMA gave to 90 percent of the incumbents seeking office, supporting only 19 challengers. Interestingly, these
challengers received higher average contributions ($5,361 compared with
$4,774), a decision probably reflecting the value of the dollars to a challenger
and the fact that many incumbents run unopposed.

The appeal of incumbents is simple: access. By providing funding for those
currently in office and likely to retain their seats, interest groups can maintain access to those policy players. When explaining their actions, *access* is
the word most often mentioned. Groups need access to affect details of policy that are important to them. Incumbents are in a better position to help
groups with these details than challengers. Sometimes conflicts appear between Washington lobbyists who want to have access to incumbents and members back home who feel that ideology is important and that the group's dollars should support like-minded challengers. Wright (1985) found that the
PAC's organization structure was important in whether the local members
or Washington lobbyists prevailed. When PACs were organized in a decentralized fashion with extensive grass-roots fundraisers, the decisions seemed
to favor local concerns emphasizing ideology and changing the membership
of Congress.

Among incumbents, PACs are most likely to give to party leaders and to
members serving on committees important to the interest group. Legislators
receiving the most health dollars tend to be those on key health committees.
Of the more than $40 million contributed to members of Congress between
1981 and 1991, 42 percent went to members who serve on four committees especially important to health: the Senate Finance and the Labor and Human
Resources Committees, and the House Ways and Means and the Energy and
Commerce Committees (Common Cause 1992). Members serving on one of
these four committees received an average of $51,668 from health interests in
1992—67 percent more than those with other committee assignments.

The largest contributions went to the leadership of these committees. Pete Stark, chair of the House Ways and Means Committee's Health Subcommittee in 1992, received more than $160,000 in PAC contributions, nearly three times the average PAC contribution to the subcommittee members. Henry Waxman, then chair of the Health and Environment Subcommittee of the Energy and Commerce Committee, received $158,000 in PAC contributions, while the remaining twenty-three members of the subcommittee averaged only $46,740 (Rubin 1993c).

Committee membership and seniority are especially important to PAC giving in House campaigns (Romer and Snyder 1994). In the Senate, PAC funding is more closely associated with party membership and voting record (Grier and Munger 1993). When no incumbent is running, interest groups often target dollars to attractive first-year members in the hope of getting more attention early in their careers. Some interest groups value ideology more than others. For example, the ANA's PAC gave more than 85 percent of its contributions to Democrats in the 1990 election, compared with 70 percent of the AHA and 51 percent of the AMA's PAC contributions. The ANA was the first major health association to endorse Bill Clinton in the 1992 election. Its support may have been rewarded with twelve seats on the forty-seven-member professional advisory review committee to Hillary Rodham Clinton's health reform task force. The AMA was not represented on the advisory review committee (Bendavid, Goldman, and Kaplan 1993).

Sometimes PACs will give to both sides and even will give after the election, as a way of "buying off a mistake" (Sabato 1985, 92). In 1982 AMPAC contributed $7,500 to the incumbent Republican Senator Harrison Schmitt of New Mexico, but after the election of his competitor, it made a $10,000 contribution to the new senator, Democrat Jeff Bingaman. The 1994 election that ushered in a Republican majority in both houses of Congress saw many PACs scrambling to retire the campaign debts of Republicans whose elections they had opposed. "When you back the wrong horses, you try to make a contribution as a token of good will," said one interest group's political director (Weisskopf 1995).

The timing of PAC giving can also be important. Not all is given during the months just before the election. Money provided early to a candidate can give legitimacy and visibility that can scare off other possible candidates and increase the likelihood of receiving even more campaign dollars from others. Another part of the explanation is that modern members of Congress collect money throughout their terms, and PAC money can be provided at any time, such as before a key vote in a committee or on a house floor. Many PACs deny giving money for "present needs" for a favorable vote or action. Rather, they say they give money based on support they may need in the future or good will that might later come in handy. Some people feel there is also a fair amount of "reward" or "thank you" money for votes previously cast in support of an interest group. Some PACs admit to "punishment" money; the PAC refuses to contribute to a candidate or gives money to his or her opponent. One highly visible example of the punishment strategy was AMPAC's spending of thousands of dollars in 1986 to unseat Representative Pete Stark, of California. (The feeling was mutual. Stark once called the AMA "greedy troglodytes" [Noah 1993, A16].) Nevertheless, such punishment is unusual and, even in Stark's case, temporary. AMPAC donated $6,000 in contributions to Stark's 1992 campaign.

PACs and the interest groups they support tend to pick their battles. For example, they prefer to support members who can help them on issues of top concern. For the nation's optometrists, when health reform is on the agenda, their top priority tends to be making sure that eye care is included in any governmental health program. That effort was worth nearly $400,000 in PAC contributions during the Clinton reform campaign. An earlier example was the 1982 effort to exempt professionals, including dentists and physicians, from regulation by the FTC. Co-sponsors of the bill averaged $1,800 more in PAC donations from the AMA and ADA than House members with similar records and reelection prospects. Legislators who cast a favorable vote received nearly $1,000 more than opponents (Sabato 1985). Yet the effect backfired when Congress Watch, a citizen group, launched a campaign highlighting the AMA's congressional operations and hinting that the AMA was "buying" votes. The citizen group put out press releases listing the AMA's contributions to cosponsors and supporters of bills "exempting doctors from FTC prosecution" and used the resulting news stories and editorials to encourage senators to vote against the bill. The six-month effort to expose the relationship between AMA money and votes succeeded when the bill lost decisively in the Senate (Pertschuk 1986; Pressman 1984).

The AMA's activities in support of congressional exemption were also criticized as reflecting "far more concern with preserving the economic health of doctors than promoting the physical health of the rest of the country" (Pressman 1984, 15). Representative Henry Waxman put it this way: "They [the AMA] were quite silent in 1981 when the Reagan administration attempted to decimate many of the national health efforts. They decided that the FTC issue was the most important matter on their minds" (Pressman 1984, 15).

Public health issues get little attention from the AMA. Sharfstein and Sharfstein (1994) found that AMPAC contributes more to candidates who opposed their own official AMA position on three major public health issues than those who supported them. Members who opposed the AMA's position on the three issues—curbs on the promotion of tobacco exports, a mandatory waiting period on handguns, and the "gag rule" that limited physicians' speech on abortion in federally funded clinics—received an average of $4,500 more than those who supported the AMA on all three issues.

What PACs Buy

There is very little evidence that PAC funding directly affects a member's vote on a given bill. Studies examining the linkage between PAC money and roll-call voting have found no relationship or a very modest correlation (Smith 1995 provides a summary of the dozens of relevant studies). Most political scientists agree that party, ideology, and constituents' attitudes are much better predictors of a member's vote than PAC contributions. Past voting records are key. Members are generally very consistent in their voting patterns and, as Grier and Munger (1993, 621) noted, "Voting records attract contributions rather than contributions determining voting records."

Campaign dollars are likely to have the best chance at influencing members when the policy under consideration is not salient, is technical or specialized, or is nonpartisan and nonideological; when there is no interest group opposition; when the contributions are accompanied by intensive lobbying; when members are facing a close election; and when the general political climate favors the objective of the interest group (Sabato 1985; Schlozman and Tierney 1986; Grenzke 1990; Wilhite 1988).

Many feel that the real value of PAC dollars is in keeping certain issues off the agenda. As Ellen Miller of the Center for Responsive Politics said, PAC money "buys silence, hearings are not held or amendments not introduced" (Matlack, Barnes, and Cohen 1990, 1479). PAC dollars may also make it more difficult to compromise, especially if both sides of an issue are providing substantial PAC funding.

There is some evidence that the money tends to be more persuasive in committee activities than on the floor, because in committees visibility is lower, there are more decisions, and there are fewer members to persuade (Keiser and Jones 1986; Hall and Wayman 1990). A member can relatively easily and without much attention table a provision or make an amendment without appearing to "sell out."

PAC money may also affect the intensity of feeling and commitment to a position. As former Representative Les Aspin put it, "There are various degrees of debate, on the floor, or in a leadership role on the floor. PAC funds can determine a member's intensity as well as position" (Green 1982, 21).

HOW INFLUENTIAL ARE INTEREST GROUPS?

Influence is affected by a variety of factors, including the type of issue, nature of the demand, availability of resources, and structure of the political conflict. In direct lobbying efforts, influence will be weaker on highly salient, visible issues that are also ideological or partisan in nature. As Denzau and Munger noted in 1986, the better informed the voters are on an issue, the less important are interest groups. Groups have more success on nonsalient, expert issues in which there is little press or public interest. If groups can tie their desired policies to strong public support, their chances of success are enhanced. To go against public support (as perceived by policymakers) is to nearly ensure policy failure, no matter how "good" the idea is. Jacobs (1993a) argues that the successful passage of Medicare—over strong interest group opposition—is best explained by the strong public preference for health care coverage for the elderly.

Interest groups are more successful on single, discrete amendments than on entire pieces of legislation and on narrow issues rather than broader, more ambitious programs. They are more successful if they can focus their lobbying effort on one or two issues. In the 1993–94 debate, it was widely acknowledged that big business with "all their wealth and power" were not effective in the shaping of health care legislation in large part because they spoke with a "fragmented voice on a variety of issues" (Stout 1994, A1).

In health, lobbyists have been successful in focusing their attention on small changes that can make a great deal of difference to them, such as the successful effort of the American College of Nurse-Midwives to be reimbursed for their services under Medicaid in 1980. However, "outside" strategies can sometimes bring issues to the public's attention and increase their salience, as the 1993–94 Harry and Louise commercials and others did with the choice of a provider, community rating, and health alliances.

Conflict also limits influence as other groups, members, the executive branch, the media, or the public fight it out. Congress responds very differently to interest groups when there is no conflict compared to situations punctuated by great resistance (Hayes 1978).

Smith (1984) emphasized the importance of timing. An interest group has a greater chance of success when pushing the passage of a conference report than when fighting an amendment on the House floor. Amendments complicate things and cause members to seek information quickly—often so quickly that interest groups cannot respond. For committed, well-informed members, such a shift is not difficult. For those not so strongly committed, the choice may be more difficult, and the result less desired by the interest group. The instability of these commitments leads to a fragility of support that Smith felt undermines interest group dominance.

Some of the nation's strongest interest groups are weakened in their bargaining ability by their membership. For groups representing a large, diverse membership, developing and maintaining a policy focus that satisfies all members can be tough. In case after case, it appears that leadership in Washington ("inside the beltway") often does not reflect the rank-and-file members. The powerful AMA facilitates member involvement by having its board of delegates review policies every six months. Such reconsideration can also lead to a change of heart, as happened in 1993 when delegates forced the association to retreat on its five-year backing of an employer mandate to cover uninsured workers. In March 1994 the board of the U.S. Chamber of Commerce reversed its one-year position supporting an employer mandate when many of its members threatened to quit over the issue. Similarly, the AHA had supported a pay-or-play proposal and then backed away from that position as the for-profit hospitals opposed the governmental regulations they feared such a plan would engender.

The clearest example of an interest group "change of heart" was the 1988 catastrophic health insurance, passed by Congress with the support of the AARP. The AARP played an insider role in the passage of the law, working closely with Congress to fashion a law that would be palatable to their constituents (Torres-Gil 1989). The strategy backfired, however. A year later an embarrassed Congress repealed the law at the insistence of a loud, committed elderly population. (Chapter 7 provides detail on the saga of catastrophic health insurance.) In the 1994 health debates, the AARP approached controversial policy positions a bit more carefully. It refused to endorse President Clinton's proposal, preferring to have its members transmit their views to their own representatives. In a statement clearly reflective of the earlier experience, the association's chair said, "When you have 33 million members, it's hard to say that every one of them feels any particular way" (Pear 1994a, A1). When later (August 1994), the AARP board endorsed two Democratic health care proposals and recommended its members support the bills, irate members flooded the phone lines to the Washington headquarters, prompting a full-page ad in the *Washington Post* in which the AARP explained its reasons for the action (Ross 1994).

Dissatisfaction can also be exhibited in other ways, such as leaving the association. The insurance industry has seen much movement, especially in the HIAA. Five large companies left the association between 1990 and 1993, a reflection of the differences in interests among large and small insurers on such issues as managed competition. Larger insurers support the idea, but small insurers fear they will be more likely to be forced out of business if they cannot select enrollees or price based on risk.

Interest Groups and the Courts

When all else fails, interest groups can still turn to the courts. Litigation can be a powerful tool for influencing policy. While often an expensive route for change, it may be the last resort for a group unable to get satisfaction through the legislative and executive branches. As Berry (1984, 197) noted, "When an industry's profits are liable to be significantly reduced by a government policy, it becomes worth the cost of litigation for a trade association to challenge the policy in court." Berry also made the case that interest groups use the courts when they feel the lack of popular support makes it fruitless for them to lobby the Congress or the executive branch. Interest groups can delay the implementation of a policy in the courts, sometimes hoping Congress or the administration will change during the delay, producing a more sympathetic body. Interest groups will sometimes use litigation as a means to force administrative action, hoping that the federal agencies will settle out of court rather than undergo uncertain court decisions. Groups representing disabled persons have been especially successful in out-of-court settlements. Using courts as a venue for policy change intensified during the 1960s, when the federal courts expanded the rules of standing so that citizen groups and trade associations could sue in court even if they had no direct economic interest in the case (Berry 1984).

Interest groups choose the judicial route (or avoid it) based on their political standing in the electoral process, the extent to which the group can frame its interests in terms of rights, and the demographic characteristics of the group. Groups turn to the courts if they are politically disadvantaged or if they have organizational resources, such as full-time staff, attorneys, financial resources to pay the legal costs, and organizational networks involving close coordination with affiliated groups or other interest groups. Groups that are often in conflict are more likely to use the judicial remedy than groups that engender no conflict. Finally, interest groups are more likely to use the courts when their areas of interest coincide with issues over which courts have clear jurisdiction (Walker 1991).

Suing has become a national pastime, even for interest groups. A 1985 survey of interest groups in Washington, D.C., found that 56 percent used the courts for some reason. Less than 10 percent said that filing amicus briefs was the extent of this involvement. Organizations representing labor and the private sector were the most likely to use the judicial strategy: 66 percent said they used the courts. More than 50 percent of the citizen groups surveyed reported using the courts to achieve policy goals (Walker 1991).

While health groups spend less time pursuing their goals in federal court than do civil liberties groups, this is not to say they do not do it at all. Delaying the implementation of regulations is one reason that health groups sue. Starr called this the "little known law of nature [that] seems to require that every move toward regulation be followed by an opposite move toward litigation" (1982, 407). He noted that the Association of American Physicians and Surgeons sued over the constitutionality of the Professional Standards Review Organizations (PSROs); the AMA sued when the proposed utilization review regulations were issued and again to block the health-planning law from being implemented. The AAMC sued over regulations imposed on medical schools.

Interest Groups' Success

Hundreds of different health interest groups participate in health policy-making today, collectively affecting a range of programs and policy issues. There are many new consumer groups and an increasing number of groups representing corporate medicine, such as prepaid health plans, hospital chains, walk-in clinics, and home-care companies. Relman (1980) referred to this body as the "new medical-industrial complex." There have also been huge increases in the number of businesses and other nonhealth corporate entities involved in health policymaking and in groups representing providers and corporate interests, which tend to have substantially more resources. These groups are more active than they were in previous years. Some 88 percent of Schlozman and Tierney's (1986) interest group respondents indicated their group had become more active over the past decade.

Despite their vast numbers, groups may, in fact, have less clout than in times past (Salisbury 1992). Part of the reason is sheer numbers. No one group can speak for "medicine" or "agriculture" as it once did. Issues are handled in small, specialized steps. Policies must be similarly specialized, such as those affecting medical school enrollment, funding for research on acquired immune deficiency syndrome (AIDS), or hospital capital pass-through formulas. Broader, more comprehensive issues involving coalitions of health groups are much harder to manage and were elusive for decades.

Most major health programs enacted over the past twenty-five years (Medicare, comprehensive health planning, PSROs, and HMOs) have been enacted despite AMA opposition to the original legislation (Tierney 1987). Hospitals and professional schools have fared no better. In 1976, for example, over the strenuous opposition of the hospital industry, Congress tightened the immigration laws to restrict the entry of alien physicians into the United States and imposed stringent constraints on the licensure of foreign medical graduates.

The once nearly invincible physician lobby has fragmented over several issues in recent years. There are now more than 115 recognized medical specialties (up from eighty-two just ten years ago). Washington representation for these groups more than doubled during that period (Kosterlitz 1992). The groups differ in many ways from the AMA in their policy preferences. For example, the American College of Surgeons supported the 1989 restrictions on Medicare payments for physicians, provided that a separate target was set for surgeons, a position in stark contrast to that of the AMA. In hearings, spokespersons for the AMA, surgeons, radiologists, internists, and family practitioners all staked out different positions on the relative value scale known as RBRVS and expenditure targets. The AMA later lost—settling for a victory in renaming spending targets "volume performance standards" and removing most of the sanctions for exceeding the standards (Kosterlitz 1992, 2429). While a victory in the sense that physicians can keep up their incomes by seeing more patients and unbundling their bills, Canadian research shows they can do this only to a limited extent, after which they actually wind up with less income under a fee schedule, such as RBRVS (Rice and Labelle 1989).

In the 1993–94 health reform debate, two key medical opponents of the AMA were the American College of Physicians and the American Academy of Family Physicians, which endorsed a national cap on spending. The Physicians for a National Health Program argued for a Canadian-like single-payer plan. Only a few days after the AMA reversed its stand supporting employer mandates, the White House brought together ten other physician groups that supported the Clinton plan, including the American Academy of Family Physicians, American College of Physicians, American Academy of Pediatrics, and American Medical Women's Association.

Similarly, the hospital associations do not speak with one voice. In addition to the AHA, hospitals are represented by the Federation of American Health Systems, National Council of Community Hospitals, Catholic Health Association of the U.S., and AAMC's Council of Teaching Hospitals. The groups often disagree on important policy issues. The Federation of American Health Systems, representing for-profit hospitals, supported the financing of HMOs, PPS, and diagnosis-related groups (DRGs). On the other hand, the AHA, representing nonprofit and community hospitals among others, opposed PPS without weighting for urban and university locations.

Yet it would probably be misleading to overstate the importance of interest groups. They have in fact kept many issues from reaching the agenda. Political scientists have long recognized the power to keep issues from being discussed and recognized as problems. For example, for years hospital overbedding was widely known and the cost implications well understood. But federal funds continued to be available to build more and more hospitals in spite of the glut of beds, largely due to the ability of provider lobbies to keep the issue off the agenda. Big businesses have successfully kept intact ERISA and restrictions on states, and teaching hospitals have protected graduate medical education (GME) dollars for years, even in light of the need for cuts in federal health spending and the desire to give states more flexibility in making policy decisions formerly concentrated in Washington. Groups have also been successful in delaying or stalling national health insurance, hospital cost controls, employer mandates, and tough quality controls on physicians and hospitals, and have reduced the size of other initiatives, including federal subsidies for HMOs.

HEALTH INTEREST GROUPS

Peterson (1993) argued that the world of health care interest groups evolved through several stages over fifty years. Until the 1950s it could be described as dominated by stakeholder groups with little competition from what he called stake challengers. In the 1960s and 1970s the stakeholders, particularly businesses, began to emerge and organize to compete with the old-guard group dominion, and by the 1980s the stake challengers had become competitive, leading to a fuller participation and more heterogeneous interest group environment. The 1990s saw a fourth, even more frantic and expansive stage bursting on the scene, launched with the election of a dark horse candidate who had run on a national health insurance platform in the Pennsylvania U.S. Senate race. Policymakers realized that the public was concerned about health care coverage, and health care became the subject of town meetings, television advertisements, and constituent mailings. It was also a focus of the 1992 presidential campaign, with the successful Democratic candidate, Bill Clinton, calling for health care reform as one of the key promises of his campaign.

Overnight, it seemed, the health interest community was activated, expanded, and the focus of massive media attention. Nearly 200 new lobbyists registered on health-related issues in 1993—a number most viewed as a serious undercount, since many lobbyists do not register (Rubin 1993a). Newspaper and television coverage was extensive. During September 1993 health issues were on the front page of the *New York Times* for twenty-two of the thirty days. The normally nonsalient, highly complex health debate had hit the big time. One public relations staffer described it this way: "In all the issues we've worked on, we've never, ever found an issue that so many different constituencies were so instantly interested in. On health care, the interest level is immediately there and it is very deep. You don't have to explain to people why they should care" (Rubin 1993a, 1084).

CONCLUSION

Interest groups are powerful actors in health policymaking, arguably second only to Congress. Yet interest groups are not all equally powerful, and even the powerful are not dominant on all issues and at all times. Interest groups are most likely to affect bills on nonsalient issues, on narrow and specialized issues, without public support, and where there is a three-part strategy that includes PAC dollars and direct, grass-roots lobbying. Similarly, interest group strategies that can target a few specific, desired changes can focus their attention in a way broader consumer groups cannot.

Changes in Congress, the presidency, the bureaucracy, the media, the public, and technology have affected interest group efforts and success rates—in many cases to reduce their influence. Some analysts now feel interest groups have more access than influence (Heinz et al. 1993), and others note that their influence, at least on the big issues, has declined (Nexon 1987; Petracca 1992a). But this view of declining power is not universally held. One widely respected journalist recently bemoaned the increasing power of interest groups (and the press) and the concomitant weakening of Congress, the presidency, and the political parties (Broder 1994a). Some academics agree that the overall influence of lobbyists and interest groups has increased over the past 30 years (Jacobson 1987). President Clinton, in his 22 September 1993 address introducing his health care proposal, acknowledged his concerns about special interests who would "bombard" Congress with information and stoutly disagree with policies of change. Events proved him correct.

What both sides of the debate might agree on is the instability of the modern policy world, including interest groups. The presidency, Congress, even the courts change in focus, institutional organization, rules, and energy over time. Those changes affect interest groups. The public is notoriously fickle, strongly supporting one policy or evidencing concern for one problem, only to move on to other problems and policies a short time later (Downs 1972). Interest groups themselves are far from stable, with the 1993–94 health care debate highlighting the changing positions and support over the months of high-level public attention to the issue.

Both sides would agree that the success of interest groups—in health and other areas—is in the details, the often complex, many times largely ignored aspects of the law or regulation that can affect millions of dollars in reimbursement or the ability of health professionals to ply their trade independently. The expertise and intensity of interest groups in the complex details is often persuasive. It is at these margins of public policy where interest groups can most effectively utilize their lobbying strategies and PAC dollars, often without the benefit of public or media scrutiny.

Both sides would also probably agree that the system in which interest groups operate is more open and more competitive than ever before. Gone are the days of "buying votes" or "wining and dining" members for favors. Congressional deliberations are almost universally conducted in full view of lobbyists, staff, the press, and the public. C-Span coverage has also widely opened the process to public view. More groups have access to policymakers, and the days of iron triangles and interest group liberalism have, for most health care issues, disappeared.

In this atmosphere, then, health interest groups seek to inform and influence national policymakers to act (or refrain from acting) in ways that benefit their memberships. They use a variety of tactics and prioritize their demands. One of the interesting aspects of the 1993–94 health care debate was the increased saliency of health issues. In the past it had often been left largely in the hands of a few expert groups. The desire to produce more primary-care practitioners (physicians and nonphysicians), which led to widespread discussions of choices of specialties, and the role of federal research dollars and graduate medical education funding, for example, are two policies formerly of low salience and little broad concern. Similarly, the inclusion of insurance reforms, malpractice relief, and possible override of state nurse practice laws are areas generally not widely debated or discussed in public forums or subjected to newspaper editorials. In 1994, they were. This increased the "scope of conflict" as nurses, medical school deans, insurance companies, and community health center directors joined the debate over the future of the nation's health system. This is a larger, more diverse chorus than the one that cheered or jeered the 1965 Medicare passage or the health debates since that time. The broadening of the debate to include issues, people, and groups that had not been involved in the issue before can be the first step to what Baumgartner and Jones (1993) called the destruction of policy monopolies and the first step toward comprehensive reform.

In the final analysis, however, it is clear that interest groups are able to play such a powerful role because they represent so well the interests of a very powerful constituency: most of us—middle- and upper middle-income Americans, shopkeepers, business executives, salaried and skilled labor, National Public Radio listeners, and even the organized staff of middle-class health and social welfare agencies delivering health care and doing other good things for poor people. From gun owners to HMOs, interest groups represent Americans who share common interests, many times—especially in the health care field—related to their source of income. As more and more health care interests come to realize that they too must be players to protect their interests, the number and variety of health care groups will continue to grow. Balance may yet be achieved as the cacophony resonates into background noise. Poor people are likely to have to count on health care interests with a stake in serving them to press their concerns regarding access, quality, and financing. But it is clear that whatever measures are taken to reduce the influence of PACs and campaign spending on health care policymaking, interest groups will still find a welcome home on Capitol Hill, at the White House, and in the health care agencies of the executive branch. They are as integral a part of the system of health care policymaking as Congress itself.

4

Bureaucracy

1965

IN THE 1965 negotiations over Medicare, one of the key players, Wilbur Cohen, was a bureaucrat. As a long-time staff member in the Federal Security Agency, the Social Security Administration (SSA), and the Department of Health, Education, and Welfare, Cohen had a hand in virtually every national health insurance proposal since the 1930s. He was well known on Capitol Hill for his knowledge of both Social Security and health insurance. In fact, Senator Paul Douglas once said that "a Social Security expert is a man with Wilbur Cohen's telephone number" (Harris 1966). Cohen helped draft the administration bill on Medicare, consulted with members on proposed bills, and was asked to summarize various proposals to the key committees. When Representative Wilbur Mills decided to combine several proposals into a "three-layer cake" (the layers were later known as Medicare Parts A and B and Medicaid), he asked Cohen to draw up legislative language to pull the pieces together, along with an analysis of the costs, within twelve hours.

But Cohen was more than a substantive expert. He was involved in meetings in the White House and on Capitol Hill to assess the standing of proposals and develop strategies to achieve legislative success. He was one of a small group of strategists who developed a plan in 1956 to prompt congressional action by persuading a well-placed member to sponsor a bill and elicit wide public concern about the health of elderly people through a media campaign sponsored by the labor union (Marmor 1970, 30). Standing outside the Senate chamber during debates on the measure in 1965, he heard rumors that labor unions were supporting an amendment the administration opposed. He called the labor representative, found out the rumor was wrong, and was able to hold the votes of liberal senators who might otherwise have been lost (Harris 1966).

Cohen served as a broker between the president and the congressional committees and among interest groups (Marmor 1970). He reported regularly to the president and transmitted the president's views back to the members. The president assigned Cohen the responsibility for working with interest groups, most notably the American Medical Association and the American Hospital Association, in implementing the newly adopted Medicare program.

Although Cohen had more access and visibility than what we might dub a typical bureaucrat, he did epitomize the importance of bureaucratic expertise and guidance to both the president and the Congress. In 1965 the presidential staff was small and typically dominated by political, rather than policy, experts. Lyndon Johnson, like presidents before him, relied on staff in the executive agencies to put presidential preferences into legislative language and to produce statistics and rationale to support the legislation. Congress too relied on the federal departments in the mid-1960s. Clapp called the executive branch "a leading source of information for the legislator" (1963, 129). Executive branch officials worked closely with congressional committees, providing them with briefings, speeches, useful documents, and strategy suggestions. While more responsive to members of the president's party, agency personnel were generally available to assist any member in drafting legislation and often even provided research to help back up a position, even if it did not reflect the thinking of the department.

In the 1960s Congress typically gave considerable discretion to the agencies in implementing the law. Wilbur Cohen negotiated actively with interest groups on many aspects of the implementation of Medicare. In the Public Welfare Amendments of 1962, Congress specified that the federal government would match 75 percent of the cost of services "prescribed" or "specified" by the secretary of the Department of Health, Education, and Welfare, words

Table 4.1. HEW/HHS and Federal Health Spending in 1965, 1981, and 1993

	1965	1981	1993
		(in Billions of Dollars)	
Federal health spending	$1.8	$66	$230
Medicare	—	39.2	130.6
Health care services	.88	21.2	86.9
Health research and training	.78	4.6	10.8
Consumer and occupational health and safety	.13	1.0	1.8
HEW/HHS* spending (without Social Security)	4.7	89.8	282.8
	1965	1981	1993
		(Percentage)	
HEW/HHS* spending as a proportion of total federal spending	4.0	13.2	20.1

Source: Data from Fiscal Year 1995 Budget of the United States.

* HEW became HHS in 1980.

that gave HEW enormous discretion in deciding the nature of the program—and its cost (Derthick 1975).

In 1965 federal health spending totaled $1.8 billion, with roughly one-half going to health care services and one-half to health research and training (table 4.1). HEW was the key health agency, accounting for 4 percent of all federal outlays (excluding Social Security). In 1965 HEW was divided into eight agencies: Administration on Aging, Food and Drug Administration, Office of Education, Social Security Administration, Public Health Service (PHS), Vocational Rehabilitation Services, St. Elizabeth's Hospital, and Welfare Administration.

1981

President Ronald Reagan was highly skeptical of the loyalty and ability of the 366,000 federal public employees working in Washington. Even though Jimmy Carter had served in office only four years, following an eight-year Republican occupation of the White House, there was a general view that the federal departments were filled with Democrats hostile to the president's desire to reduce the size and power of government. Reagan's skepticism led him to adopt a very careful hiring policy, putting in place cabinet and subcabinet appointees and other top officials who were often highly ideological and very loyal to the president—to the extreme in cases involving an Environmental Protection Agency (EPA) director and a Department of the Interior secretary who were forced to resign early in their assignments over questionable decisions and clear preferences to business. The Reagan administration reached down further into the operations of agencies, filling a higher proportion of noncareer senior executive positions than in any other modern presidential administration.

In addition to "stacking the deck" with like-thinking employees, the White House also encouraged these appointees to use their administrative powers to advance White House objectives (Salamon and Abramson 1984). They were encouraged to reinterpret the conduct of agency business to the extent possible, reduce regulatory action, and reduce the negative impact of regulations on business. There were layoffs in many agencies, called reductions in force. Some 12,000 federal employees lost their jobs from RIFs in fiscal years 1981 and 1982.

In 1981 the relationship between the executive agency staff and Congress was very different from the days of the Johnson presidency. With the dramatic increase in congressional staff, there was less call on agency staff to assist in drafting laws and less need for agency help in plotting political strategies. There was still a need, however, for some agency expertise, particularly statistics, evaluations, simulations, and informed estimations of the effect of current and proposed programs. A congressional staff person, usually new to the job and often to the issue, could rely on a seasoned agency expert to help in preparing speeches, testimony, committee reports, and sections of the bill—and often did. To gain expertise, a congressional committee would often "borrow" federal agency employees for temporary assignment. Such an arrangement benefited all parties. For the Congress, it was an opportunity to get top-flight expertise; for the staff person on loan, it was an opportunity to directly affect policy; for the agency, it was a way to build good will and strong bonds with congressional members and staff.

In 1980 a new Department of Education was formed and HEW became the Department of Health and Human Services. There were four operating agencies within HHS: Public Health Service, Social Security Administration, Office of Human Development Services, and Health Care Financing Administration. By 1981 HHS accounted for some 13 percent of total federal outlays, with total spending of nearly $90 billion. Federal health spending was more than $66 billion—with health care services and Medicare making up more than 90 percent of the total.

1993

In size, the federal bureaucracy facing Bill Clinton was similar to that in the time of Lyndon Johnson and Ronald Reagan. There was growth in the number of public employees between 1965 and 1993, but it was largely in the state and local sector, which grew by more than 40 percent. The health bureaucracy played a key role in Hillary Rodham Clinton's health reform task force. Early in the new administration, a key advisor in health, Judith Feder, was named principal deputy assistant secretary for planning and evaluation/health, indicating that HHS was likely to be highly involved in the formation of any health policy initiative. Yet, in fact, the key decisions about the makeup of the Clinton health package were made in the White House. HHS Secretary Donna Shalala took a back seat to both the first lady and White House advisor Ira Magaziner, who directed and coordinated the efforts of the 500-member task force assembled in the early months of the Clinton presidency. Federal agency personnel were actively involved in the task force deliberations but were outnumbered by congressional staff and outside advisors. Some 137 HHS staff members participated in the health care reform work groups— about one-third of the number of total government employees (including congressional staff and representatives of other federal agencies) and more than one-fourth of the total membership of the committees. While White House officials were busy crafting a comprehensive health plan, HHS officials, working with the Congress, drafted a $1.4 billion entitlement program to provide vaccines to state Medicaid programs for uninsured children, enacted in the summer of 1993.

Vice President Al Gore headed an effort to make government more efficient called the National Performance Review. The effort produced hundreds of recommendations designed to save $108 billion over five years. In the first year the National Performance Review claimed to have reduced the federal work force by 71,000 positions and saved $47 billion. Early in his presidency, Bill Clinton announced that he intended to provide more flexibility to states in launching innovations in Medicaid and Aid to Families with Dependent Children. The Health Care Financing Administration soon set about implementing the policy, which broadened the scope of the research and demonstration waivers, allowing their use for a series of statewide demonstrations in 1993 and 1994.

In 1993 HHS accounted for some 20 percent of all federal spending—more than $280 billion. Health care services and Medicare made up 95 percent of the total federal spending on health. There were now four operating agencies in HHS. Three were the same as in 1980: Public Health Service, Social Security Administration, and Health Care Financing Administration. The new agency was the Administration for Children and Families.

UNDERSTANDING THE PUBLIC BUREAUCRACY

The president, members of Congress, and the courts, the traditional triumvirate of power in the United States, tend to overshadow another policymaker, one that is clearly more important in the day-to-day operation and working of government—the public employees who work for federal, state, and local governments. There are more than 17 million public employees—most, 10 million, at the local level. States have 4 million, the federal government a little more than 3 million civilian employees. While the term bureaucracy encompasses both public- and private-sector organizations that are large, hierarchically organized, and highly specialized, in common parlance, bureaucracy has come to mean publicly funded agencies and offices. Public-sector employees are called, usually derisively, bureaucrats.

Bureaucracy conjures up images of inefficiency, waste, and red tape. Yet the evidence is not so clear cut. For example, *red tape*, clearly understood in the abstract, is difficult to pin down. Appleby described red tape as "that part of my business that you don't know anything about" (1945, 64). A study by Kaufman (1977) concluded that while citizens object to the weight of red tape, everyone likes some portion of that total weight. What is to one person red tape is to another an important consideration that could not be omitted. While many local officials feel that regulations associated with the rights of disabled people are excessive, expensive, and unnecessary, to disabled individuals these requirements are essential.

There is also the vague but widespread feeling that government is out of control. Only 20 percent of Americans trust the federal government to do the right thing most of the time, down from 76 percent in the 1960s (Gore 1994). Approximately 65 percent believe that people in the government waste a lot of the money we pay in taxes (Dubnick and Romzek 1991). However, studies of welfare recipients, unemployment insurance recipients, and the postal service have found dissatisfaction levels of less than one-third (Goodsell 1994).

In the United States, the standing of public administrators is much lower than that in European and many Asian countries. In part this is a function of history. There is no mention of administration or bureaucracy or federal agencies in the U.S. Constitution, and the development of the modern administrative state came only recently, somewhere between the two Roosevelt administrations (Morone 1990). In many European countries, the bureaucracy developed before the governmental system and plays a strong institutional role in developing and implementing policy. The rather weak position of U.S. public bureaucracy has forced federal agencies to build independent political bases "to provide sustenance to their pursuit of organizational goals" (Nelson 1982, 774).

Political Appointees versus Careerists

The top-level policymaking jobs in federal and state governments are generally filled with appointees of the president or governor. At the federal level, the president fills about 2,000 jobs, from HHS secretary and deputy assistant to Office of Management and Budget deputy to members of the Federal Communications Commission and other independent commissions. Only 275 of these positions require Senate confirmation (Stillman 1987). In some states, governors make many appointments; in others, appointments are limited. Public appointees tend to be short-timers in federal and state government—the mean tenure for a Washington political appointee is around two years. When the president leaves, so do these people, to be replaced by appointees of the new administration. Heclo dubbed public appointees, birds of passage, who understand that they will not be around long and who must act quickly if they expect to accomplish anything (1977, 103). Most public employees are civil servants, personnel who are hired and rewarded on a merit system and whose tenure does not rely on any one political party or officeholder.

Robinson (1991) gave examples of conflicts that can arise between political appointees who are pursuing a presidential goal (in the 1980s it was holding down costs) and careerists who want to continue or expand programs they feel are worthy. The Reagan administration wanted to drastically reduce support for PSROs. One career agency official dedicated to keeping the program launched a campaign lobbying Congress on its value. While his supervisors knew what he was doing and objected to it, they could not stop him.

Sometimes members will try to separate careerists from the political aspects of the department by contacting them directly. According to Robinson (1991), some congressional committees sent packages of materials to the HCFA with instructions that political appointees were not to see the material. The committee wanted technical assistance but did not want to release the information to political appointees of the opposite political party.

Bureaucratic Power

When many people think of power, defined simply as the ability to act or the capability of producing an effect, they probably do not think of the bureaucracy. But they are wrong. As Norton Long noted over a half-century ago, "the lifeblood of administration is power" (1949, 257). Public employees are armed with the ability to influence legislation, interpret it, implement it, evaluate it. They work closely with most of the key actors in the policymaking process and make linkages between them. They have their own motivations and act accordingly.

Bureaucratic power has long rested on expertise. No matter how many staff people Congress and the president may add, that staff will likely not be expert in every programmatic aspect of an issue. In contrast, agencies staffed with personnel whose jobs are to deal with the details of a program and who have been doing so for years and years will still have the advantage. Bureaucratic expertise is "indispensable for the effective operation of any modern political system" (Rourke 1984, 15).

Sparer and Brown (1993) provided evidence of how Medicaid staffs in the states use their expertise to guide policy development. Minnesota's Medicaid staff helped draft legislative language, lobby, and otherwise "quarterback" the state's prenatal initiatives, the children's health plan, and an innovative and comprehensive MinnesotaCare Plan first adopted in 1992. Similarly, New York's Medicaid staff helped launch an innovative home care program by acting as intermediaries among elected officials, industry representatives, and client advocates, drafting legislation, testifying before legislative committees, and "generally pushing for action in a contentious area" (Sparer and Brown 1993, 294). Their knowledge of the programs, their strengths and potential, provided them with the basis for their standing in the policy debate.

Bureaucrats in state and federal governments also have the advantage of staying power. While executive-branch political appointees come and go, and congressional staff are highly transient, by definition careerists stay. They stay and learn and remember. Often the institutional memory of what was proposed and adopted in earlier years is a valuable commodity in an issue like health, in which many "new" proposals have actually been introduced several times over.

Bureaucratic power also rests on what Rourke (1984) called political mobilization and Long (1949) called political astuteness—the ability of an agency to garner support from recipients or beneficiaries of the agency's programs. As Rourke put it, "in the United States, it is fair to say, strength in a constituency is no less an asset for an administrator than it is for a politician, and some agencies have succeeded in building outside support as formidable as that of any political organization" (1984, 48).

It is important to keep in mind that power does not reside solely in the top leaders of the organization, but, as Long (1949, 258) said, "it flows in from the sides of an organization . . . it also flows up the organization to the center from the constituent parts." Power is not just a friendly lunch between the department secretary and the chair of the House Energy and Commerce Committee. It is also the friendship between congressional committee staff and a staffer at the Health Care Financing Administration's Office of Legislation and Policy, and the support from interest groups and recipients who want to make certain that Medicare and Medicaid are well staffed and well funded—a goal shared with the agency personnel.

Agencies often try hard to obtain positive and strong public support. They do it with good service, good media relations, advertisements ("Be the Best You Can Be"), education campaigns in public schools, and public involvement on commissions, boards, or contests. They especially desire strong support of "attentives," those people and groups who directly benefit from or otherwise support the agency's mission. The National Institutes of Health, for example, is supported by the research community of health professional schools and laboratories, high-tech industries, and broad-based organizations supporting specific diseases (such as the American Cancer Society). In the case of NIH and other agencies, many of these groups benefit from research dollars available from the agency directly or indirectly. Some agencies have a specific, highly targeted clientele, such as veterans. Organizations of veterans have been highly vocal, and extremely effective, in maintaining programs and increasing funding for the Veterans Administration.

Some feel that bureaucrats are getting more powerful. Morone (1993) noted that bureaucrats are playing a greater role in formulating health care and implementing laws with less deference. Others disagree. Rourke (1991) argued that the role of expertise has diminished in recent years as the public's confidence in experts has declined. There are simply too many experts—and they disagree too often. Whether it is "expert" testimony over the psychological profile of the defendant in a murder trial, the disagreements of scientists over the extent of the problem with ozone, or the disagreements of statisticians over the prevalence and incidence of the AIDS crisis, the point is the same. President Bush's Chief of Staff John Sununu put it succinctly in the debate over acid rain when he talked about "our" experts and "their" experts. Whom is the public to believe?

The Political Environment

The political environment of agencies can vary enormously. Wilson (1989) categorized agencies into four types based on whether the benefits they provide are narrow or wide and whether the costs they impose are narrow or wide.

For agencies providing narrow benefits and imposing narrow costs, their political environment can be categorized as interest group politics, best described by having interest groups on both sides of issues. A good example of this interest group agency is the Occupational Safety and Health Administration: labor and business often clash over the agency's actions, and the agency finds it hard to please both with its activities and its choices. At the other extreme, some agencies that distribute broad benefits and impose broad costs have little interest group involvement and may be called majoritarian agencies. The Centers for Disease Control (CDC) is one such agency. Reduced interest group participation might seem enviable at first glance, but it might prove problematic in times of budget cutbacks when the agency can find it hard to muster outside support.

An agency whose programs grant broad benefits while imposing costs only narrowly is not in an enviable position, because interest groups might coalesce to fight the costs and oppose the agency's goals. Few have much at stake in the benefits, but those suffering the costs are big losers. The Food and Drug Administration is a perfect example of this type of agency, called an entrepreneurial agency. Its mission is to broadly protect the public interest. But doing so means battling food and drug manufacturers that are financially harmed by the agency's actions. With millions of dollars at stake, the effort and cost of marshaling powerful coalitions to fight the agency are a good investment for the drugmakers.

The final category of agency politics is those whose benefits accrue to a few and the costs are widespread. Health manpower agencies, such as the Bureau of Health Professions, are examples of these client agencies. Their programs directly benefit medical and nursing schools, with costs widely spread across most of the population. Such an agency is a good candidate for "capture" by interest groups, because the goals of the agency and the goals of the groups are likely to be closely aligned. Opponents are hard to find and unlikely to invest the effort to form an interest group to oppose the agency's actions because the costs are so widespread and small to each payer.

Bureaucratic Behavior

Rationality is a important goal of public administration. It has many meanings, but Waldo's (1955) concept of rational action is appropriate to public administration: action correctly calculated to realize given desired goals with minimal loss to the realization of other desired goals. Yet clearly not all decisions are rational because few decision makers have the full information, time, and resources necessary to know the consequences of each alternative with certainty. More likely, for public decision makers, is that they are under time and resource constraints. Full knowledge about the alternatives and their consequences is nearly impossible to attain. Instead, public decision makers "satisfice," or make the best decision given the constraints. Simon (1945) described a "satisficing" decision maker as one who does not examine all possible alternatives, ignores most of the complex interrelationships of the real world, and makes decisions by applying relatively simple general rules. Another way Simon described it was that the decision maker applied "bounded rationality" to decisions.

Simon (1960) talked about two types of decision: programmed and nonprogrammed. Programmed decisions are those that recur frequently and can be handled by standard operating procedures (SOPs), the rules of operation followed by all employees in the same situation, rather than consideration of alternatives or their merits. SOPs can be viewed as a way to limit bureaucratic power and force staff to conform to organizational goals (Rourke 1984). They are also the only practical way to run a large organization. The regional offices of federal agencies make many decisions on a daily basis about what is acceptable and unacceptable behavior from grantees and recipients. SOPs help ensure uniformity among these offices and their counterparts in Washington. The emphasis on SOPs is not arbitrary or necessarily convenient. As Peters (1981, 76) put it, "They are responsible for public money and act in the name of the people and must therefore be accountable to the public. Accountability, in turn, may force the bureaucrat to protect himself against possible complaints, and the protection comes through adherence to rules and procedures."

Nevertheless, SOPs can prove annoying to presidents, Congress, and others who prefer a quick response without going through the normal channels of operation. Allison's (1971) analysis of the Cuban Missile Crisis recounted developments when Secretary of Defense Robert McNamara wanted to make certain that the Navy's actions during the blockade of Cuba were in line with the president's desires to avoid confrontation. He questioned the chief of Naval Operations about the procedures to be employed. Smugly, the officer picked up the Navy's *Manual of Naval Regulations* and confidently asserted that it provided all necessary guidance. The president might be commander in chief, but the Navy knew how run a blockade, thank you.

Nonprogrammed decisions are those that are novel, unstructured, and consequential. They cannot be handled with SOPs but must be dealt with using the staff's discretion buttressed with training, judgment, and rules of thumb. Decisions related to the drafting of regulations, allocation of resources, and implementation of new programs are examples of nonprogrammed decisions.

Missions, or commonly held goals of an agency, are important to that agency's survival. In health the NIH is an example of an agency with a strong sense of mission—biomedical research—that has remained constant over decades. In contrast the Public Health Service has seen its mission change from caring for merchant sailors to environmental and preventive medical activities to responsibility for the delivery of care to targeted populations, preventive care, and health manpower. While agencies must be somewhat flexible to survive, such major organizational personality changes can strip an agency of its identity and leave it floundering. As Greenberg (1975) described the PHS, it seems little more than a shell for a variety of categorical programs, without an overall concern for the general public health.

NIH, on the other hand, holds so strongly to its mission that it has repeatedly successfully resisted efforts by powerful health committee and subcommittee chairs to add new agencies with a statistical and social science focus. When one was slipped in—the National Institute on Aging—its director (despite his own training as a psychiatrist) quickly realized that his agency must focus on the biological aspects of aging rather than social science concerns if it was to thrive in the NIH environment.

Sometimes what Mosher (1982) called dominant professions can disagree over an agency's mission in a way that weakens its allegiance to the mission. Public Health Service officials, in a 1960 response to congressional pressure to deal more directly with environmental issues, established a new Bureau of Environmental Health to enforce pollution standards on the states. Immediately a fight broke out between the agency's physicians and engineers over who would control the new bureau. Each was concerned with pollution but their approaches were quite different. The physicians won initially, and the engineers complained to Congress. Congress responded by moving the new bureau to the Food and Drug Administration, a newly named agency headed by an engineer. By 1969, said Greenberg (1975), two separate agencies within a single Public Health Service bureau were formed to accommodate both professions. But it was too late. Congress had lost patience and established a separate environmental agency: the Environmental Protection Agency, to which pollution programs formerly under HEW were transferred.

THE PUBLIC BUREAUCRACY AND POLICYMAKING

In the early years of public administration, politician and public employee were seen as distinct and clearly defined roles. Elected officials were responsible for political decisions or making policy; appointed officials handled administrative matters and the implementation of political actions. Such a distinction, known as the politics-administration dichotomy, now seems naive and outdated. Today's public bureaucrat is involved in all aspects of policymaking, setting the agenda, formulating solutions, and implementing the policy, including translating sometimes vague congressional directions into concrete, workable programs.

Setting the Agenda

Items get on the health care policy agenda by rising from the primeval policy soup described in Kingdon (1984). Public bureaucrats help. They are the factotums, providing information and statistics that define problems in a way that can move them to the forefront of public attention. They can make its dimensions and severity known to the Congress, the White House, and the press. Kelman (1980) attributed the rise of occupational safety and health to the presidential and congressional agendas to a bureaucrat in an HEW research unit who worked on occupational safety and health issues and whose brother wrote speeches for President Johnson. The brother occasionally slipped occupational safety and health issues into the president's speeches. The staff of the secretary of labor, looking for new legislative proposals, noticed the references and proposed legislation on the issue in 1968.

Robinson (1991) recounted that a midlevel civil servant in the Health Care Financing Administration was assigned to respond to a letter to the president from a retired, single teacher in California who discovered that her state medical insurance was not available to retirees and that she was not eligible for Medicare. The letter alerted the staffer to a problem that could be solved with a change in the Medicare statutes to include state and local employees. He persuaded others in HCFA, the White House, and eventually Congress. His proposal, prompted by the letter to the president, became law. Nelson (1978) noted in her study of child abuse how the Children's Bureau supported research to legitimize an issue and gain the attention of the media and policymakers.

Formulating Health Care Policy

Medicare and community mental health programs are examples of health care policies generated within the bureaucracy (Peters 1981). A more recent example is the Medicare Prospective Payment System, which flowed from over a decade of HCFA-sponsored research and demonstration projects to develop a more effective administrative mechanism for controlling health care costs. HCFA funded eight state demonstration projects in 1975 to try out mandatory and voluntary health cost-control programs. Seven years later, Congress required HCFA to develop a legislative proposal for Medicare payment to hospitals, skilled nursing facilities, and other providers on a prospective basis. Following the advice of a task force composed of HCFA staff and experts from outside the government, the HCFA administrator proposed a hospital prospective payment plan based on the latest PPS demonstration project, one operating in New Jersey. The plan was enacted virtually intact by the Congress three months after it was submitted (Morone and Dunham 1985).

When Congress considers measures to provide insurance for the uninsured, it needs to know how many Americans are uninsured, where they reside, and why they are uninsured. HHS can provide that information. The agency is even more successful in helping develop the administration's policy agenda than one for Congress. Robinson (1991) said that 89 percent of executive-generated Medicare legislation in 1987 could be traced to HCFA.

Nonetheless, reliance on the federal bureaucracy for ideas and legislative language is not as heavy as it once was. Homegrown expertise in Congress and the White House has increased dramatically over the past twenty years, allowing them to be more independent and reducing the role of bureaucratic knowledge. In 1967, 73 percent of legislatively adopted provisions came from the executive branch and only 5 percent from the Congress. But a more recent count found that only 36 percent of the legislative provisions in the 1987 Medicare hospital legislation had their origin in the executive branch (Robinson 1991). Bureaucratic expertise is still valuable, particularly in filling in the details of a congressional or White House plan and stopping potentially naive or bad ideas. But when the president wants to make heavy use of health care expertise to forge a political strategy for health care policy, he recruits it to the White House staff—as President Bush did when he promoted HCFA administrator Gail Wilensky to the White House when health heated up as a campaign issue.

Implementing Health Policy

Implementation may be defined as the set of activities directed toward putting a program into effect or what happens after laws are passed authorizing a program policy, benefit, or some other tangible output (Ripley and Franklin 1986). Peters (1981, 77) argued that, to a great extent, "the 'real' policy of government is that policy which is implemented, rather than that policy which is adopted by the legislature." Yet implementation is an area not widely understood, even by policymakers. Nathan (1993, 122) called it the "shadow land" or the neglected dimension of U.S. governance. A 1993 report of the National Commission on the State and Local Public Service called implementation the short suit of American government. So much time is devoted to what should be done that little energy remains for the question of how to do it. The commission felt that the frustrations of the American public about government stem from unsuccessful implementation—the failure of government to turn promises into performance.

Implementation begins when Congress delegates the policy it wants carried out to federal agencies through a series of instructions, sometimes specific, sometimes less specific. The federal agency then carries out those instructions. While seemingly straightforward, many things can happen to impede successful implementation:

—agencies responsible for implementation may be less than enthusiastic, not well staffed, or without the expertise or resources needed to carry out their responsibilities;

—the congressional instructions may be so vague that the federal agency must make many key assumptions, such as designating which state programs are "acceptable" or what is "reasonable cost";

—there may be multiple congressional goals or conflicting instructions that make it difficult for agencies to carry out their assignments;

—interagency rivalries may cause problems with agency staff fighting one another over the interpretation of the law and resource issues;

—the recipients (for example, state or local governments) may be uncooperative or demand different interpretations;

—the number of people involved may slow the process (if there are several federal agencies and several state and local agencies that must serve as "clearance points," the eventual success will be adversely affected);

—time can be a problem (for complicated measures, such as clean air and clean water, the process of collecting information, writing draft regulations, and encouraging public comment can add years to the process of rule making);

—state and local agencies, communities, or recipients of the program can slow the implementation if they disagree with any aspect of it.

An example of a poorly implemented program due to lack of resources was the National Center for Health Care Technology (NCHCT), authorized in law in 1978 but without any appropriations. The agency limped along for several months with borrowed staff and offices. Finally, a small amount of money was shifted from another HHS agency. A short time later, the center's mission was transferred to the National Center for Health Services Research, which later became the Agency for Health Care Policy and Research (AHCPR). Downs (1967) would say that the NCHCT never overcame the initial survival threshold necessary for a thriving agency.

Congressional ambiguity can cause enormous problems in a program's implementation. The Early and Periodic Screening, Diagnosis, and Treatment (EPSDT) program was enacted in 1967 without clear language specifying whom the program would serve, how much it would cost, or which agency would administer it. In this case, the ambiguity was due not to inability to reach agreement but rather to congressional indifference. As Foltz (1975, 49) put it, the United States' "first policy mandating preventive health services for needy children, a kind of health insurance for the poor" was enacted without much ado in the Congress. Indeed, the tough question of whether it was a health or a welfare program—a question key to its implementation in both Washington and the states—was left unanswered in the legislation. It was left to the secretary of HEW to make the tough calls over administration, eligibility, and costs.

Congress gives broad discretion to federal agencies to implement its laws for a variety of reasons: because it is impossible (and unwise) for Congress to write a law so detailed that it can be put in place immediately; sometimes members do not want to deal with a touchy or difficult issue and passing it on to federal agencies gets them off the hook; the complexity of many issues prevents Congress from fully understanding enough to write details; and the experimental nature of policymaking is promoted with bureaucratic discretion. It is easier for administrators to change or revise a troublesome provision than for the Congress to reconsider the matter.

Sometimes the delegation of authority is quite broad. In Medicare, for example, it was left to the HEW officials to determine what the Congress meant by "reasonable costs" of providing hospital care. Since hospitals were key to the success of the new program, Social Security officials agreed to depreciation and capital development provisions that were quite generous and contributed to rapidly increasing hospital costs in the 1970s (Feder 1977). The law setting up OSHA said the agency should foster healthful working conditions "so far as possible" and deal with toxic substances "to the extent feasible" (Thompson 1983, 219, 221). States too give health experts plenty of leeway in conducting their business. Medicaid officials in New York placed a limit on the number of visits to physicians and dentists and on laboratory procedures that the program would reimburse. The state court invalidated the regulations as "unauthorized by law," but the legislature later adopted the limitations, and they were carried out (Sparer and Brown 1993, 288). In day-to-day implementation of state and federal Medicaid policy, state officials' discretion can lead to big differences in provision of service delivery (Weissert 1994).

Congress does not treat all agencies equally. The amount of discretion afforded an agency depends on several factors, including the agency's resources (such as political support, expertise, and leadership) and tolerance of other actors, especially interest groups. Meier (1985) described an agency's decisions as falling within or outside a zone of acceptance. If the agency's decision falls within the zone of acceptance to Congress, the president, and the courts, the agency will be afforded more autonomy. Agencies dealing with salient issues that are not complex are most likely to have smaller zones of acceptance, and Congress is most likely to intervene. Sometimes the Congress has little choice but to provide discretion to agencies, especially on complicated, politically volatile issues. But it can still provide specific guidance to these agencies. For example, while delegating the authority to set new physician fees in RBRVS to HCFA, the Congress placed two constraints on HCFA's decisions: the payment levels had to reflect production costs and had to be budget neutral (Balla 1995).

In recent years there has been a trend for more specificity and less discretion in enabling legislation guiding federal agencies. Altman and Sapolsky (1976, 423) noted the trend in the 1970s, saying that "Congress has become the focal point of health legislation activity." They quoted a congressional staffer as saying in 1975, "Congress has begun to turn the tables. . . . Legislation will change not only in content but in form . . . legislation will look much more to you like *Federal Register* notices" (423).

The congressional tendency to limit an agency's discretion flourished in the 1980s thanks to distrust between a Democratic Congress and a Republican White House. The Democratic Congress wanted to make certain that their version of the legislation was implemented by including detailed instructions, definitions, and guidance in the law. Congress decided it liked this detailed brand of legislation so well that even when a Democratic president took over in 1993, the micromanagement continued. Such direction had become not only possible but also commonplace because Congress now had the staff to oversee agency activity. One example of the micromanagement was a congressional order to add another layer of bureaucracy in the AIDS office. "There isn't a scientist in the country who thought that [this personnel change] would give us better science," complained HHS Secretary Donna Shalala, "but it certainly responds to a political need" (Broder and Barr 1993, 31).

Regulation

The single most important bureaucratic task in implementation is issuing regulations for carrying out the law. Drafting regulations or rule making follows procedures required by the federal Administrative Procedure Act. This act requires notice that a department plans to issue a rule. The notice must be published in the *Federal Register,* the official notification document of the federal government. Interested parties are allowed an opportunity to participate in the proceedings by presenting written or oral information. Hearings are often held on salient rules of great interest to many people. Final regulations are then published. Some agencies are required by law to hold hearings and base final rules on the evidence in the record. Legislation delegating the assignment to set new Medicare physician payment levels under RVRBS to HCFA required the agency to publish preliminary payment levels in the *Federal Register,* providing physicians ample opportunity to comment. Nearly 100,000 physicians did so (Balla 1995). Most states have similar sets of procedures for the promulgation of regulations. (Cities and counties do too, but they frequently override them by invoking provisions of their charters that permit the declaration of an emergency, though it is often difficult to see how a zoning change can constitute a real emergency.)

Before writing an initial draft rule, agencies often convene task forces and commission issue papers to best inform themselves on the issues involved. In drafting regulations for the 1973 Health Maintenance Organizations Act, for example, HEW set up eight task forces involving bureaucrats and representatives of interest groups and others knowledgeable on the subject. The task forces' recommendations were submitted to a decision policy group, which formulated issue specifications and passed their work on to a technical staff, which translated the specifications into legal language. Only then was a draft notice of proposed rule making published (Altman and Sapolsky 1976).

Yet the attention afforded to the HMO regulations was not really typical. For regulations accompanying legislation that is more routine or that involves incremental changes in areas where agency staff are highly expert, regulation writing is often done internally, by overworked staff members pressured by deadlines and without much outside participation in the initial stages, either because they lack time and resources or because the agency feels fully competent to act on its own. An example of the latter is the health-planning legislation of 1974. Altman and Sapolsky (1976, 429) quoted one HEW official as saying, "We've been in the business of planning and developing health areas before and we are accustomed to dealing with the conflicts that arise from federal-state-local relations." HEW limited feedback to written comments, which for nonnational organizations were submitted to and summarized by HEW's ten regional offices. As it turned out, the HEW official overstated the routine nature of the 1974 planning program. The states, working primarily through the National Governors' Conference, argued that the law was an important federalism issue and their views had to be considered more forcefully in the process. HEW agreed to fund states to research and organize their views on the regulations, hold private meetings with state representatives, and sponsor public meetings throughout the country to discuss the regulations (Altman and Sapolsky 1976).

The assumption is that agencies will do whatever Congress asks and do it well. This is not always the case. RBRVS is a case in point. HCFA had been directed by Congress not to reduce payments to physicians as a group. Yet when the regulations emerged, payments had dropped by 16 percent—a reflection in part of the bureaucracy's dual masters (Morone 1993). HCFA and other federal agencies are accountable to both the Congress and the White House, entities whose goals may be quite different. The White House often demands that the agency hold down costs and reduce paperwork or administrative burdens on hospitals, physicians, or businesses. Congress is often more expansionary, calling for more programs, to more recipients, at more cost, and with more paperwork.

Such a dilemma arose when HHS dragged its feet on payment adjustments under Medicare's prospective payment system for disproportionate-share hospitals, or those serving a high percentage of low-income and Medicare patients. Although the 1983 legislation mandated that the HHS secretary provide special treatment for such hospitals, the initial regulations reflected no such provisions. To the White House, special treatment meant more money. This was not what they had in mind. The following year, the Congress again signaled its intention for disproportionate-share hospitals to get special treatment, this time setting a deadline of 31 December 1984 for the receipt of a report describing the criteria developed by HHS to classify these hospitals and to list hospitals so classified. HHS finally complied.

When an issue enters the regulation-writing stage, politics is not cast aside. Rather, interest groups understand the bureaucracy to be another venue for achieving policy goals. For example, as a result of demands from the American Hospital Association and the Federation of American Hospitals, HCFA in 1983 revised the final regulations on prospective payment review to remove outlier payments from the calculations of the hospital portion of the PPS.

Sometimes interest groups try to obtain in regulation what they failed to achieve in the congressional process. In the HMO Act of 1973, labor "lost" when the law ordered employers to do something that labor would rather keep on the bargaining table: a mandate for employers to include an HMO option if they employed twenty-five or more workers, pay minimum wage, and offer health benefits. Labor representatives argued that the requirement undercut the role of collective bargaining. They also said it posed a threat to the economic well-being of large labor trust funds, which they said could be dissipated by HMO health benefit plans over which the union had little control. The initial draft regulations gave only minor concessions to labor's preferences. As the regulation moved up the line in HEW, the decision was made to allow collective bargaining representatives to "pass judgment" on HMO offers. However, that position was reversed by HEW Secretary Caspar Weinberger, who supported the earlier, tougher version. Months later, he reversed himself, and the version giving collective bargaining agents more control was adopted.

Labor's success during a Republican administration is no doubt partly explained by the American Medical Association, which also opposed the provision because it would have aided HMO development. But the workability of the regulations was a factor too. The agency understood that it was the local companies, bargaining units, and workers influenced by their physicians who would make the law a reality. The regulations had to accommodate these groups' influences or risk being stymied or ignored. One HEW official quoted by Altman and Sapolsky (1976) said that regulatory decisions must be subjected to the "rational man" criterion: regulations must protect the statute but make reasonable adjustments where implementation demands.

Another example of HEW adjusting legislative intent to make a program work was the health-planning law of 1974. It required a variety of new state and planning agency responsibilities without additional money to pay for them. To ease the burden, the regulations limited the activities of the health systems' agencies and omitted several rate-setting experiments mandated in the law (433).

While many regulatory decisions are complex, detailed, and of interest to only a few affected groups, some are of broad public interest. In 1994 when the Occupational Safety and Health Administration published draft rules that would ban smoking in the workplace, more than 700 organizations and individuals wanted to testify. The hearings continued for three months (Swoboda and Hamilton 1994).

There is often considerable delay between legislative enactment and the issuance of final regulations. The EPSDT program of the Social Security Act was enacted in 1967, but final regulations were not issued for five years. Implementation took another year. Ambiguities in the federal law, including which agency would administer the program, the costs of the program, and eligibility for and scope of service caused the HEW to spend years hammering out answers with interest groups, community organizations, and states, which were the real implementors of the program (Foltz 1975).

Congress can and does intervene in the regulatory process if it does not approve of the regulations. Public Health Service rules intended to discourage an excess of hospital beds brought a quick response from Congress. The regulations said that rural hospitals should deliver at least 500 babies annually if they were to maintain a maternity ward and delivery room. Occupancy of 80 percent or less was defined as an indicator of excess capacity. The House unanimously adopted a resolution clearly indicating to HEW that the final rules needed to be more lenient on rural areas. HEW got the message.

Regulators pushed the industry further than it wanted to go in rules for a 1978 congressionally mandated system of hospital uniform reporting under Medicare and Medicaid. Unhappy with the 500-page manual produced by HEW, the hospitals complained to Congress that the agency was on an expensive "fishing expedition" for information at the hospitals' expense. The House held hearings, then voted to cut off funds to implement the program. The Senate asked for a General Accounting Office evaluation. A compromise was reached in 1980 to collect data not felt to be too intrusive by hospitals (Thompson 1983). In 1995 the Congress launched an effort to curb what many members felt was excessive regulation with the Senate proposing to review and possibly overturn new regulations. Such a change would greatly expand the congressional oversight role of the federal regulatory process.

In past years it was common in political science to talk about agencies being "captured" by interests, an event most likely to occur in agencies whose tasks involved providing benefits to a narrow group of interests—a client agency in Wilson's (1989) terminology like the Veterans Administration. The idea was that because the agency's survival depended in large part on the support of its constituents, the agency could not be impartial but would accommodate the needs of the constituents, regulating to protect their interests. In recent years empirical studies testing the regulatory capture theory have debunked the idea for most regulatory agencies. In fact the studies have shown how agencies continue to regulate an industry vigorously rather than be increasingly sympathetic to it (Quirk 1981; Meier 1985). Recent work has highlighted a more pluralistic interest group model in which many interest groups form advocacy coalitions but find their influence curbed by external pressures from other actors and groups and by internal structure, professionalism, and leadership (Gormley 1982; Meier 1985).

The courts do not get involved in writing regulations, but they do respond when a group or person challenges the legality of a regulation. The Administrative Procedure Act provides for judicial review of any agency's action by a person or corporation wronged by the agency or with a grievance. Under this act, citizens can use the courts to prod agencies into action. When federal agencies fail to issue regulations expeditiously or within congressional deadlines, they may be sued and the plaintiffs may prevail. Some federal agencies have their regulations taken to court with some regularity. OSHA and EPA routinely see their regulatory products questioned in court.

Where the Rubber Hits the Road

Simply issuing the regulations does not get the agency home free. Bureaucrats must encourage, cajole, and otherwise urge providers or other governments to which the money will flow for the provision of service to act in an expeditious way, faithful to the law and regulations. Sometimes getting a high level of compliance is not so easy. Since much of the money goes to state and local governments, they are the primary focus of much of this activity. Control by federal bureaucracy over state and local officials is quite limited: Washington agencies can urge, educate, provide their state and local counterparts with financial incentives, or threaten them with the loss of federal grant money, but they cannot force perfect compliance or timeliness. The relationship can best be described as bargaining, under which the federal government, by offering a grant, achieves only the opportunity to bargain with the states (Ingram 1977). "Instead of a federal master dangling a carrot in front of a state donkey, the more apt image reveals a rich merchant haggling on equal terms with a sly, bargain-hunting consumer" (499).

HCFA may have characterized California as something of a stubborn donkey in the late 1980s when the nation's largest state balked at implementing 1987 nursing home standards adopted by Congress. California argued that their state standards were better than those proposed by HCFA and the imposition of the federal standards would cost the state nearly one-half billion dollars. After HCFA threatened the state with the loss of federal Medicaid dollars, California's Republican governor appealed to the Republican president. A short time later, the state and HCFA reached a compromise. HCFA eased its demands that states use a lengthy and complicated survey process in return for California's agreement to begin inspecting nursing homes using HCFA guidelines. California did not win in the long run, however. While Sacramento and Washington argued, a group of providers went to court over implementation of the law and forced California's Medicaid program to pay an extra $2 per day per bed to meet the nursing homes' costs of complying with the law.

Thompson (1983) noted the difficulties in implementing EPSDT. To encourage (or coerce) states to participate, Congress passed legislation threatening to reduce AFDC payments for failure to carry out EPSDT. To be compliant (and avoid the loss of federal dollars), states had to inform parents of eligible children at least once a year that services were available, make certain those who wanted screening received it within sixty days, and guarantee treatment within sixty days of the screening. The states largely ignored the order, and HEW resisted imposing the penalty.

More successful have been efforts in which federal health officials work with the states to reach a compromise solution. Thompson (1983) gave the example of Medicaid error rates as one in which the regulations reflected several compromises with states over the data base and tolerable error rate. There were also provisions permitting state appeals over disallowance, thus providing more state flexibility and the opportunity to argue for their own unique situation. Some in Congress objected to the apparent capitulation; "just too doggone mealymouth," was how one member quoted by Thompson (1983, 141) put it. But HEW was trying to avoid more trouble and get a program implemented. It was well aware of what might be called the Derthick rule of specificity: the more specific the language of the federal requirement, the lower the federal capacity to adapt to state peculiarities and the greater the danger that the limitations of the federal capacity to force conformance might be exposed to view (Derthick 1970).

Agencies must also keep Congress happy. While much of the congressional oversight fits the "fire alarm" analogy discussed in Chapter 1, all it takes is one senator to become concerned over a program, and press conferences will be called, hearings held, and the agency generally held to task. In 1994 several senators were unhappy about the progress of a new program to supply vaccine to the nation's poor children. Arkansas Senator Dale Bumpers at a Senate Appropriations HHS Subcommittee hearing lambasted the Centers for Disease Control for assigning the General Services Administration management responsibility for storing the nation's supply of vaccine. While the agency spokespersons tried to convince the senators of the safety of the plan and the competence of the GSA to manage it, the Senate Appropriations Committee voted to cut off funding for the program unless CDC officials could prove they could safely implement it. A few weeks later, the administration scrapped the GSA warehouse and launched a private-sector program to supply vaccines.

Few headlines can be gained in hearings focused on which agency is to administer the program or feasible scopes of work and timetables. On the other hand, the spectacle of hapless bureaucrats cringing before an arm-waving member is inherently photogenic, and the member gets to take an active role in casting blame on someone else.

One avenue key to oversight is the evaluation of health programs. Most federal programs are evaluated by outside groups of consultants or academics, and the General Accounting Office also serves as an important evaluator for the Congress.

Regulatory Agencies

In addition to "line" agencies within HHS, such as the Social Security Administration, Bureau of Health Professions Education, and HCFA, which are responsible for issuing regulations and for program management, there are agencies whose entire role is regulating economic or social activities. The three key regulatory agencies with authority over health issues are the Food and Drug Administration, the Federal Trade Commission, and the Occupational Safety and Health Administration. A fourth regulatory agency, the Environmental Protection Agency, deals with environmental issues.

The FDA regulates drugs, cosmetics, medical devices, and food, but its primary function is the approval of drugs. A new drug must undergo an extensive testing procedure, and some eight to nine years generally pass before it is accepted for marketing in this country. The agency is proud of its careful, comprehensive premarketing procedures and harkens back to efforts by one of its employees to keep thalidomide, a tranquilizer that led to deformed children in Europe, off the American market, despite strong efforts by an American drug company that wanted to market it here. Nevertheless, the agency's cumbersome and lengthy procedures for drug approval are also controversial among drugmakers and groups who might benefit from new drugs, such as AIDS victims. The FDA also has jurisdiction over food regulation, including the regulation of food additives and programs that specify the content of labeling. In the 1980s and 1990s the FDA was frequently in the news targeting smoking among young people, ill effects of passive smoking, and efforts by cigarette makers to hide the ill effects of their product. But the most controversial recent FDA action was its 1995 pronouncement that the nicotine in cigarettes should be declared an addictive drug, followed by a series of proposals aimed at curbing smoking by young people. Tobacco companies immediately filed suit in federal court arguing that the FDA had exceeded its authority.

The FTC was established in 1914 to prohibit unfair competition and prevent unfair and deceptive trade practices. In 1982 the FTC won a U.S. Supreme Court case upholding its regulation of physicians. In the 1990s the big issue is how to balance concerns over antitrust with the trend toward managed competition. Managed competition relies on efficient networks of providers competing for health care business. But FTC guidelines view arrangements allowing one competitor or a unified network of competitors to have too much market share as restraining competition. Advertising and price fixing remain important issues in the 1990s, as evidenced by the commission's 1993 action to bar the California Dental Association from preventing certain classes of price advertising (such as senior citizen discounts) and prohibiting the advertising of special patient services.

OSHA was established in 1970 with the passage of the Occupational Safety and Health Act. Its director also holds the title of assistant secretary of labor. OSHA's rule-making power is broader than that of most other regulatory agencies. For example, OSHA can adopt temporary emergency rules outside the Administrative Procedure Act and was allowed to promulgate consensus industry standards as rules in the agency's first two years (Meier 1985). OSHA may undertake rule-making processes on its own initiative or in response to an individual petition. In its early years OSHA concentrated mainly on safety issues, until a 1975 House Committee on Appropriations directed the agency to shift its emphasis from safety to health-standards enforcement (Thompson 1983). Two years later its administrator announced that the agency would change its policies to focus on health.

OSHA's relationship with Congress and businesses has been rocky. In its first six years a hundred bills a year were introduced that would have restricted the agency, many involving exemptions of farms and other small businesses. The courts are similarly engaged in the agency's activities. According to Meier (1985), every major health regulation issued by the agency (except its first on asbestos) has been challenged in court, often by both business and labor. It fared very poorly in the Reagan and Bush administrations, which targeted the agency for cuts and reduction in monitoring. However, under the Clinton administration, the agency stepped up its enforcement of workplace safety laws and strongly supported a major revision of the OSHA law—the first time since its initial passage in 1970.

The primary regulation in the environmental area comes from the EPA, which regulates air pollution, water pollution, hazardous wastes, and pesticides. During the Bush administration, the role of developing environmental regulations was shared by EPA and the President's Council on Competitiveness, whose purpose was to make certain that new regulations issued by the government were not unduly burdensome to business and industry and were not injurious to the national economy. Drafting regulations for the 1990 Clean Air Act was controversial in that some environmental groups claimed that the competitiveness council, chaired by Vice President Dan Quayle, was making concessions to industry in regulations that had been explicitly rejected by Congress (Weisskopf 1991).

THE MANY MASTERS OF THE BUREAUCRACY

In recent years political scientists have argued among themselves about bureaucratic accountability and control. Some (Weingast and Moran 1983; Fiorina 1981; Calvert, Moran, and Weingast 1987) argue that the Congress is the real master of the bureaucracy. Its longstanding ability to authorize programs, appropriate agency funding, approve executive appointments, and monitor activities has been amplified with its tendency to micromanage the implementation of programs and to conduct highly publicized hearings on any agency actions. Thus, say some, Congress clearly holds many of the puppeteer's strings. A counterargument is that the president is the primary overseer of the bureaucracy, through the appointment process and budgetary and regulatory direction (Moe 1985; West and Cooper 1989–90; Rockman 1984).

Others argue that the existence of so many masters undercuts the power of any one and that the bureaucracy is relatively autonomous because Congress and the president are simply too busy or too bored to adequately oversee its activities (Wilson 1989). Hammond and Knott (1992) concluded that there are some conditions in which each situation fits. They argued that one institutional actor cannot determine the policy outcome, but rather that the results flow from the product of interactions among the president, the House, the Senate, and their committees.

The Bureaucracy and Congress

The Congress is important to federal agencies, because it authorizes the legislation setting up the programs and outlining the duties of the federal bureaus, and it appropriates funds to carry out the programs and staff the agencies. With these laws, Congress must decide how much discretion to give agencies, whether to "hardwire" or "softwire" the process (Epstein and O'Halloran 1994). When the Congress hardwires the program, it provides detailed directions to the agency. Softwiring the program means the Congress gives the agency considerable discretion in carrying out its will. Although many citizens and politicians complain about bureaucratic insensitivity, the evidence runs counter to this notion. Study after study has documented the responsiveness or willingness of the federal bureaucracy to respond to Congress, the president, and other elected officials.

While the bureaucracy is responsive to the concerns of Congress and others, the Congress is often unresponsive to bureaucracy and unwilling to acknowledge agencies' needs and capabilities. Despite its willingness to oversee and even ridicule administrative implementation efforts, Congress does little up front to make certain that implementation goes smoothly. Derthick (1990), in a case study of two programs in the Social Security Administration, highlighted the congressional lack of concern over administrative problems. Congress has little interest in the capabilities of the implementing agency or department or in problems that might arise among agencies or among federal agencies and their state and local counterparts. "It does not occur to presidential and congressional participants that the law should be tailored to the limits of organizational capacity. Nor do they seriously inquire what the limits of that capacity might be" (Derthick 1990, 184). Congress changed its mind several times in the months prior to the implementation of the Supplemental Security Income (SSI) program. On the day before the law was to take effect on 1 January 1974, a bill was signed by the president increasing benefits and changing the program for a last time before the checks were mailed.

An example of congressional lack of concern about an agency's capability was the 1973 HMO legislation, which housed the program in an agency that had previously administered only poverty programs. The first "middle-class" program of the Health Services Administration (HSA) was the controversial and innovative HMO program (Altman and Sapolsky 1976, 427).

The Bureaucracy and the Presidency

One of the assignments given to the president in the Constitution is to make certain that the laws are faithfully executed, notably by the bureaucracy. The president can do this in several ways. The first, and perhaps most important, is through the appointment of the agency's leadership. The president also has some leverage over agencies through the development of the president's budget. While Congress must finally dispose of the budget, an agency will generally want to receive a maintenance, if not increasing, budgetary allocation. The president has leverage in that agency's priorities, and its goals are expected to reflect those of the president. While some exceptions occur at the individual level, an agency's leadership will bring its considerable forces to bear in testimony and meetings with the Hill to pursue a program desired by the president. Finally, the president has leverage over agencies through the role of White House staff, particularly the Office of Management and Budget. OMB oversees the issuance of regulations and agency policies that affect the budget.

Often agencies and OMB disagree on what the administration's official position should be. OMB typically supports reduction in funding in its effort to hold down costs. The agency will usually argue on the side of the continuation or expansion of programs, particularly those it administers. In the 1980s OMB became quite strong and won many internal skirmishes with agencies over legislative support and the issuance of regulations. In the 1970s the opponents were better matched, and HHS sometimes won. For example, in 1974 OMB argued that the existing program providing capitated grants to medical schools should be terminated, because its goal of increasing the number of medical graduates had been reached (Behn and Sperduto 1979). Further, it was widely agreed that the country had a surplus of physicians, so there was little reason to provide incentives to produce more. Reason seemed to be on OMB's side, but politics were not. Interestingly, HEW's argument against termination was not based on the merits of the proposal. Instead, the agency argued that Congress was going to renew the program anyway, and if the administration held out for its termination, it would have "no influence on the type of bill that Congress eventually passes" (Behn and Sperduto 1979, 59). HEW won. The administration decided to support the program, and it was eventually reauthorized.

The relationship between the president and the federal bureaucracy is often adversarial—at least on the part of the president. Harry Truman was reported to have complained, "I thought I was President but when it comes to these bureaucrats, I can't do a damn thing" (Nathan 1983, 3). Richard Nixon in his second term tried to control the bureaucracy by putting Nixon loyalists into key policymaking roles in federal agencies. Ronald Reagan adopted a jigsaw puzzle management approach, whereby information was given to career bureaucrats only in pieces so they would not be able to contribute to the larger picture or puzzle (Pfiffner 1987). There has also been a trend toward placing political appointees further and further down the policy chain as a way of ensuring compliance (Rourke 1991). But there is little evidence of deliberate bureaucratic sabotage. Rather, career bureaucrats tend to want to please newly elected presidents, even those with whom they may not agree. As Wilson (1989, 275) put it, "What is surprising is not that bureaucrats sometimes can defy the President but that they support his programs as much as they do."

Once a measure becomes law, the president's interest often wanes. Only on rare occasions (for example, when a regulation is controversial, highly valued by an important interest group ally, or potentially counter to other goals, such as cost-cutting) will the president inject himself into regulation writing or other implementation processes. There are some exceptions, however. Jimmy Carter, in 1978, concerned about inflation, ordered the weakening of the regulations protecting workers from cotton dust (Thompson 1983, 22). Similarly, the Reagan and Bush administrations were concerned about the impact of environmental and health regulations on businesses.

The Bureaucracy and the Courts

The judiciary plays an important role in bureaucratic policymaking, a relationship Rosenbloom (1981, 31) quoted Judge David Bazelon as calling "an involuntary partnership." The court oversees bureaucratic actions to make certain that they are not violating due process, legislative intent, individual liberties, or equal protection of the law. Many regulatory agencies often spend years developing legal theories, collecting data, and preparing analyses that will stand up in court (West 1984).

In the past decade courts have stepped up their oversight of administrative regulatory decisions, often questioning both the process and the substance of administrative activities, abandoning their traditional deference to bureaucratic expertise (Melnick 1983). In 1976 a federal district court ruled that error levels specified by HEW in regulations were arbitrary and capricious *(Maryland v. Mathes)*. In 1978 the fifth district court of appeals set aside an OSHA requirement that the concentration of benzene in air not exceed one part per million parts of air "in the absence of substantial evidence indicating that measurable benefits to be achieved . . . bore a reasonable relationship to cost." It also noted that OSHA had acted using "dated, inconclusive data" (Thompson 1983, 238). The ruling was upheld in the U.S. Supreme Court two years later, with the court saying that OSHA had failed to present sufficient evidence that the proposed reduction in exposure to benzene was "reasonably necessary . . . to provide safe and healthful employment" (238).

The courts are also concerned with what Rosenblatt (1993, 439) called "right-enforcing roles": a tendency to consider recipients' entitlement to benefits as a right, rather than a privilege that may be withdrawn or diminished at any time. This emphasis on beneficiaries' rights has led to a greater concern about an agency's use of discretion over Medicaid, cash assistance, housing assistance, and other federal programs and to more specific court guidelines for action. Horowitz (1977) provided a partial list of areas in which these specific guidelines were applied: food handling, hospitals' operations, recreation facilities, inmate employment and education, sanitation and laundry, painting, lighting, plumbing, and renovation in some prisons. Courts have ordered the equalization of school expenditures on teachers' salaries, established hearing procedures for public school discipline cases, decided that bilingual education must be provided, and suspended the use of the National Teacher Examination and of comparable tests for school supervisors by school boards. They have called for the construction of roads and bridges and suspended performance requirements for air bags and tires. They have told the Farmers Home Administration to restore a disaster loan program, the Forest Service to stop clear-cutting trees, and the Corps of Engineers to maintain the nation's nonnavigable waterways (Horowitz 1977). Apart from the intrusiveness of the courts in daily management issues, these decisions usually cost governments money—often millions of dollars.

One of the most far-reaching court cases affecting the administration of a health program, and one costing states a great deal of money, was *Wilder v. Virginia Hospital Association*, a 1990 U.S. Supreme Court case that found that hospitals and nursing homes were the intended beneficiaries of the Medicaid law and had standing to sue in court. That case reaffirmed the rights-affirming role adopted by earlier courts that the statute "creates a 'binding obligation' on a government agency to do something" (Rosenblatt 1993, 459). Following the Supreme Court's lead, courts in Washington, New York, Michigan, and other states found reimbursements were less than "reasonable and adequate" and ordered higher state spending, totaling $70 million in a year in Michigan alone. Other state agencies settled out of court with nursing homes and hospitals at a cost of $65 million over two years to Oregon. In another example, a district court order in Alabama raised that state's spending on mental hospitals from $14 million in 1971 to $58 million in 1973 (Horowitz 1977).

One of the criticisms of this increased judicial activity, also dubbed "imperial judiciary" (Glazer 1975), is that court mandates have come to dominate the activities of federal and state agencies, particularly those most likely to be sued in court. The EPA, for example, must make decisions among competing priorities, and with few exceptions, court mandates take top priority in the EPA, even ahead of congressional directives (O'Leary 1989). O'Leary concluded that courts have reduced the discretion, autonomy, power, and authority of EPA administrators. She also concluded that the emphasis on responding to courts increases the power and authority of attorneys within the EPA while decreasing the power and authority of scientists.

For the states, one of most troublesome rulings of the court has been over the interpretation of the federal Employee Retirement Income Security Act. The courts have ruled that the 1974 law preempts state laws that relate to employee benefit plans, including their health coverage. Until 1995, the U.S. Supreme Court interpreted ERISA very broadly to include laws that affect employee health plans, even if their purpose is not directed at such plans. ERISA prohibits or severely curtails state activities in a number of areas crucial to state health reform efforts, including financing employer mandates, provider rate setting and global budgets, insurance reform, and the collection of data (Butler 1994).

Agencies are not simply victims of the courts but, in fact, use the courts to uphold their pronouncements or punish those who violate federal regulations. The EPA, for example, often brings civil suits against companies that fail to comply with the Clean Air Act. Some state agencies use the courts to get increased funding from their legislatures (Rosenberg 1991). If agency directors' pleas for more money fall on deaf ears in the legislative appropriations process, a court order mandating spending to ameliorate the program will provide the needed funds.

The Health Bureaucracy

The primary health agency in the federal government is the Department of Health and Human Services, although at least fifteen other federal agencies have health care–related outlays. In 1993 HHS's budget was nearly $283 billion (excluding Social Security), of which more than 80 percent was spent on health.

The two key health agencies within HHS are PHS and HCFA (figure 4.1). The Administration for Children and Families administers AFDC and other federal welfare programs. While PHS and HCFA look like roughly equal agencies in figure 4.1, the budget for HCFA dwarfs that of PHS. In 1994 HCFA spent nearly $239 billion; PHS spent only $17 billion.

The oldest federal health agency is the Public Health Service, whose lineage dates back to the 1798 Marine Hospital Service. It became the Public Health Service in 1912. PHS was housed in the Treasury Department, a location that made sense because customs collectors in U.S. ports historically

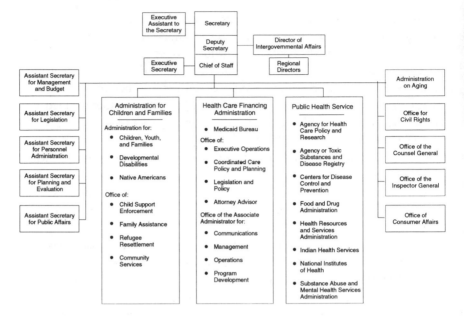

Figure 4.1 The Department of Health and Human Services

Source: 1994 Government Manual, detail 1995.

provided medical care to merchant sailors. In 1939 the Public Health Service, Social Security Board, and Office of Education were merged into the Federal Security Agency. A year later the FDA was transferred from the Agriculture Department. The PHS was primarily concerned with the provision of medical care to federal beneficiaries, such as the Coast Guard, and with technical assistance to states to deal with infectious and communicable diseases (Feingold and Greenberg 1984). After World War II, when the federal government stepped up its activities in health, the PHS was forced to broaden its scope to include hospital construction and support for biomedical research.

A turning point for PHS came in 1965, when the newly created Medicare and Medicaid programs were housed in different agencies. Medicare went to Social Security and Medicaid to the Social and Rehabilitation Services. Indeed, in the 1960s the HEW secretary expressed dissatisfaction with the rigidity and lack of imagination of the PHS commissioned corps and its head, the surgeon general. He took the control of the PHS away from the surgeon general (without abolishing the job) and gave it to the assistant secretary for health and scientific affairs, a political appointee. Subsequent reorganizations ensued, and the PHS has persisted as an entity, although in a rather weak form. The Office of the Assistant Secretary for Health provides funds for PHS staff and public health programs dealing with disease prevention and health promotion, health of minority groups, physical fitness and sports, and vaccine and HIV program coordination. In the president's budget the PHS appears as an item under the assistant secretary for health and scientific affairs rather than under its own heading (as do the other three components of HHS).

Other early federal health agencies were the National Hygienic Laboratory, established in 1887 (which became the National Institutes of Health in 1930); the Food and Drug Administration, established by law in 1907; and the Children's Bureau, established in 1912. These early agencies were primarily concerned with public health. The interest in children's issues, evidenced by the establishment of the Children's Bureau and the passage of the Sheppard-Towner Act of 1922 providing funding to states for personal health services to pregnant women and children, was a turning point in federal governmental duties and responsibilities—away from public health and toward personal health services.

Until the 1950s there was no overall, comprehensive health agency. Departments operated independently, reporting to Congress and the White House. In 1953 the Department of Health, Education, and Welfare was created. Interestingly, President Truman had attempted to create this consolidated agency for several years but had been thwarted by interest groups, including the American Medical Association. The AMA agreed not to oppose it when President Dwight D. Eisenhower promised that the government would "stay out of medical affairs" and that the AMA could choose the department's special assistant for medical affairs (Harris 1966, 65).

While some view the bureaucracy as an unchanging leviathan, nothing could be further from the truth. As table 4.2 illustrates, the health bureaucracy changed with some regularity over a thirty-year period, with consolidations, reorganizations, and agency elimination regularly reframing the bureaucracy over time.

Among the federal health agencies, HCFA, which administers Medicare and Medicaid, is by far the biggest spender, accounting for more than $230 billion in fiscal year 1992 alone. The distant second in health agency spending is the National Institutes of Health, the principal biomedical research agency of the government, which spent $8.4 billion in 1992. NIH is made up of the following institutes:

—National Cancer Institute
—National Heart, Lung, and Blood Institute

—National Institute of Diabetes and Digestive and Kidney Diseases
—National Institute of Allergy and Infectious Diseases
—National Institute of Child Health and Human Development
—National Institute on Deafness and Other Communications Disorders
—National Institute on Dental Research
—National Institute of Environmental Health Sciences
—National Institute of General Medical Sciences
—National Institute of Neurological Disorders and Stroke
—National Eye Institute
—National Institute on Aging
—National Institute of Alcohol Abuse and Alcoholism
—National Institute of Arthritis and Musculoskeletal and Skin Diseases
—National Institute on Drug Abuse
—National Institute of Mental Health
—National Institute of Nursing Research

Also within the NIH are the National Library of Medicine and the National Center for Human Genome Research. The National Cancer Institute receives the most funding, nearly $2 billion in 1992; the National Institute of Nursing Research, one of the newest, received only $49 million that year. The National Institute on Dental Research spent $161 million; the National Eye Institute, $276 million; and the National Institute on Deafness and Other Communications Disorders, $151 million.

The National Cancer Institute is the oldest institute, created in 1937, predating the formation of NIH by seven years. Its organization is more autonomous than the other institutes, with the director reporting directly to the president, through OMB, bypassing the NIH director and HHS secretary (Epstein 1979). The unusual organizational system was put in place in 1971 federal legislation launching a national effort to cure cancer. As Epstein (1979) noted in *The Politics of Cancer,* the effort was sold to Congress in a campaign that the cure for cancer was imminent and needed only a massively funded national effort to conquer the disease by America's 200th birthday. The National Cancer Institute's autonomy was so important that it should be "removed from the 'bureaucracy' of NIH" and be free to find the cure for cancer (326). The organization suited President Nixon, who was suspicious of federal agencies and preferred a direct relationship to the rejuvenated and well-funded agency. The cure for cancer still evades us, but the National Cancer Institute remains the only institute directly accountable to the president.

Table 4.2. Chronicling Bureaucratic Change: A Sample of Activity, 1965–1993

Year	Action
1966	National Institute of Mental Health (NIMH) became independent of other NIH institutes
1968	HEW reorganized from eight operating agencies to six
	HSMHA and Social and Rehabilitative Services (SRS) created
	PHS broken into three units
	PHS removed from the surgeon general to the assistant secretary for health and scientific affairs
	NIMH becomes part of the HSMHA
	Consumer Protection and Environmental Health Service (CPEHS) established within HEW
	FDA placed under CPEHS
1970	CPEHS eliminated
	Environmental Health Service (EHS) created
	FDA restored to operating agency status
1972–73	EHS disbanded
1973–74	Major reorganization of HEW
	NIH, FDA, CDC, Health Resources Administration (HRA), and HSA subsumed under PHS, which is under ASHSA
	SRS and SSA remain autonomous and report directly to HEW secretary
	HSMHA divided into three parts: CDC—combining the CDC and National Institute for Occupational Safety and Health (NIOSH)—HRA, and HSA
	NIMH renamed Alcohol, Drug Abuse, and Mental Health Administration (ADAMHA)
1977	HCFA created by taking Medicare and Medicaid financing away from SSA and SRS
	PHS financing responsibilities given to HCFA
1980	HEW split into HHS and the Department of Education
1982	HRA and HSA combined into Health Resources and Services Administration (HRSA)

Table 4.2. *(cont.)*

1983	Agency for Toxic Substances and Disease Registry created
1991	Administration for Children and Families created
1992–93	Office of Human Development Services (OHDS) eliminated
	AHCPR formed
	ADAMHA becomes SAMHSA, which had charge of service delivery including mental health; the research component returned to NIH and became NIMH

In 1995 the Social Security Administration was severed from HHS and became an independent agency; its director also reports directly to the president.

One of the most recent changes was the recasting and restructuring of the National Center for Health Services Research (NCHSR) into the Agency for Health Care Policy and Research, with a new mission, in 1989. The new agency was formed to showcase and more generously fund health services research, in particular research on the outcomes of diagnostic and therapeutic interventions. The funding for the parent agency, NCHSR, had been rather stagnant, and proposals had been made to move the agency to NIH or other agencies within PHS. AHCPR funding started at $85 million in fiscal year 1990 and increased to $185 million in 1994. NCHSR's proposed 1990 funding was $78 million (Gray 1992).

CONCLUSION

Unlike the situation in many other countries, a life of public service in the executive branch has never been highly regarded in the United States. Rather, bureaucrats are often the butt of jokes, cartoons, and snide remarks from friends, family, and customers. Nevertheless, bureaucrats are key actors in forming, implementing, and evaluating policy in health as in almost every other area of public concern. Bureaucrats provide the expertise and institutional history that are essential to Congress and the presidency, which may have ideas but little sense of how they might actually work in the real world. The linkage they provide, between truth and power, is essential. Nevertheless, the health bureaucracy, like its legislative and presidential counterparts in other areas, is suffering under a public skepticism about government and governmental programs. The role as scapegoat, especially useful to members of Congress, state legislators, and presidential candidates, has hurt them in the public's perception. Many people worry that the unattractiveness of the public sector will repel the best and brightest young people and lead to a weakening of governmental expertise (National Commission on the Public Service 1989).

In health, bureaucrats have helped draft such major legislation as Medicare and Medicaid, have offered such solutions as DRGs, and have been responsible for implementing every national health program since 1887. They regulate the operation of the health care industry, safeguard the health of the nation's workplace, and protect consumers from unsafe food and drugs. At the state level, they oversee the insurance industry, license health care professionals, and monitor provider services and facilities. Bureaucrats work closely with the Congress, president, and interest groups but are also policy actors in their own right, with their own preferences and goals and basis of expertise and political support.

Some people feel that as turnover increases in the federal and state legislative branches through term limits in states and public desire for "new blood" in Washington, the bureaucratic role in policymaking will be strengthened. With this turnover will come the loss of congressional specialists in health and other areas, forcing new members to look elsewhere, such as the bureaucracy, for substantive guidance. The inability of comprehensive health reform to successfully make it through Washington's legislative maze may strengthen the bureaucrat's hands as well. Incremental change—often made outside the bright policy lights—is typically more influenced by bureaucratic knowledge and expertise than broader, more salient change. On the other hand, the wide availability of expertise, technological advances allowing members to obtain data quickly and in an assessable form, the proliferation of specialized health lobbies armed with detailed information and technical analyses, the difficulties in attracting smart new employees, and budgetary constraints may negatively affect a stronger bureaucratic role in policymaking.

5

States and Health Care Reform

A LOOK BACK

1965

IN THE EARLY 1960s state governance was largely embarrassing. Governors were generally elected every two years or were allowed only one four-year term and had little power when they did assume office. Thanks to citizens' concerns about vesting too much power in a few persons, states had successfully spread decision making over a spate of agencies, commissions, and boards that were not directly accountable to anyone. Daniel Evans, on taking office as governor of Washington in 1965, called a cabinet meeting and sixty people came (Sanford 1967). Legislatures were even more poorly prepared to deal with state problems. Legislative pay was a pittance, there were no or very few staff members, and the legislature was in session on a few days every other year. The state was often run by special interests. In some states, railroad interests dominated; in some, it was power companies or race tracks, oil companies or insurance companies.

Cities were often ignored by legislatures composed largely of members representing rural parts of the state. In 1960 more than 6 million people lived in Los Angeles County and fewer than 15,000 lived in a rural county in northern California's mountains, yet each was represented by one senator. In Vermont a town with a population of thirty-eight had the same representation as the city of Burlington, with 35,531. Translated into legislative control, 11 percent of the people in California could control the state senate; 12 percent of the people in Vermont could control the state house (Grant and Omdahl 1993). The reason for this maldistribution was twofold. First, many states had not changed their legislative district lines (or redistricted) for decades. In 1963 twenty-seven states had not redistricted their legislatures in twenty-five years, and eight states had not redistricted in more than fifty years (Sanford 1967). The Vermont house had not redistricted since 1793. Second, many states copied the federal legislative model, with an upper house based on geographic units (states in the U.S. Senate). For states, the obvious geographic units were counties, and states often assigned one senator for each county.

Problems were often ignored by state officials. As Sanford (1967, 35) put it, "The states . . . have failed to advance with their citizens into the modern world." He continued, "When twentieth-century growth began to overtake us, the machinery of state government was outmoded, revenue resources were outstripped, and the state executive was denied the tools of leadership long supplied the President of the United States" (36–37).

Despite their lackluster leadership, states were key players in health in the early 1960s, serving as the primary providers of mental health and (with local government) public health services. By 1965 change was in the air. States were scrambling to reapportion their legislative bodies to respond to the Supreme Court decisions in *Baker v. Carr* in 1962 and *Reynolds v. Simms* in 1964, which applied the principle of one person/one vote to both houses of every state legislature. In 1967 more than one-half of the states had constitutional revisions on their ballots to reorganize the legislatures, make changes in the executive branch, improve the judicial branch, and change the relationship between states and their local governments.

Between 1965 and 1975 states underwent a remarkable transformation. Their legislative, judicial, and executive offices became vibrant and responsive. Their state employees were energized, and state capitals became places where exciting programs were launched and carried out, thus attracting many of the brightest and the best young people to Albany, Lansing, and Tallahassee. Changes were made in state constitutions to unshackle local government and to balance the state's tax system so it would weather economic difficulties and maintain equity among its citizenry. States began to tackle the tough issues they had often avoided in previous years—from environment to economic development, from education reform to controlling health care costs.

1980

By the 1980s state legislatures had greatly improved their staffing and more adequately represented all citizens of the state. There were more women and minorities in the legislature, and compared with the 1960s, there was greater partisan competition, with Republicans picking up seats in the South and Democrats in the North. There was a tremendous jump in the number of women serving in state legislatures between 1969 and 1980, increasing from a total of around 300 to nearly 800 (Patterson 1983). Membership in legislatures for ethnic and minority groups also increased during this time, although their proportion of all legislators was small—around 4 percent. State after state strengthened the powers granted to governors, giving them longer terms of office, the ability to serve multiple terms, stronger budgetary authority, and the ability to appoint more cabinet members and to have a strong item veto (Beyle 1989). Overall, states had made a remarkable, but not widely heralded, recovery in their ability to deal with tough problems. Indeed, in 1985 the Advisory Commission on Intergovernmental Relations (ACIR) described states as moving from fallen arches to arch supports of the system. The ACIR noted that states are "more representative, more responsive, more activist and more professional in their operations than they ever have been" (364).

Further, states were the sources of innovative policies, particularly in health. In the 1970s and 1980s states became concerned about the rapidly increasing costs of health care to their budgets and instituted reforms, such as rate-setting systems, negotiated contracting, and diagnosis-related groups. They also adopted risk pools for health insurance, right-to-die acts, and mandatory seat belt laws.

1993

The makeup of state legislatures in 1992 was much more representative of the population in gender and occupation than in earlier decades. In 1993

Table 5.1. Percentage of Women Serving in the U.S. House, State Houses, and State Senates

	1975	1981 (Percentage)	1994
U. S. House	4.4%	4.4%	11.0%
State houses	9.3	14.0	21.8
State senates	4.5	7.0	17.3

Source: Data from the Center for the American Woman and Politics, Eagleton Institute of Politics, Rutgers University, and Ornstein, Mann, and Malbin (1994).

more than 20 percent of the 7,424 state legislators were women, five times as many as in the 1960s (Thaemert 1994). In five states—Arizona, Colorado, New Hampshire, Vermont, and Washington—women held more than one-third of the legislative seats. In others, women were still somewhat rare. In Alabama, Kentucky, Louisiana, Oklahoma, and Pennsylvania, women made up less than 10 percent of the total (the percentage of women serving in the U.S. Congress in that year). Compared with the U.S. House of Representatives and with previous years, female representation on state legislatures was greatly enhanced (see table 5.1). State legislatures had fewer attorneys, business owners, and farmers in 1994 than in the 1960s and more legislators whose service comprised their full-time job. Some 15 percent of all state legislators in 1994 were full-time, up from 3 percent in 1976.

In 1992 a sitting governor was elected to the presidency—the first time since Governor Franklin Roosevelt was elected in 1932. President Bill Clinton, governor of Arkansas, not only understood state governance but also was actively involved as a spokesperson for states through the National Governors' Association, which he headed and served as leader in the development of several policy positions, including those on welfare reform and health care.

States had become increasingly active players in the health care field. Ideas discussed in Washington in 1993–94 were already in place in several innovative states; other states were considering such ideas as a single-payer system, generally viewed as too radical for national consideration. The role of states in health reform was more than a parochial concern but was identified as a key issue in congressional hearings, news conferences, and Sunday morning talk shows. It was clear that Washington could not monitor and implement the program on its own. It needed states.

OVERVIEW

The states' role in health is broad. One analyst called the scope of state activities in the health area "truly awesome and capable of reaching into almost every facet of health care delivery" (Clarke 1981, 61). States are responsible for funding and coordinating public health functions, the financing and delivery of personal health services (including Medicaid, mental health, public hospitals, and health departments), environmental protection, the regulation of providers of medical care and the technology they employ, the regulation of the sale of health insurance, state rate setting and licensing, and cost control. States provide health insurance for their own employees and retirees and play a pivotal role in educating and credentialing health care professionals. Some 20 percent of state budgets are allocated to health (U.S. GAO 1992).

State institutions are similar to national entities in their structure and purpose. However, several differences are also key in understanding why state and federal policies can be so divergent, including the requirement for a state balanced budget, direct democracy, and the very muted role of the press in state capitols. States differ from one another in significant ways, including their willingness to enact innovative legislation and in their implementation of the Medicaid program. In recent years states have provided innovative solutions to a slew of health problems yet are constrained by federal law from making some changes (especially by ERISA, which limits states' ability to make comprehensive state reforms).

FEDERALISM AND INTERGOVERNMENTAL RELATIONS

To understand states and health policy, one must understand federalism and intergovernmental relations that define the states' roles and responsibilities in health and other areas.

In the earliest years of this country, we were governed by the Articles of Confederation, which set up a weak national government and strong states. The national body (unicameral, with equal representation from the states) had no power to tax, enter into commercial treaties, retaliate against discriminatory foreign trade policies, or enforce the provisions of existing treaties. The Congress relied on states to act, and it needed state cooperation to discharge any functions. There was no national government, but rather the United States "consisted solely in the congregation of envoys from the separate states for the accommodation of certain specified matters under terms prescribed by the federal treaty" (Diamond 1985, 30).

The states issued their own money and had their own trade policies with other states. When there were interstate disagreements, the Congress was virtually powerless to deal with them.

While acknowledging that the confederation did not work, the delegates to the Constitutional Convention of 1789 were not yet ready to establish a fully national government. They compromised in the wording of the Constitution, which divides responsibilities between the two levels of government. Certain functions, such as interstate commerce and national defense, were assigned to the national government, while others, such as the selection of presidential electors who were to select the president, were left to states. The strongest language in favor of states came in the Tenth Amendment, which says that "powers not delegated to the United States by the Constitution, nor prohibited by it to the states, are reserved to the states respectively, or to the people."

On the other hand, the same Constitution authorizes the national Congress to "provide for the general welfare" and to "make all Laws which shall be necessary and proper" for executing this and other powers given to the legislature. The commerce clause is also key: anything defined as interstate commerce, or crossing state lines, is in the federal domain. Finally, the supremacy clause clearly states that if federal and state laws are incompatible, the federal law will prevail.

The broad parameters allocating powers between the national and state government soon led to the important role of the courts in defining those powers. The first major decision on this, *McCullough v. Maryland,* in 1819, was brought when Maryland leaders questioned the power of the federal government to establish a national bank in Baltimore, a power not specifically listed in the Constitution. This celebrated decision established the notion of "implied powers," that the national government was not limited to those powers clearly outlined in the Constitution, but that the Congress could also become involved in areas that were "implied" in such vague phrases as "providing for the general welfare" or "necessary and proper." By so broadly construing the intent of the Constitution, the Supreme Court allowed the responsibilities of the federal government to encompass a broad array of activities and programs. Over the years, the court has come down strongly on the side of the federal government.

A key point to keep in mind about federalism is that it is a system of rules for the division of public policy responsibilities among a number of autonomous governmental entities (Anton 1989). In the United States these entities are the national and state governments. The autonomous nature of the relationship is key. In this country states are not administrative units of Washington but have their own responsibilities and duties, many of them overlapping those of Washington. The relationship was once described as cooperative federalism, in which federal and state governments work to achieve common goals through the interactions of both. The metaphor commonly used is a marble cake, with the governmental units representing the cake layers and programmatic activities, such as education, welfare, and health, "marbling" through the cake.

Ronald Reagan, in his vision of "New Federalism," preferred a different view of the relationship between federal and state governments. His call for a sorting out of responsibilities, whereby the national government would handle only those functions purely national and the states would handle most other areas, was similar to dual federalism, a system with another cake metaphor—a layer cake—in which one layer represents the responsibilities of one government and the other those of another, with little overlapping. The models differ in the extensiveness of the federal role; they share the view, established in the Constitution, of state sovereignty.

The point, then, is that the important role of states is established in the U.S. Constitution and ratified by history. Like most dynamic relationships, there are changes over time. The 1960s and 1970s were primarily times when Washington was very strong and states rather weak in capacity and resources. In the 1980s and 1990s the federal government was fiscally constrained with a $3-trillion budget debt, while the states were reasonably fiscally secure and administratively capable to take on problems, including health.

Federal Grants

For the first century of this country, government at any level did very little. The people did not particularly desire governmental services, and governments had few taxes from which to obtain the resources to provide services. The federal governmental role was largely restricted to "war and danger" and some limited pork-barrel funding. States were more active, particularly in economic-development activities. States built roads and bridges, dredged canals, set forth civil and property rights, family and criminal laws, and provided education (Walker 1995). For the federal government, a turning point was the imposition of the income tax in 1913. Finally, there were resources.

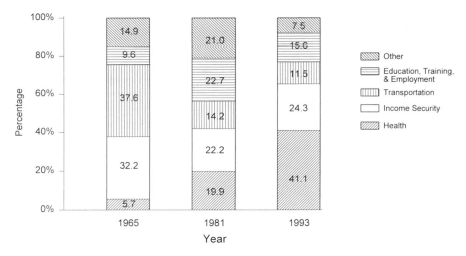

Figure 5.1 Federal Grants by Function as a Percentage of Total Federal Grants

With the coming of the New Deal, Franklin Roosevelt's effort at overcoming the Depression, there was also a cause. The federal government wanted to help citizens find jobs, bring home a salary, and put them on the road to financial recovery. Yet it could not do this solely from Washington. Rather, it was easiest for Washington to give grants to states and localities so they could provide the services. Thus in the 1930s began the age of the federal grant. Between 1933 and 1938 sixteen federal grant programs were enacted.

If the 1930s saw the development of the federal grant, the 1960s and 1970s were their heyday. Again, the federal government wanted action: to alleviate poverty, to equalize educational opportunities, to clean the nation's air and water, and to ensure adequate health care for underserved populations. But it could not be done from Washington. In the 1960s the Congress enacted hundreds of new federal grants. In 1965 alone more than 150 grants were enacted. Between 1965 and 1970 the dollars provided in federal grants doubled; the total doubled again between 1970 and 1975, and nearly doubled again over the next five years (table 5.2). In 1979 for the first time, the rate of increase slowed, and the heyday of federal grants was over. In 1985 grants were 11 percent less than they were in 1980 in adjusted dollars.

The nearly $220 billion provided to states and localities in 1994 went to programs ranging from highway beautification to Aid to Families with Dependent Children, from Head Start to water purification. The biggest federal grant program in health is Medicaid, which accounted for $76 billion in federal spending in 1993. Other federal health programs are much smaller: sub-

Table 5.2. Federal Grants, 1965–93

Year	Amount (in Billions of Dollars)	Percentage of State and Local Outlays	Percentage of Federal Outlays	Constant Dollars (1987)	Grants to Individuals as a Percentage of the Total
1965	$ 11	15%	9%	$ 42	34%
1970	24	19	12	73	36
1975	50	23	15	105	34
1980	92	26	16	128	36
1985	106	21	11	113	47
1990	136	19	11	120	57
1994	217	—	15	169	65

Source: Data from Walker (1995).

stance abuse grants totalled $1.4 billion; community health centers, $558 million; maternal and child grants, $665 million; and family planning, $173 million. Health grants account for more than 40 percent of all federal grants—up from 5.7 percent in 1965 and 20 percent in 1980 (see figure 5.1).

Federal grants were a boon to states and localities because they provided the resources to pay for services that could not, or would not, have been offered without the additional money. They helped professionalize state and local work forces in many areas, including health. States increased the salaries of employees and challenged them with innovative and meaningful programs funded in part by federal dollars. They also helped equalize services in a way that states could not do on their own. Medicaid, AFDC, and other federal grants are designed especially to assist poor states or states with poor citizens and few natural resources to tax.

Most federal grants are categorical; money is provided to states and localities, which must perform rather specific functions, from funding black lung clinics to providing curriculum assistance in health professions. Sometimes the grants are competitive; states and localities must submit proposals, and only a small number will be funded. More often, the grants are distributed to all states or localities based on a formula that includes such "need" measures as the number of poor persons, rural highways, waterfront land, or dilapidated housing.

In 1966 a new type of grant came into existence, a block grant, which allowed states and localities more discretion over how the dollars could be used. Generally, the Congress would specify the area in which the funds could be spent, but recipients could decide within those broad categories which programs best fit their own needs. The first block grant was in health, the Partnership for Health Act in 1966. Other health block grants were for maternal and child health; alcohol, drug abuse, and mental health; and preventive health. While states and localities liked block grants, the Congress was generally less enthusiastic because it was much harder for members to take credit for programs funded under this grant device and oversight was difficult. The biggest push for block grants was in 1981 when the Omnibus Budget Reconciliation Act consolidated more than fifty categorical grants into nine block grants and reduced federal funding by 12 percent. In the mid-1990s block grants were again on the public agenda as congressional Republicans pursued "blocking" a variety of existing grant programs to give more discretion to state governments with less money.

While the $220 billion in federal grants may seem at first glance to be a substantial funding source, several things should be kept in mind. First, the total of federal grants in 1993 was only slightly more than the interest on the national debt. Second, in adjusted dollars the amounts have stabilized for states and significantly dropped for most localities. Third, the dollars are going to people—not places. In other words, the money passes through the state budgets on the way to the recipients, but the state cannot use the money for other priority programs or policies. Finally, the desire for a reduction in the federal budget deficit has focused attention on possible areas in the budget to cut, and federal grants, unlike entitlement programs discussed earlier, are appropriated yearly and can be zeroed out or reduced. Thus they seem to be a likely target for efforts to slow federal spending. Indeed, as a result of the 1993 budget agreement, the total federal discretionary spending is expected to decrease by nearly $2 billion between 1994 and 1999 (Dearborn 1994).

Regulatory Federalism

In the 1980s when federal budgetary restraints began to take hold, new federal grant spending became a liability, and federal regulation—under which states and localities could be coerced into acting in certain ways—became more appealing. Regulations and requirements have long been a part of federal grants, going back to the Hatch Act of 1939, which prohibited partisan political activity by federal employees and by state and local employees funded with federal grant dollars. Nevertheless, the past few decades have seen a new type of regulation in which Washington enlists state and local governments in national efforts on behalf of particular disadvantaged groups or to advance certain policies, such as environmental protection. Four types of intergovernmental regulation are popular: cross-cutting requirements, crossover sanctions, partial preemption, and direct orders or mandates.

Cross-cutting requirements are general policy provisions that apply across all federal grants in such areas as discrimination, wage rates, and environmental protection. A recent example is the Drug-Free Workplace Act put into effect in 1989, which requires all federal contractors, grant recipients, and state agencies awarded contracts or grants of $25,000 or more to certify that they will provide a drug-free work environment.

Crossover sanctions are newer regulatory mechanisms that impose a financial penalty on one problem based on the defects of another. Particularly popular are imposing penalties from the highway trust fund if states do not make desired federal changes. While early crossover sanctions dealt with transportation (e.g., lowering the speed limit and changing the minimum drinking age), more recent laws have tied the loss of a state's highway trust fund monies to nontransportation issues, such as the control of junkyards and clean municipal air. States now face a total of thirteen different financial penalties under which they can lose from 5 to 100 percent of their highway trust funds for failure to comply with federal requirements.

Partial preemption is where the national government establishes rules and regulations calling for minimum national standards. States can administer the program if they follow the standards. If they fail or do not wish to do so, federal agencies will administer the program in their states. This type of intergovernmental mandate is often used in the environmental area in such laws as safe drinking water, surface mining, and clean air amendments. It also applies to state occupational health and safety. Half the states have chosen to administer that program; half have not.

Direct orders or mandates are where the federal government orders lower governments to take certain types of actions. More than 50 percent of all federal statutes preempting state and local authority enacted in our 200-year history have been enacted during the past two decades. The amendments to the Medicaid law in the 1980s requiring states to cover certain services and groups under the program are mandates that states must follow. Between 1984 and 1990 some thirty-two mandates were enacted to expand Medicaid eligibility and services. A 1994 mandate required states to cover under Medicaid poor women impregnated by rape or incest, even though a half-dozen states had constitutional provisions or laws prohibiting such coverage. Other examples of mandates include recent federal laws:

—requiring employers (including most states) to offer terminated employees the option to buy health insurance identical to what was provided before the termination;

—requiring state licensure boards to compile and distribute to all nonbaccalaureate schools data on their pass/fail ratios for students who take licensure exams;

—mandating states to evaluate the competency of nurse's aides, maintain a register of those who pass the exam, and establish a mechanism for handling complaints.

Particularly troublesome for states is the tendency for Washington to mandate without federal financial assistance to pay for the newly required service. By one count, some 174 unfunded mandates have been enacted over the past twenty years—ninety-two of these between 1981 and 1988 (Zimmerman 1991). The cost to states and localities is immense. The cost to localities alone between 1993 and 1998 is estimated at $90 billion (Suskind 1993). Ohio Governor George Voinovich estimated that unfunded mandates cost his state nearly $2 billion between 1992 and 1995 (Will 1994).

Many of these mandates are in the area of environmental protection. While states pay some environmental costs, the burden is largely shifted to local governments. Some 87 percent of government outlays in environment are expected to be paid by local budgets in the year 2000 (Arrandale 1994). The effect on smaller jurisdictions can be devastating. An Environmental Protection Agency mandate requiring localities to monitor a particular substance in sewage discharge is costing a small North Carolina town of 3,000 residents more than $30,000 a year—an amount equal to a six-cent increase in the property tax. Boston residents saw their water rates go up a whopping 600 percent in the late 1980s to pay for a huge waste-treatment plant to clean up Boston Harbor, mandated by the EPA.

The 1990 Americans with Disabilities Act is another unfunded mandate costing states and localities billions of dollars—dollars that could have been spent elsewhere. One California mayor noted that the $400,000 his city spent on new playground equipment to comply with the mandates was "taken right out of child-care facilities, out of after-school programs for disadvantaged youth" (Will 1994). Philadelphia Mayor Edward Rendell estimated that the costs to his city of altering curbs and building ramps will take one-third of his city's public works budget for street paving and repair (Suskind 1993).

But the largest federal mandate is Medicaid. Congress has substantially broadened the scope and reach of the program over the past decade, at an estimated cost of some $16 billion to the cost of Medicaid in 1992 alone (Morgan 1994, 8).

As congressional budget procedures make it difficult to enact new programs, the mandate route gets more and more attractive. It allows the member of Congress to have services or programs provided but without the incentive of federal dollars. Indeed, in the 102nd Congress, more than 125 bills were introduced containing unfunded mandates, and more than twenty of the most expensive were introduced by the Democratic leadership. While presidents like to place the blame entirely on the Congress, none of the laws containing mandates was enacted over a presidential veto during the Reagan or Bush administrations (Hinds 1992).

One of the first measures to pass the Republican-controlled Congress in 1995 was a bill to limit unfunded mandates. The 1995 law provided that any proposed bill is out of order if it will cost state and local governments more than $50 million. The provision can be overruled with a majority vote. Mandates in place in 1995 were not affected by the law. While clearly a step forward in the eyes of many state and local officials, it does not guarantee federal mandates will end; in fact as many as two-thirds of the major mandates that Congress imposes on states are exempt from the bill. Some fear that Congress will now simply make certain desired activities a condition of federal aid or fund a program for a few years, then withdraw the funding, actions not prohibited by the law.

Most observers of federalism would describe the American model as nationally dominant—that is, with the national government having key leadership responsibility. However, problems caused by the $4-trillion federal debt and political changes in Washington and the states in 1995 have led to some leveling of the playing field. Members of Congress were serious in their effort to return power (and less money) to states at the same time states seemed eager to take more control over welfare, food stamps, job training, and school lunches. And there was more willingness on the part of the federal program administrators to "bend" as well. In December 1994, the EPA—one of the federal agencies that imposes many (unwanted) mandates on states and localities—announced it would give states more leeway in designing their clean air strategy and backed off requiring states to use a high-tech, centralized emission control program initially demanded by the agency.

UNDERSTANDING THE DIFFERENCES BETWEEN FEDERAL AND STATE GOVERNMENTS

States are similar to and different from the federal government and one another in ways that affect their policymaking in health and other areas. They are similar to the federal government in their organization, structure, and policymaking processes. They are different in three key areas: budget constraints, direct democracy, and media coverage.

State government is structured and run in a manner similar to the federal government. Every state has a state constitution that contains a bill of rights and provisions setting forth the structure and function of states and of local governments. All have three branches of government, and forty-nine have two houses. Like Congress, state legislatures are organized by the dominant political party, and forty-nine states have bipartisan membership (only Nebraska is unicameral and nonpartisan). Every state has a governor with duties roughly analogous to those of the president, including administering state government and initiating a policy agenda. Like the president, governors appoint members of a cabinet, although in a number of states several important cabinet positions are elected or appointed by commission. Every state has a judiciary that includes both trial and appellate levels.

The duties of the three branches are nearly identical between federal and state governmental levels. In both the legislature passes laws, provides appropriations, and oversees the executive branch. Federal and state legislatures are organized by parties, use committees as key decision makers, and have nearly identical flow charts illustrating "how a bill becomes a law." In both the chief elected official of the executive branch sets the agenda, oversees the running of the government, and handles relationships outside the capitol. The judiciary in both determines the constitutionality of laws, adjudicates violations of law, and protects the well-being of individual citizens. Both levels of government are lobbied by interest groups and provided funding by PACs. And, importantly, both governments are sovereign and operate by virtue of the power of the people. Each citizen is subject to at least two governments, under which some rights are identical and some are very different.

States and the federal government differ in their revenue sources and their spending priorities. The big spending area for states has traditionally been education (both K–12 and higher education). In the past decade, corrections and Medicaid have become big-ticket items, often displacing education, transportation, and other areas of spending. Primary and secondary education is the largest single category of spending (30 percent); higher education makes up 12 percent of state spending. Corrections and Medicaid funding increased dramatically in the 1980s. In 1976 Medicaid accounted for only $0.33 of the $5.96 in total state spending per $100 of personal income; by 1991 Medicaid had more than doubled, accounting for $0.79 of the total spending per $100 in personal income. Similarly, spending for corrections more than doubled during that period. Spending for elementary and secondary education and for health and hospitals remained fairly stable; spending for higher education, welfare, and highways decreased, welfare the most dramatically (Gold 1992).

Both states and the federal government use the income tax as a major source of revenue. For the states, however, it is one of a number of lucrative taxes and is second to the sales tax in revenue generation. Sales taxes (both general taxes and taxes on certain items like gasoline, cigarettes, and liquor) make up nearly one-half of a state's tax revenue; individual income taxes account for nearly one-third. The states also obtain substantial revenues from corporate income taxes, lotteries, motor vehicle and operators' licenses, and gift and estate taxes. Washington relies overwhelmingly on the income tax, which accounts for nearly two-thirds of the total revenue.

Balancing the State Budget

One of the key things to understand about states is that unlike Washington, states cannot operate in deficit. By constitution or statute, the state budget must be balanced at the end of each fiscal year in forty-nine states (only Vermont allows a deficit by law, and it discourages it by custom). Unlike the federal government, states have capital budgets for financing infrastructure projects, such as roads and buildings. States also have many special accounts, often funded with earmarked taxes, which are not subject to limitations and have semiautonomous agencies that can use their own borrowing authority. Most states are prohibited from borrowing money for operating expenses, such as payrolls or benefit checks. While this provision has caused many states difficulty, particularly in times of economic downturn, it has also forced them to make tough choices much earlier than their Washington counterparts and to stay within limited resources in meeting their citizens' needs.

If, midway through a fiscal year, state officials realize that the budget will not be balanced (i.e., spending is exceeding expected revenues), those officials must either cut an existing program or enact a tax. (There are, of course, some stopgap measures, such as delaying the payment to state employees and welfare recipients, but these delays usually raise little money and are often unpopular.) The choice of program cuts or tax increases is not welcome, and legislators prefer to make careful choices in the initial budget to getting into this unwelcome situation.

States can and do enter a new fiscal year with a budget surplus, but politically, officials are generally careful not to carry over too much money, since the media and citizens will demand tax cuts, even if the surpluses can be useful in tiding over the state in future years. To avoid some of the "feast or famine" choices facing them, thirty-three states have established rainy day funds in which a certain small proportion of state revenues is set aside in good economic times to help fund possible shortfalls in tighter economic times.

For many states, unfunded federal mandates, especially such expensive ones as Medicaid, can wreak havoc with their attempts to balance budgets and can force them to make cuts in long-standing state programs in elementary and secondary education, public colleges and universities, welfare, and transportation.

Ironically, this seeming constraint on state spending may be one of the states' strengths compared to Washington. While state choices are often excruciatingly tough, especially in recessions when demands for state programs increase at the same time revenues from sales and income taxes fall, they put states in a good fiscal position when economic conditions improve. For example, unlike the federal government, which, with its $4.4-trillion debt and yearly deficits of more than $255 billion, is limited in its efforts to fund new programs, states entered the 1990s in relatively strong fiscal condition, without debt or deficit repayments, and largely able to launch and adequately fund innovative programs, including efforts to make health care available for all their citizens.

Direct Democracy

Democracy is much more direct in many states, where citizens can initiate, endorse, or recall a law or elected official. In more than one-half of the states, the people play a key role in ratifying or proposing legislation. Twenty-four states offer voters the ability to propose legislation or constitutional

Table 5.3. States with Constitutional and Statutory Initiative Processes

States with Constitutional Initiatives	States with Statutory Initiatives
Arizona	Alaska
Arkansas	Arizona
California	Arkansas
Colorado	California
Florida	Colorado
Illinois	Idaho
Massachusetts*	Illinois
Michigan	Maine*
Missouri	Massachusetts*
Montana	Michigan*
Nebraska	Mississippi
Nevada	Missouri
North Dakota	Montana
Ohio	Nebraska
Oklahoma	Nevada*
Oregon	North Dakota
South Dakota	Ohio*
	Oklahoma
	Oregon
	South Dakota
	Utah*
	Washington*
	Wyoming*

Source: Data from Council of State Governments (1992).
*These states use an indirect method whereby after the signatures are collected, the proposal goes to the legislature. If the legislature fails to act on the measure or rejects it, it goes to the ballot. If the legislature enacts a different proposal, both versions go on the ballot.

amendments through an initiative process (see table 5.3). Twenty-four states use the referendum, whereby citizens can petition for a vote on statutes or ordinances the legislature has passed and, if they so vote, reject them. Fifteen states have a recall provision that allows voters to remove a state elected official from office. Together, the three—initiative, referendum, and recall—are referred to as direct democracy.

Direct democracy forms a type of accountability and responsiveness unmatched in Washington. It allows citizens to organize to support or fight an issue or person. Legislators and governors (and local officials) are aware of the latent power of the initiative, referendum, and recall, and know they are accountable for individual decisions in a way a member of Congress is not. For example, in 1983 two Democratic members of the Michigan Senate were recalled because they voted for a major tax increase (to balance a badly out-of-kilter, recession-affected state budget). Members of Congress might vote for a similar tax increase with the hope that two (or six) years hence voters will have forgotten the transgression or wish to vote for the member for his or her position on other issues.

Initiatives are very popular and are increasingly being used for major environmental and health issues. Toxic chemicals, toxic cleanup, nuclear waste, gun control, AIDS, Medicaid spending for abortions, and right-to-die laws have appeared on the ballot in states across the country. In the 1990s California voters considered (and rejected) initiatives requiring an employer-mandated health insurance system and setting up the nation's first single-payer health system, headed by an elected commissioner of health care.

The possibility of an initiative or referendum affects the kind of law proposed by the legislature. Unlike the Congress, which has no public mechanism for expressing approval or disapproval of individual laws, in states, a legislator might see a long-sought law up for public approval, sometimes brought by a petition-signing effort sponsored by interest groups defeated in the initial legislation. The possibility of such a reassessment, and of bringing up original bills, affects the design, strategy, and politics of state legislation, particularly those in highly salient issue areas.

The Press and the State Legislature

A major difference between most state legislatures and the Congress concerns media coverage. As discussed earlier, members of Congress have become masters at manipulating the media through making clever pronouncements in the thirty-second sound bite and writing press releases and editorials that are often used verbatim in hometown newspapers. News coverage, especially local coverage, is widely available and highly useful to members. Press secretaries are important staffers, often highly influential in both formulating and packaging members' policy positions.

In states the media coverage and press staffing are markedly different. Relatively few reporters cover the state house, and what coverage there is tends to be focused on the governor and a few legislative leaders and to highlight partisan bickering and embarrassing or ridiculous situations. Most state legislators do not have much access to public relations staffs, and even those who do are often unsuccessful in their efforts to make the six o'clock news. In "professional" state legislatures, press functions are often handled by party caucus staffs, although recently three Michigan senators hired their own press secretaries—a movement noted with alarm by some observers.

News directors and city editors often view state politics as dull and unappealing to viewers and readers. There are few exciting "photo opportunities," and the issues are often complex and not easily explained in a sound bite. Further, most state capitals are located in small towns relatively remote from the state's largest media centers. Thus, Albany, Sacramento, Lansing, Tallahassee, and Springfield may seem unimportant to the lives of the media—and the people they serve.

Television coverage of state government is especially poor. A 1985 survey found that twenty-three states had no full-time television bureau in the state capital, and no television bureau had more than one reporter (Brooks and Gassaway 1990). The nation's largest state, California, has no television news bureau (outside of the Sacramento stations) covering the capital.

The simple fact is that state political coverage does not fare well in the stations' periodic "sweeps," which determine advertising rates and assess the popularity of shows and news coverage. As Kurtz (1990, 10) put it, "Television doesn't cover legislatures because people are not interested in state government." But, he suggested, people are not interested in state government because television does not cover it well (10). One exception to the rather abysmal press coverage is that provided by public television. Several public television stations feature legislative coverage regularly, and some have gavel-to-gavel coverage similar to the popular C-Span coverage of the Congress and other events in Washington.

This overall lack of coverage allows state policymaking to take place in a setting without widespread public input and press coverage. The process is more closed, dominated more by those with special interests and concerns than in Washington, not because of a state's intent or differences in state legislative rules or procedures but rather because of the media coverage, or lack thereof.

INTERSTATE DIFFERENCES

The similarities among the states are legion and unmistakable. A transplant from Rhode Island walking into the North Carolina state house would have little difficulty finding her way around or understanding the process, language, and operation of the legislative body. (Only in Nebraska would a visitor be confused: it has the country's only unicameral legislature.) Similarly, governors' offices, executive branch agencies, and lobbies operate roughly in the same manner across the fifty states. However, it would be a mistake to think that state legislatures are identical from Maine to New Mexico. They differ in many ways, among the foremost in what is known as their professionalism.

While every state in the country modernized to some extent in the 1970s, adding staff, increasing time in session, adopting procedures to expedite and streamline the legislative process, increasing salaries, and adding technology linking legislators to one another, to state agencies, and to the public, not every state made the same level of progress. Eight states can be referred to as professional—those with many specialized and personal staffs, with relatively generous levels of compensation, and in session nearly full-time. At the other end of the spectrum are seventeen nonprofessional or citizen legislatures, which have few staffs, low pay, and limited sessions. Twenty-five states are hybrids, having some of the characteristics of each (Kurtz 1989).

Table 5.4 shows the range of professionalization of states, characterized by time in session, legislative salaries, and staffing. The level reflects how closely each state legislature approximates the Congress in the three areas. The measure shown is the mean for each state of the percentage of the congressional standard the state achieves for each of the three measures (time, staffing, and salaries). The table illustrates the enormous diversity of the states in their levels of professionalization. New York, the most professionalized state legislature, has a professionalization level some 66 percent of that of the Congress. At the other extreme, New Hampshire's legislature has a professionalization level less than 5 percent of that of the Congress (Squire 1992). It is interesting that even the largest states have professionalization levels less than two-thirds of that of the Congress. Also noteworthy is the big gap between the top four states (New York, Michigan, California, and Massachusetts) and the fifth state (Pennsylvania, with only around one-third of the professionalization level of Congress). Clearly, state legislatures still retain their nonprofessional nature—at least compared with their national counterparts.

State legislatures also differ substantially in their levels of partisanship. Nebraska is the only state where legislators do not run on a party label. Parties are generally important in identifying members to the electorate and in organizing legislative activities. Hawaii has long been one of the most Democratic legislatures, with only two Republican senators out of twenty-five

Table 5.4. State Levels of Professionalization Compared with the U.S. Congress

>50 Percent That of Congress		30–49 Percent That of Congress		20–29 Percent That of Congress		10–19 Percent That of Congress		<10 Percent That of Congress	
New York	66%	Pennsylvania	34%	Missouri	29%	Delaware	19%	North Dakota	8%
Michigan	65	Ohio	33	Hawaii	28	Louisiana	19	South Dakota	8
California	63	Alaska	31	Wisconsin	27	Nebraska	19	Utah	8
Massachusetts	61	Colorado	30	Florida	26	Oregon	18	Wyoming	6
		Illinois	30	New Jersey	26	South Carolina	18	New Hampshire	4
				Arizona	25	Virginia	17		
				Oklahoma	25	Alabama	16		
				Connecticut	23	Maine	16		
				Iowa	23	Mississippi	16		
				Washington	23	Nevada	16		
				Texas	21	Kansas	15		
				Maryland	20	Rhode Island	15		
				Minnesota	20	Vermont	15		
				North Carolina	20	Indiana	14		
						Tennessee	14		
						Georgia	13		
						West Virginia	13		
						Idaho	12		
						Arkansas	11		
						Montana	11		
						Kentucky	10		
						New Mexico	10		

Source: Data from Squire (1992).

members and seven Republican members in a fifty-one-member house. Louisiana is also a strong Democratic stronghold, with only six of its thirty-nine state senators in the Republican party. At the other extreme, Idaho is highly Republican, with only thirteen Democratic members of the seventy-member house and eight Democrats in the thirty-five-member senate. In other states, parties are more competitive, with party control shifting with some regularity or with party control shared in some way. In New York, for example, there has been split party control for decades. The Republicans have had control over the Senate for more than thirty years and the Democrats the assembly (the lower house) for twenty-two straight years. Until 1995, Michigan, Illinois, and Pennsylvania legislatures had been split between the parties for a number of years.

The 1994 elections saw Republicans win big in state houses across the country. In 1995 Republicans gained control over seven senates and nine houses and swept seats all over the country. In one election, the percentage of total state legislative seats went from 60 percent Democratic, 40 percent Republican to fifty-fifty. The number of states where both chambers were controlled by Republicans went from eight in 1994 to eighteen in 1995. In fourteen states, including Michigan, Illinois, Ohio, and Wisconsin, Republican governors oversaw Republican majorities in both houses.

When no party can claim a majority in a legislative house, innovative measures can ensue. The 1992 legislative elections produced ties in the lower house in Michigan and in the upper houses in Florida and Alaska. Michigan opted for a shared-power scheme, with Democratic and Republican cospeakers who alternated monthly as floor leader. Committees also had cochairs and also alternated, but with the party in control of the floor serving as minority committee chair. Florida chose a system under which one party had control for the first year of the session and the second party, the second year.

A final way state legislatures differ from one another that has a large potential effect on state policymaking is term limits. Twenty states now have term limits on their state legislators. Since these initiatives amended the state constitutions, which outline the qualifications of elected state officials, there are few questions about their legality. More in question is the application of term limits to congressional delegates. In 1994 the Arkansas supreme court and a federal district court in Washington found the limitations on congressional terms unconstitutional, and the U.S. Supreme Court in 1995 agreed with the lower courts.

Although term limits are too recent for their impact to be quantified, we can expect several changes in legislative behavior. For legislators under term limits, usually six to eight years in one house, there is less time for an apprenticeship or learning the job before taking an active role in introducing bills and participating in the give-and-take of lawmaking. While this increased activity might be good, it might also lead to an unwillingness to compromise and a concern for short-term, rather than long-term, issues. The limit on service might also curtail legislative expertise, gained over years in the legislature, and thus increase reliance on expertise outside the legislature, particularly that of interest groups and state agency officials. Finally, term limits might affect the type of person attracted to legislative service and career patterns. One might expect to see legislators serving the maximum in one house, moving to the next house, and then to the congressional elections in a more lockstep pattern than previously experienced. Or some legislators might choose to take several years away from their professional lives to serve only briefly in the legislature and then return to their former lives.

Gubernatorial power too varies across the fifty states. Governors' formal powers—those outlined specifically in state constitutions or statutes—include the length of the term, possibility of serving multiple terms, role in shaping the state's budget, ability to appoint cabinet members, and ability to reorganize state agencies. Some governors have relatively little formal power, limited to two terms with few cabinet appointments and without the power to revamp the state bureaucracy without legislative approval. Other governors can serve many terms, have a large slate of possible appointments, and can make changes in state agencies with minimal legislative interference.

State judiciaries differ in how they are selected. States use three methods of choosing judges and some states use a combination of several (i.e., one process for supreme court justices and another for lower trial judges). State judges are often elected by the citizens, usually on nonpartisan tickets. In a number of states, judges are appointed by the legislature and/or the governor. Nearly one-half of the states have adopted a modified merit approach, called the Missouri Plan, where judges are initially appointed by the governor based on recommendations by a blue ribbon committee and after a short time in service must face the voters in an election.

State executive agencies also differ markedly. Some states have large, professional bureaucracies dominated by civil service rules, and others have fewer, more generalist officials not uniformly hired or protected by merit-based nonpartisan rules. State agencies in some states work closely with the legislature in drafting and producing legislation; agencies in other states might work in a more "arms-length" fashion, meeting only occasionally with legislative staff and others.

Finally, the importance of lobbyists varies from state to state. While every state has seen the number of lobbyists increase in a fashion similar to that which occurred in Washington over the past twenty years, the style of lobbying and the effect of lobbying on the legislative product can vary considerably (Thomas and Hrebenar 1990). In some states interest groups are more influential than political parties in helping recruit and elect candidates as well as shape legislation. Especially in citizen legislatures, lobbyists serve to provide valuable information on both substance and political issues. Rules vary regarding who is considered a lobbyist and to what extent lobbyists must report their activities. In Iowa lobbyists must register which bills they intend to support or oppose. In many states multiclient lobby firms are the norm—a handful of lobbyists serve dozens of corporate and association clients (Rosenthal 1993). Finally, states differ in lobbying styles. In New Jersey lobbying can be confrontational and loud; in Iowa effective lobbying can be accomplished by correspondence (Browne 1985).

The variations in state process and policy are, of course, not random, but depend on large variations in citizens' wealth and education, the states' businesses and industries, and the residents' expectations, ideologies, and views of government. A large body of political science research has considered the role of political and economic factors and measures of "need" on state policy choice and found that all are important but that there are differences across policy areas. The variables that successfully predict why states are generous in welfare or Medicaid payments or eligibility criteria are not necessarily good predictors of what state policies will be enacted in water pollution or education or health professions education. Political variables, particularly, seem to weigh more heavily in some kinds of policy choices than in others (Lambert and McGuire 1990; Mueller 1992; Weissert, Knott, and Stieber 1994).

Also key is the presence of a policy entrepreneur who will sell and continue to push the idea through innumerable hurdles and who has the standing to make things happen. Governors are often very effective policy entrepreneurs who can put issues on the agenda, work with legislative leaders and interest groups to shape the plan, and obtain the public's backing for the plan. Most of the comprehensive state health reforms of 1992–94 were spearheaded by governors who were committed to change and politically astute enough to help engineer reform past innumerable objections (Brown 1993).

The diffusion of state policies has long been of interest to political scientists. Early research indicated that diffusion was largely regional, with states within a region looking to "leader" states for guidance in handling similar problems (Walker 1969). With improved technology and the expansion of sources of information and networking, states now tend to reach more broadly for their ideas, often as likely as not to try out an idea of a state unlike theirs in population, wealth, and ideology. Many state legislative staffs communicate with one another, and organizations like the National Conference of State Legislatures and the National Governors' Association provide opportunities for face-to-face meetings with counterparts across the country to obtain up-to-date information about what other states are doing, including legislative language and technical assessments.

Nevertheless, some states pride themselves on being more innovative than others. One long-time intergovernmental observer, John Shannon, of the Urban Institute, likened states to convoys. No state wants to be too far ahead; similarly, no state wants to be in a vulnerable position in the rear. But some like to be among the first to try new programs. States like Maine, Vermont, Minnesota, and Oregon have often led the way in new approaches to dealing with problems in health, environment, criminal justice, and other areas. On the other hand, states like Virginia feel more comfortable with other states trying out ideas and working out the problems. There are some noteworthy exceptions, however. In 1993 Tennessee, generally comfortable in the middle of the convoy, launched an innovative health care program that was examined and copied by states across the country. But innovative states are often not innovative in all areas. In one study of health professions education, for example, states like Maine, Massachusetts, and New Jersey, often innovative, were not (Weissert, Knott, and Stieber 1994).

Finally, the tendency of states to innovate can be traced to the state's political tradition or culture. In some states the populace feel that government should be proactive, providing "good" to its citizens who are actively involved in the political process. Other states have the opposite view, thinking that government should be avoided, that the political process should be dominated by a few knowledgeable people, and that citizens' roles should be limited.

Elazar (1984) divided states into three political cultures. The traditionalistic culture, where government intervention is not generally desirable and where citizen participation is minimal, is best exemplified by the southern states. The moralistic culture, where government is viewed as a positive instrument to advance the public interest and where citizen participation is encouraged, can be illustrated by Minnesota, Vermont, and Wisconsin. The individualistic culture, where the role of government is primarily to encourage private initiative and where citizen involvement is encouraged only to the extent that it promotes economic concerns, can be found in Illinois, Indiana, and Ohio. States with moralistic cultures are often the most innovative; those with traditionalistic cultures often do not value innovation involving governmental action (Johnson 1976; Sigelman and Smith 1980; Sigelman, Roder, and Sigelman 1981). Some states are a mixture, such as Florida (traditionalistic and individualistic) and California (moralistic and individualistic), making predictions based on political culture difficult. Nevertheless, the political culture provides some explanation for state activities and policy choice.

STATES AND HEALTH

The state role in health goes back long before the New Deal. Social legislation, especially programs protecting the public's health and assisting poor and disabled persons, was initiated in many states in the early years of the century. States and localities were the traditional source of health care for poor people until World War II. States provided the money to build hospitals and adopted scores of public health measures.

State regulation of health providers goes back to before the country was established. The first state law licensing physicians was in 1639 in Virginia. State mental institutions trace their history to the early 1800s in Virginia and Kentucky; in the early 1950s states began to establish departments of mental health. In the 1960s the governmental role in health significantly expanded.

In the 1960s and 1970s the federal government stepped up its spending in many health areas, including mental health, substance abuse, environment, and public health, and states took a back seat in many of these areas. The biggest changes in the national arena were the enactment of Medicare and Medicaid in 1965, actions that "altered the entire nature of public policy decisions" (Piore, Lieberman, and Linnane 1977, 19) and "profoundly changed the parameters for the financing and organization of health services in the nation" (26). Medicare and Medicaid put the federal government in the role of a major purchaser of health care and, as such, a shaper of the way that care is delivered.

A look at governmental spending in health shows the impact of Medicaid on federal and state-local health spending. In 1965, the year Medicaid was enacted but not yet implemented, federal health spending totaled $3.7 billion, a shade less than the state-local total of $4.1 billion. Ten years later, governmental spending for health had risen to $27 billion in Washington and $28 billion in states and localities. Over the next ten years, health spending more than doubled again—to $68 billion in Washington and nearly $70 billion in states and localities.

Medicaid

Medicaid has been called "the PAC-Man of state budgets" (Weissert 1992, 93), taking up larger and larger proportions of state budgets held in check by state-balanced budget restrictions. Table 5.5 shows the increase in Medicaid

Table 5.5. Medicaid Spending, 1970–93

Year	Total	Federal (in Billions of Dollars)	State
1970	$ 5.3	$ 2.9	$ 2.5
1980	26.1	14.5	11.6
1985	41.3	22.8	18.4
1990	75.4	42.7	32.7
1993	117.9	76.1	41.8

Source: Data from Levit et al. (1994).

spending from its inception through 1993. The growth is phenomenal, expanding fivefold between 1970 and 1980 and nearly threefold between 1980 and 1990. The early 1990s saw an explosion in spending—doubling over the first three years of the decade. Medicaid is the largest single item of state health spending, making up 17 percent of total state spending in 1992. In some states the percentages are higher. For example, in 1992 state Medicaid expenditures took up 34 percent of the state budget in New Hampshire, 28 percent in Rhode Island, 24 percent in Tennessee, 23 percent in New York and Louisiana, and 21 percent in Indiana and Missouri (National Association of State Budget Officers 1992). By fiscal year 1993 the mean state spending for Medicaid exceeded state spending for higher education, a traditional state responsibility, by $2 billion (Eckl, Hayes, and Perez 1993).

Under Medicaid, the federal government sets minimum requirements for benefits, eligibility, and reimbursement of health care providers, sets standards for participating providers, and establishes rules that must be followed by states in administering the program. Federal law requires that certain groups are covered and certain services provided to them. However, states can expand those eligible to include persons who are "medically needy." States can also offer a number of additional services from a list of optional services provided in federal law. States have flexibility in determining the reimbursement policies for most providers. Federal rules set forth administrative requirements in such areas as the designation of a state plan, provider certification, timeliness of provider payments, and quality control.

The 28 million recipients of Medicaid are largely children and adults in families with dependent children. However, this group is not the category responsible for the greatest spending. Aged people make up 15 percent of the recipients but use nearly 60 percent of all expenditures. Mentally retarded persons, who make up less than 1 percent of the recipients, accounted for 12 percent of the spending in 1989 (National Center for Health Statistics 1993).

Until recently, eligibility for Medicaid was tied to two welfare programs: Aid to Families with Dependent Children and Supplemental Security Income. To be eligible, persons had to meet the requirements of cash assistance in terms of age, blindness, disability, or membership in a family with dependent children.

In the late 1980s the link between Medicaid and AFDC and SSI was weakened when states were allowed to set income levels for Medicaid eligibility (up to the poverty level) separate from those used to establish AFDC and SSI eligibility. Further, the cutoff for pregnant women and children utilizes a national income standard that means that many recipients in poorer states will qualify for the program. Households with children making 133 percent of the national poverty-line income are now eligible for Medicaid. The Congress in 1984 moved to expand Medicaid coverage to a variety of groups and to all poor children under the age of eighteen. As of 1990 federal law requires Medicaid to cover all pregnant women, infants, and children under the age of six whose family income does not exceed 133 percent of the federal poverty level. By the year 2001, states are expected to phase in coverage of all children between the ages of six and nineteen in families below the national poverty line. However, states were given the option to extend coverage to pregnant women and infants with family income up to 185 percent of poverty, and many have done so. In 1992 nearly one-half of the states (twenty-four) had expanded to the 185 percent of poverty standard (Holahan et al. 1993).

While it is easy to conclude that the increase in Medicaid costs in the early 1990s was a direct result of the expansion of the program, such a conclusion would be misguided. While some 2.5 million children and 1 million pregnant woman were added to Medicaid between 1988 and 1992, this expansion accounted for less than 11 percent of the spending growth in that time.

Other factors affecting the spending were an increased expenditure per enrollee, which accounted for one-third of the total spending growth, medical price inflation, which caused more than one-fourth of the growth, and the expansion of other enrollment groups, such as SSI and AIDS patients. Medicaid pays for an estimated 40 percent of the total spent on the care of persons with AIDS (Holahan et al. 1993). Court decisions challenging the reasonableness of Medicaid payment rates to providers have resulted in an increase of hospital-related spending. The Boren Amendment passed by Congress in the mid-1980s allows hospitals and nursing homes to challenge their Medicaid reimbursements as not "reasonable and adequate." Dozens of cases have been filed on behalf of hospitals and nursing homes. A 1991 Michigan court ordered the state to spend an additional $70 million, and an Indiana court required that state to spend an additional $120 million on nursing homes. Oregon settled out of court, agreeing to provide an increase in reimbursement to nursing homes amounting to $65 million over two years.

A final factor is the tendency of states to use Medicaid to provide funding for programs formerly provided by states. By shifting such recipients to Medicaid, the state can save money by having Washington pay around one-half of the costs, a process known as Medicaid maximization (Holahan et al. 1993, 188), which is so commonplace that it has become a verb, "to Medicaid" programs, meaning to use Medicaid to support ongoing state activities (Fossett 1993).

Another strategy commonly used by states was innovative financing techniques, such as imposing provider taxes or seeking provider "contributions" in exchange for rate increases. Under such a scheme, hospitals are repaid for their contributions, and the federal government pays their portion of the bill. The states' costs are offset by the provider contributions, and they can use that money to support other Medicaid spending or spending for other programs. The Congress curtailed the scheme in 1992, but states can use broad-based health care–related taxes, which meet specified federal requirements, and in 1993 thirty-five states supplemented general revenue expenditures for Medicaid with provider taxes (Eckl, Hayes, and Perez 1993).

Despite these seemingly successful examples of game playing, state officials have complained vociferously about the increasing burdens of Medicaid on their states and the congressional proclivity to add more mandates to the program. One reason for the states' sensitivity is that the effect of Medicaid increases on state budgets is direct. When the costs of Medicaid escalate, states must cut the program, increase taxes to pay for it, or take money from other programs to pay for the Medicaid increases. Between fiscal year 1993 and 1994, state spending for Medicaid went up an average of 12 percent, compared with overall state spending of 5 percent (Eckl, Hayes, and Perez 1993).

During the 1970s states adopted a number of innovations and administrative improvements in the Medicaid program, such as prior authorization, Medicaid Management Information Systems, provider profiles, and computerized billing. A number of states established successful programs to control hospital costs, including rate setting based on prospective payment. The Arizona Health Care Cost Containment System (AHCCCS) set up a statewide managed-care network, using the bidding process to select providers. For the first few years, AHCCCS delivered only acute care; in the early 1990s it expanded the program to cover long-term care, home health care, and mental health care. States also began using managed care in the Medicaid program in the 1980s and 1990s to curb costs.

Medicaid, while important, is not the only health program in states or the only area in which innovations have occurred. In the 1980s, with more concern for federal-spending patterns and efforts to reduce federal grants and other programmatic funding, states began to assume leadership in public health, mental health, substance abuse, environment, and health services delivery mechanisms and to offer innovative approaches to providing services yet controlling costs.

State Innovations

State innovations in health and other key areas are very useful in that they can serve as test cases, working out problems and highlighting consequences before national imposition. The use of the states as "laboratories of democracies" has a long history in this country. The 1921 Sheppard-Towner Act, providing social and medical assistance to pregnant women and babies, was copied from a Connecticut law. States provided models for the 1935 Social Security Act, the 1973 Supplemental Security Income programs, and dozens of health measures (Silver 1991). More recently, Medicare's payment system based on diagnosis-related groups was modeled on a program in New Jersey. In fact, New York Governor Nelson Rockefeller once noted that "those elements of the New Deal which failed, were largely in areas *not* tested by prior experience at the state level" (Silver 1991, 445).

In recent years states have launched innovative programs to establish universal coverage, to reform small-group health insurance and establish risk pools for those for whom insurance is difficult to obtain, to mandate community rating, to develop new ways of delivering services to Medicaid recipients and state employees, and more (see table 5.6).

Universal Coverage

As Washington was considering ways to ensure universal coverage of health care to all Americans in 1993 and 1994, state after state was acting. Several—Hawaii, Washington, Minnesota, Oregon, and Florida—adopted wide-reaching programs designed to provide health care to all state residents within the next decade.

Table 5.6. Innovative State Health Policies, 1965–95

Date	Action
1965	New York adopts certificate of need
1974	Hawaii passes state-mandated, employer-sponsored insurance
	Rhode Island enacts catastrophic health insurance plan
1975	Indiana enacts comprehensive medical malpractice act
	Connecticut establishes risk pool for the uninsured
1976	Maryland establishes an all-payer system for hospitals
1977	New Mexico adopts right-to-die act
	New York adopts nursing home without walls program
1978	New Jersey extends rate setting to all payers and hospitals
1981	Oregon receives Medicaid home- and community-based care waiver
1982	California enables PPOs to do business in the state
	Arizona launches capitated program for Medicaid
	New York develops uncompensated care pool for sharing hospital revenues
1983	Virginia adopts a natural death law
	Oregon contracts with providers on prepaid capitation basis for Medicaid patients
1984	Florida taxes hospitals to supplement state match for Medicaid expansion
	New Jersey reimburses hospitals using DRGs
	New York enacts mandatory seat-belt use law
	Washington makes basic health services available for low-income residents in five areas of state
1988	Massachusetts passes first pay-or-play employer mandate
	Kansas enacts broad employee wellness program
1989	Oregon enacts legislation establishing rationing system
	Rhode Island passes "bare bones" insurance plans for small businesses
	Arizona launches capitated long-term care program for elderly
1990	Maine introduces practice guidelines to reduce medical liability
	Maine introduces RBRVS into Medicaid
	Connecticut enacts small-group insurance market reform
1991	Connecticut receives clearance for state-endorsed, long-term care insurance
	New York phases in requirement that 50 percent of Medicaid (AFDC) recipients be in managed care
1992	Minnesota attempts universal coverage through integrated service networks
	Vermont requires community-rated health insurance.

Table 5.6. *(cont.)*

1993	Washington and Florida adopt managed competition programs
	Tennessee expands Medicaid program to cover categorically ineligible people above poverty
	Missouri passes medical savings account law
1994	Mississippi and Florida sue to recover state dollars spent on tobacco-related illness
	Oregon voters adopt assisted-suicide measure
	Kentucky establishes a statewide alliance based on public employees
	California and Maryland adopt bans on smoking in any enclosed space that is also a place of employment
1995	Maryland passes antidumping law for nursing home residents

Source: Data from *State Health Notes*, 1980–95, Intergovernmental Health Policy Project and interviews with IHPP staff.

Hawaii's universal health plan is the oldest, enacted in 1974. The state has the country's only operating program of state-mandated, employer-sponsored health insurance, which covers most of the employed workers (but not their dependents). In 1990 the state established a new program to provide coverage for dependents and part-time employees working less than twenty hours a week. In 1993 it launched a third effort, HealthQuest, a mandatory Medicaid managed-care system for those up to 300 percent of the federal poverty level with sliding premiums. An estimated 98 percent of Hawaii's citizens are covered by health insurance (Lewin 1992).

Three states acting in 1992 and 1993 established managed-competition systems; one with mandatory participation, two relying on volunteerism. The state of Washington's plan, adopted in 1993, set up a mandatory employer mandate. But employers do have a choice: they can run their own certified health plan (if larger than 7,000 employees), contract directly with certified health plans, directly purchase basic health plan coverage at full cost, or join one of four health insurance purchasing cooperatives. The state has also expanded its basic health plan, which provides health care to individuals at or below 200 percent of the federal poverty level, to provide universal access by 1998. In 1995 the state repealed several key elements of the 1993 reforms including employer mandates, the comprehensive uniform benefits package, and insurance premium caps. The 1995 law did expand the popular basic health plan.

Minnesota's new system, put in place by laws in 1992 and 1993, established a system of integrated service networks (ISNs) that are responsible for arranging or delivering a full array of services to a defined population for a fixed price. Employers choosing not to enroll in a network were covered by an all-payer system and must abide by price ceilings. In 1995 the legislature repealed the all-payer system, modified the definition of universal coverage, and established requirements for the ISNs. It did authorize implementation of a federal waiver covering acute and long-term care and continued MinnesotaCare, the subsidized insurance program for uninsured Minnesotans.

Florida's 1992 law established eleven community-health purchasing alliances available to small employers, state employees, and Medicaid recipients. If all residents of the state do not have access to an affordable basic benefit package by a given date, a state-run program will go into effect. Florida also expanded health coverage for persons with income below 250 percent of the federal poverty level. In 1995 the political tides turned in Florida as the legislature refused to implement a federal waiver that allowed it to add more than 1 million adults and children to its Medicaid program and turned down the governor's proposal to subsidize private health insurance for the working poor.

Oregon's reforms in 1987 and 1989 sought to achieve universal access by broadening Medicaid coverage and putting in place a "pay or play" component. The first part of the plan got national attention as the "rationing" scheme, whereby the state established a priority list of services that would be available to Medicaid beneficiaries. Thanks in part to federal insistence, the state was able to eliminate or "ration" only a few marginal medical services, saving little money. The second part of the plan was delayed until 1998 due to resistance by small business owners. In 1994 the state struggled to find the money to pay for essentially the same Medicaid services for an expanded number of recipients, and the employer mandate was delayed indefinitely. The Oregon case is noteworthy because it was the first government to raise questions about the efficacy of treatment and to attempt to answer tough questions of how to best allocate health dollars. It is also illustrative of how difficult comprehensive reform at a state level can be.

Massachusetts is a good example of where one road to universal access—employer mandate—did not work. In 1988 the state became the first to enact a "pay or play" scheme, whereby employers must provide specified health coverage for their employees or pay the consequences. In Massachusetts the "pay" constituted a 12 percent surtax on firms failing to provide employees with insurance. Signed with fanfare by a popular governor then running for president, Michael Dukakis, it was delayed two years later in an effort spearheaded by a new governor who felt the program was bad for the state's ailing economy.

In 1995 the state repealed its employer mandate and launched a new effort providing tax credits for employers and subsidies for low-income workers. Several states have taken a more incremental approach to universal coverage through expanding coverage for near-poor people or providing a type of Medicaid buy-in. Connecticut, Florida, Maine, Minnesota, New York, and Vermont initiated health care coverage for children. Washington and Maine expanded Medicaid coverage to some low-income people (U.S. GAO 1992, 87).

One of the most daring and controversial reforms of 1993 was the establishment of TennCare, Tennessee's dramatic expansion of Medicaid to all uninsured residents of the state. To cover the additional residents without additional cost to the state, TennCare relies on an extensive managed-care system and closely monitors the costs. The state makes a flat per-patient payment, or capitation rate, to the twelve managed-care organizations, which then negotiate rates with physicians, hospitals, and other providers. The program is available to those with incomes between 100 and 199 percent of poverty, with copayments and premiums based on a sliding fee scale. No deductibles or copayments are required for preventive services. To ensure good-quality care, physicians who provide care for state and local employees through Blue Cross/Blue Shield must also serve TennCare patients. The policy, called cram down, is the source of many complaints from the state's physicians, who call it blackmail, extortion, or worse (Demkovich 1994, 2).

The implementation of TennCare was difficult. The Medicaid waiver from Washington allowing the state to go forward was approved only six weeks before the start-up date. In addition, the demand was enormous. In the first three months, applications for coverage were eight times the number planners had anticipated (Demkovich 1994). Physicians in the state were angry that they were not consulted, and many boycotted the program in the early weeks. Specialists are especially unhappy with low rates, estimated from 30 to 60 percent less than Medicaid rates, and some refused referrals from TennCare primary care providers. The Tennessee Medical Association took the state to court, claiming that the state's failure to develop the capitation rate in public violated the state's administrative procedures act.

The TennCare proposal is also noteworthy for its genesis. It was put in place by the governor's executive order. Only minor changes, encompassing only a page and a half in legislative language, were put into law. While it dramatically increases access to health care in the state, covering 25 percent of the state's population, it began as an effort to control Medicaid costs, which in 1993 accounted for more than 26 percent of the state's budget. The choices, said the governor, were to raise taxes, slash medical benefits for poor people, or try something new. He proposed the last (Lemov 1994).

Reforming Small-Group Insurance

States have the primary responsibility for regulating the insurance industry. Unlike automobile, life, and other insurance issued in the state, state regulators are limited in their authority over health insurance by a federal law, the Employee Retirement Income Security Act of 1974, which excludes from state regulation the health insurance provided by firms that have elected to self-insure their health plans. Only around one-fourth (24 percent) of health care is paid for by private health insurance regulated by state insurance departments (U.S. GAO 1994, 2). Nevertheless, small businesses, those most likely not to provide insurance coverage for their employees, do operate under state regulation.

In the 1990s states were active to protect citizens from unreasonable or expensive insurance provisions. Some forty-three states adopted one or more regulatory insurance reforms that affect small insurers, such as placing restrictions on rules regarding preexisting conditions and waiting periods, prohibitions against cancellation due to medical history, guarantee of continuation of coverage when employees change employers or employers change insurers, and restrictions on rate increases. More than one-half of the states established high-risk pools for individuals who are denied coverage and small-employer pools in which small businesses band together to purchase health insurance (U.S. GAO 1992). New York and Vermont enacted community rating laws allowing few or no adjustments based on demographic factors.

New Service Delivery Systems

In the early 1980s California replaced its fee-for-service system with one relying on negotiation, and Arizona set up a system for competitively bid fixed-price arrangements for Medicaid. Four states—Maryland, New York, Massachusetts, and New Jersey—adopted all-payer hospital reimbursement systems under which the cost of uncompensated care is distributed proportionally across all payers. An all-payer system determines each hospital's rates by the types and volume of services it provides to patients. The system requires that all payers, both public and private, pay nearly identical rates for services. Maryland, the state with the most successful experience in holding down costs using an all-payer system, recently expanded its system to include physicians' payments.

Beginning in the 1980s states began to utilize managed care in Medicaid.

Under this system, states set a predetermined fee for a health facility, often a health maintenance organization, to provide care for each patient. Other managed-care programs include prepaid health plans, preferred provider arrangements, and selective contracts. More than thirty states had experimented with managed care in the Medicaid program by 1992.

A number of states have also considered a single-payer system. Vermont and Montana asked commissions to design a single-payer model that could be implemented by subsequent legislatures. Vermont later decided that the single-payer system and the $750 million in new income and payroll taxes that would be involved was simply not possible. Montana considered a single-payer system, along with a plan relying on competition among private health care providers in 1995. New York launched a single-payer demonstration project establishing a single payer for hospitals (U.S. GAO 1992, 73).

Other Issues

While garnering most of the attention, efforts to provide universal coverage and respond to insurance deficiencies were not the entirety of states' scope of health care reforms in the 1990s.

States have purchased private health insurance for those with AIDS, prohibited discriminatory practices and protected confidentiality in testing, organized special facilities to provide targeted care, and provided their own funding for the treatment of the disease.

States have directed state medical schools to change their curricula, admissions policies, and faculty priorities to produce more primary-care physicians. They have also directed additional money to family practice programs, nurse practice programs, scholarships, and loan-forgiveness programs for providers willing to serve in underserved areas, and have provided tax and other incentives for young primary-care providers to work in rural and inner-city areas in the state. New York has an innovative approach to encouraging more primary-care physicians by weighting graduate medical education dollars toward primary-care training programs.

Long-term care, an area where federal policy has floundered, has been the focus of several state efforts. States have led the way in providing home- and community-based care programs in an effort to provide more choices for needy elderly persons. The state of Washington has authorized demonstration projects of social HMOs to bring a full range of health and social services for elderly people under one organization. Connecticut funded a program to encourage the purchase of long-term care insurance.

Table 5.7. State Health Agencies' Programmatic Responsibilities

Responsibility	Number of State Agencies*
Public health	51
Institutional licensing	41
Children with special health care needs	39
Health planning and development	22
Institutions/hospitals	16
Environment (lead agency)	15
Professional licensing	10
Medicaid (single state agency)	5
Mental health	4

Source: Data compiled from Centers for Disease Control (1991).
*Includes the District of Columbia.

A number of states have limited malpractice awards, setting caps on punitive damages. Other states have required plaintiffs to obtain a certificate from a medical expert that the suit has merit, as a way of reducing the likelihood of frivolous cases and reducing costs. Maine's innovative approach to malpractice reform was to provide physicians who follow specified practice guidelines protection in malpractice suits.

State public health efforts include drives to ensure that children have proper immunizations, assessments of community health status, efforts to reduce violence and abuse, and smoking cessation. As part of its reform effort, Washington State set aside $20 million for public health and the development of a public health plan. Michigan set aside money from its new cigarette tax for a new public health initiative. Maryland's Partners in Prevention Program delivers preventive health care services to residents of medically underserved communities.

A number of states have adopted workers' compensation reforms. Washington and Oregon have consolidated their workers' compensation programs with the state's system of managed competition (Washington) or group health insurance (Oregon). Massachusetts law provides for innovative labor-management carve-outs or agreements outside the workers' compensation system. Other states, including California, have enacted measures to curb abuse and reduce the costs of the program.

Thus, in the late 1980s and early 1990s every state did something to reform health care, from restructuring malpractice to ensuring fairer treatment by insurers, from setting up a new system of regional health care providers to attempting to make tough choices about what services should reasonably be provided. In 1995 a number of states pulled back from some of their comprehensive reforms, particularly provisions guaranteeing universal access, setting global budgets, and mandating employers to provide insurance coverage. However, it is noteworthy that a few states, such as Kentucky, launched new health reforms in 1995 and even those states serving as early health reform leaders, such as Florida, Washington, and Minnesota, which did retreat somewhat from broad, comprehensive reforms, continued, even expanded, their efforts to provide health care to the working poor.

State Health Agencies

Every state has at least one agency that oversees health programs, but the scope and purpose of the agencies vary, and many states have health responsibilities shared by many. A typical state health agency is responsible for quality control, including licensure and regulation of standards of practice for health care professionals, licensure and certification for Medicare and Medicaid reimbursement of hospitals, nursing homes, and other providers, monitoring laboratories, health-related services, and environmental and sanitation conditions. It collects and analyzes data, evaluates and assesses health services, conducts health-planning activities, coordinates with other agencies and providers, issues vital records, and sometimes provides services in underserved areas and regions. It often administers the Medicaid program (but many times does not). In most states, other health services are administered by different agencies. These include professional licensure and regulation (often independent boards), health insurance regulation (insurance commissions or departments), mental disability programs (mental health and mental retardation departments), health personnel education (higher education), health facilities construction (direct appropriations and independent financing authorities), and cost-control activities (sometimes in independent commissions). Table 5.7 lists the responsibilities of the fifty-one state health agencies (including the District of Columbia).

The fifty state health departments work closely with more than 3,000 local health departments charged with assessing the public health needs of their communities, developing policies to meet those needs, and ensuring that primary and preventive care is available to all residents who need it. In recent years local health departments have moved more and more toward providing care to medically underserved persons. In a 1990 survey 92 percent of all health departments reported that they provide immunizations, 84 percent provide other health services, and nearly 60 percent provide prenatal care (National Association of County Health Officials 1990).

Constraints on State Innovation

While the innovations and reforms are impressive, there might be more but for two important constraints: the ERISA and federal Medicaid and Medicare laws.

ERISA preempts state regulation of health insurance provided by large companies that self-insure or provide health insurance for their workers instead of buying coverage. State law cannot require these employers to cover certain procedures, insure high-risk groups, or adopt measures to reduce health care plans. Most important, states cannot impose taxes on self-insured companies to finance care for uninsured people in the state. Virtually every comprehensive health care reform law runs afoul of ERISA. In 1974 when the law was passed, a small number of health plans were self-insured; today it is between 50 and 60 percent and even higher in some states (Polzer 1992).

The courts have generally strictly construed the language of the federal law to stymie state efforts at including self-insured companies in health care reform. For example, a 1992 New Jersey court found that state's surcharge on hospital bills to fund an uncompensated care trust fund a violation of ERISA and struck it down. (A later court overturned the decision, but the state had already changed its financing scheme.) A 1994 court decision in Connecticut knocked down a tax on Connecticut hospitals to finance uncompensated care. A 1994 New York court held that New York's assessment of hospital surcharges violated ERISA. However, a federal district judge in Minnesota in 1994 upheld that state's 2 percent tax on doctors and hospitals which subsidizes the Minnesota program. In a 1994 New York court case, commercial insurers and HMOs challenged that the state's community rating pools violated ERISA because the costs of employer benefit plans are divided up by the pooling arrangement.

In a move surprising to many, in 1995 the U.S. Supreme Court ruled that New York's surcharges levied on hospital bills did not violate federal ERISA laws. The case reopened the possibility for states of imposing hospital taxes or surcharges on providers to fund care for the poor. Indeed, within a month of the decision, Connecticut's governor asked the state legislature to reinstate a hospital tax the state had abandoned after two lower court decisions declared the surcharge illegal. Other elements of potential ERISA preemption including employer and individual mandates and single-payer plans were not dealt with in the New York case.

The court role in ERISA is important because changes in the legislation have been stalled for decades by business and labor interests that prefer uniformity in health insurance across the states. A Coalition for the Preservation of the ERISA Preemption, consisting of more than 100 self-insured employers and trade groups, was formed to prevent any change in the law (Chirba-Martin and Brennan 1994). Indeed, when two states that passed employer mandate laws in 1993 (Washington and Florida) sought ERISA exemptions from Congress, they were unsuccessful. The only state with an employer mandate in operation, Hawaii, was exempted from ERISA by congressional law. New York received a two-year exemption in 1993 through a provision in the budget bill sponsored by its senator and chair of the Senate Finance Committee, Daniel Patrick Moynihan. The New York provision says that if a self-insured company does not abide by New York's rate-setting system, the company has to forgo all tax deductions in its health insurance plans (Wagar 1994).

Medicaid and Medicare waivers are easier to get than ERISA waivers (they can be obtained through an administrative decision of the HHS secretary). In 1994 the Clinton administration announced a policy of expedited attention to the waivers as a way of encouraging state reform. By mid-1995, more than one-half the states were developing, had submitted, or had received HCFA approval for waivers under Section 1115 of the Social Security Act, which allowed them to modify their Medicaid programs as statewide demonstrations. States used the waivers to make changes in the eligibility, benefit, and service delivery components of their programs. A number of states expanded those eligible to include the working poor and the unemployed and required beneficiaries to select a managed care plan. In 1995 several states obtained waivers to integrate acute and long-term care for elderly eligible for Medicaid and Medicare and to include the SSI disabled population in managed care.

CONCLUSION

Few would question the role of state governments as key actors in health care in this country. They serve as the providers, financiers, administrators, initiators, and regulators of health care delivery. Their reach cuts across traditional health providers, insurers, businesses, educational institutions, and, of course, citizens. State governments are capable of adequately performing all their roles and representing all the groups and citizens they serve. They are the innovators and creators of many of the most promising ideas considered today in Washington and elsewhere. They are probably the most pivotal governmental actor in health care because they implement and help define federal policies, define and implement their own policies, and define and oversee local health-related activities as well.

Nathan (1989) argued that there is a cyclicality in the role of state governments, based on the political ideology of the nation's citizens. In conservative periods, when there is a skepticism and pulling back from an activist federal government, the states' role is enhanced relative to the federal government. Interest groups turn more willingly to states for assistance and innovation flourishes. In more liberal periods of national mood, the activism tends to be focused on Washington, with increased intensity in federal laws and regulations. Nathan argued that in the early years of the twentieth century, states were the source of progressive policies, such as unemployment insurance, public assistance, and workers' compensation. Indeed, before World War I, there was intense interest in many states in adopting a compulsory health insurance program funded by employers, employees, and the public. At least sixteen states introduced health insurance bills based on a model bill prepared by the American Association for Labor Legislation, a group that had led the successful drive for workers' compensation (Anderson 1990). In the 1930s through the 1960s, the states provided key health services but were generally not leaders in innovation or responsiveness to the public.

The 1970s and 1980s witnessed a spurt of innovation and activity in the states and a pulling back in Washington from pushing a progressive health agenda. In health care, innovations in financing health care, designing new forms of health care delivery, and developing systems so that citizens could make the tough "rationing" choices were developed at the state level, and in 1992 and 1993 the states put into place the ideas of managed competition, global budgets, and major insurance reforms. With the popularity of neo-Reaganism in 1995 and the failure of any national health reform package, the focus again turned to the states in the second part of the 1990s. Both Nathan's model and the practicalities of failed federal action seemed to presage state leadership in health reform.

Part II

Health and the Policy Process

6

Health Care Policy and
Problem Definition

Two ELDERLY WOMEN are admitted to a large Chicago hospital. Both worry about their illness, and though they know that with Medicare they should not have to worry about the costs of their care, they do. Both will have to pay for the first day of their stay. Medicare policy requires a deductible. One of the two women is more worried than the other, because her doctor has said that Medicare may refuse to pay for her hospital stay since she was readmitted so soon after her last stay for the same disease. But the other is worried, too. Even though she bought a private "Medigap" insurance policy to pay her deductible and some other charges, she knows that some charges will not be covered by it either and that if she needs a nursing home after her hospital stay, Medicare and her Medigap policy may pay for little or none of it. It could be worse: her son is out of work, under age sixty-five, and has no insurance at all. If he were in the hospital, worry about the cost would be enough to drive him crazy. Indeed, with no one to pay, he would be lucky to get into a hospital at all.

This is health care policy: what services get paid for, the share the individual pays, what types of health care are covered, who is and is not eligible to receive subsidized care, who can render it and get paid for rendering it, what procedures will be paid for, what government does and does not do when a private party needs care but does not have the money to pay for it, who gets financial help with medical care training, what nurses can and cannot do for patients, the width of doorways on the hospital's bathrooms, and much, much more.

THE EVOLUTION OF PUBLIC POLICY

The Ambiguity and Consequences of Public Policy

It would be naive to think that the purpose of health care or other public policy is always obvious. Policy is formed by compromise. Things are left deliberately vague so that many people with different perspectives can see their views represented in the same ambiguity. For this reason (and also because of incompetence, uncertainty, time pressures, and bad writing), even though policy always has a purpose, it may not always be easy to figure out. Program evaluators find this out early in health care and every other type of program. Asked to evaluate programs against their goals, more often than not, the evaluators discover the program does not seem to have any goals. Sometimes it has too many goals and they often conflict. That a program has been running for several months or years on some vaguely worded rationale may be disturbing to evaluators, but it rarely seems to get in the way of the actors. So the evaluator quickly learns that goals must often be translated from something implicit in the actions taken by the actors. Wilson (1989) made a similar argument regarding the implementation of public policy by bureaucracies (discussed in Chapter 4).

At other times, ambiguity can be quite troubling. Smits, Feder, and Scanlon (1982) showed that Medicare policy toward skilled nursing home coverage after a hospital stay was actually no single policy at all but rather a wide range of policies varying from one part of the country to another. Vaguely worded regulations specifying the conditions under which a Medicare patient's posthospital stay would be covered led to widely differing interpretations by the private employees working for the Medicare fiscal intermediaries (the government-contracted insurance companies that enforce governmental payment rules) contracted to interpret the law and decide which nursing home claims to pay. Smits, Feder, and Scanlon described nine hypothetical cases to each fiscal intermediary. Each interpreted the rules differently, disagreeing widely on whether cases were covered or not. Even when the intermediaries agreed on coverage, they often gave different reasons for their decisions.

Policy action in health care and other fields often differs, sometimes painfully, from intention. Health care policymakers intended to improve the quality of nursing home care for publicly subsidized patients when they wrote new standards for participation in the Medicaid program in the 1960s and 1970s. While that purpose was accomplished for many patients, for others—low-income, privately paying patients living in facilities too poor to meet the new standards—life was probably made worse when facilities dropped out of Medicaid because they could not afford to comply with the new standards.

Similar dilemmas face those who would upgrade fire and sanitation standards for poor inner-city apartment buildings and hotels (flop houses). Tenants too poor to pay higher rent for the improvements move to settings worse than they inhabited before the government decided to help them. Indeed, in health care policy, much of the problem is trying to resolve the inherent tension between reform efforts aimed at improved quality and their unintended consequences for access to care by poor people or between cost-containment strategies and reduced quality or access.

Public versus Private Health Care Policy

Health care policies are not unique to government. Hospitals have their own private policies; for example, medical records may not be removed from the medical records room without special authorization, or infants under five pounds at birth must be kept in the hospital till they gain weight, or this hospital will not operate a drug detoxification center. These private policies share many characteristics with public policies. They differ in that they do not usually have an explicit public purpose, and they are not compelled by public authority. People do not go to jail for violating a corporate policy (but they may be fired). The real difference, however, is that governmental policies are made by government and, as such, are the product of the political process (see box 6.1).

Policies evolve. Ask any nursing home operator what Medicaid's specific policy is on the quality of care in general or on the prevention and care of decubitus ulcers and the maintenance of skin condition. The answer you get will take a long time. By the end, the operator will probably have worked himself or herself into a bit of a pique. The last thing said is likely to be "You tell me," or "Do you mean this week or next?"

Box 6.1 Defining Public Policy

Public policy has been defined as "what government does." But Anderson (1994) and others ask who is government? (a member of Congress? the president? the chair of the Physician Payment Review Commission?) And what does *does* mean? (a law? a proposal? a speech? a proposed regulation? a ruling? a conference report recommendation? writing a Medicare check to pay a hospital?) Simon (1960) called check writing and similar activities "programmed" decisions because they are repetitive, routine, and based on standard operating procedure. He said that policy involves discretion, making choices that are novel, unstructured, and consequential.

Dye (1984, 1) said that public policy is "whatever government chooses to do or not to do." That captures the kind of power lobbyists are best at: keeping unwanted proposals from being adopted or even debated. But not addressed is the difference between nominal policy and actual policy. Medicaid law requires "statewideness" (no urban-rural differences in access to Medicaid-subsidized services). But who would argue that there are no differences? Nonetheless, the law gives rural dwellers a legitimate claim that efforts be made on their behalf to try to mitigate those differences. Sometimes nominal policy is the goal, while actual policy is the route being followed toward that goal.

Policy is not written in stone. It is dynamic, a potpourri of laws (often vague), regulations (often late, ambiguous, changing), government officials' interpretations (often conflicting, sometimes wrong), court decisions (sometimes bizarre), and, in the final analysis, the level of compliance of providers, fiscal intermediaries, and patients themselves, who sometimes find ways to systematically alter policy by, for example, giving away their assets instead of spending them for care in lieu of public subsidy. Policies evolve and change because they reflect the negotiated preferences of many parties over differing periods of time. They change because the world changes, and the policies must reflect the private sector and the everyday activities of consumers. They change and evolve because they must to be effective and reflect changing demands.

In health care, as in every other field, policies come from demands for action or for deliberate inaction. Poor people want access to care. Physicians want a new procedure paid for by Medicare (the federal health financing program for elderly people). Hospitals want a place to send patients who cannot find a Medicaid nursing home bed or relief from antitrust enforcement, which makes it risky to talk about mergers with other providers. Federal agencies want to constrain Medicare spending, and state agencies want to allow provider "contributions" to count in their Medicaid match. Nursing homes want federal quality-of-care surveyors to come less often; Citizens for Better Care, a patients' advocacy group, wants them to come more often. Claims may be specific or general, demand that something be done or that something very specific be done. The demand may inspire new health care policy or give existing policy content, direction, or interpretation. The form of the policy may be a law, a change in an existing law, a regulation, a court decision, or a supervisor's memo interpreting policy to the field staff.

Whatever the genesis, the demand is important to the success of any public policy. Who participates, what resources that person or group possesses, and how that group translated its resources into influence are all important elements of policy development (Hayes 1992). In addition to the important role of interest groups (see Chapter 3), informal groups of experts in academia, think tanks, and agencies can also play an important role in helping policymakers understand issues and come up with reasonable solutions. These actors—part of what Kingdon (1984) calls the policy community—constitute their own attentive public that can actively aid the progress of an idea. When this community is integrated and in agreement on the nature of the problem and its optimal solution, it can play an important role in policy development. If it is fragmented or multiple groups claim policy community standing, its influence is diminished, and the likelihood of successful comprehensive policies is lessened.

The Public and Public Policy

An important distinction in public policy is that it reflects the public's concerns. Members of Congress and the president (and their counterparts in the fifty states) do not make policy in a vacuum. They listen to their constituents, interest groups, colleagues, and (increasingly) rely on polls and focus groups for policy guidance in answering such questions as: Is there really a health care crisis? Are health care costs too high? Are there too many medical specialists? Experts can help answer these questions, but expert advice alone is not the key to policy initiation. The public must perceive a crisis—and for a while in 1993, it did.

The pattern of public support for health reform closely follows what Downs (1972) calls the issue attention cycle, in which the public becomes interested in an issue (or problem) and, for a while, their attention grows as the issue gains salience, is covered by the media, and is the focus of congressional hearings and presidential speeches. At some point, however, it becomes clear that the problem is not to be easily solved, that it will likely involve great expense, and that some groups will be hurt by proposed solutions. By that time, the public may begin to lose interest, and policymakers lose support for making tough decisions to solve the problem. The public may then go on to be concerned over another issue, and the Congress moves on as well. The 1993–94 debate on national health care reform seemed to fit the pattern. In the spring of 1994, health was the top concern of the public; a few months later, it had been replaced by crime.

While Downs's model is pessimistic about the possibility of major reforms, others believe that actions can be taken within the cycle that will perpetuate the interest and promote long-term reform. Baumgartner and Jones (1993) argue that "even [a] short-lived spurt of (public) interest may leave an institutional legacy" (87), such as an office, group, or staff committed to the issue.

Getting on the public agenda is not necessarily easy, however. There is enormous competition for space on the crowded public agenda, requiring the work of an army of public relations specialists and a concerted effort by leaders to make the rounds of the Sunday and morning news shows. Events, consequently, may play a less important role than ideas (Peters and Hogwood 1985).

The public is very susceptible to symbolism, and politicians are often successful at manipulating value-laden issues like patriotism or universal coverage to seek public support. When President Clinton promoted national health reform as "health security" for everybody, assuring portability from job to job and coverage of existing conditions rather than focusing on the problem of the uninsured, he was trying to "widen the scope of conflict" in Schattschneider's (1960) term. He wanted to make average Americans feel they had something to lose if health care policy did not undergo reform. The public likes symbols that oversimplify and often find comfort in their use (Edelman 1964).

The public (and policymakers) also tend to choose problems for consideration that can be solved. As Wildavsky (1979, 42) put it, "a difficulty is a problem only if something can be done about it." Problems that tend to defy solution, according to Downs, are those for which:

—a numerical minority (not necessarily ethnic) is suffering the problem;
—suffering is caused by social arrangements providing benefits to the majority or a powerful minority of the population;
—the problem has no exciting qualities (or is no longer seen as exciting).

Consumed as entertainment, the news must stay lively to keep its viewers. If the problem is of national scope and objectively a major concern, it may sporadically recapture interest or attach itself to another problem dominating center stage. When it does so, it will usually receive a higher level of attention, effort, and concern than problems still in the prediscovery stage. As Schon (1971, 42) put it, "old questions are not answered—they only go out of fashion."

Categories of Public Policy

Policies can be categorized in a variety of ways. They can be grouped by issue (say, health work force) or target audiences (medical students). They change over time and so may also be categorized as post–World War II policy, or Clinton-era policy, or current policy. Some policies emanate from the state, others from the federal government, others from the 82,000-plus local jurisdictions making policy on everything from AIDS screening to water quality.

Policies also vary between substantive and procedural. Substantive policies do things like improve health care, protect the environment, or regulate employment practices. Procedural policies are concerned with how the government is doing it. The Administrative Procedures Act of 1946 is the quintessence of a procedural policy or set of procedural policies. It requires that governmental regulatory and administrative actions be taken only after notice of proposed rule making, an opportunity for comment, publication before becoming effective, explicit procedures for relief and appeal, and more. The National Environmental Policy Act requires environmental impact statements before government agencies can act. Title XIX of the Social Security Act (Medicaid) requires states to adopt a state plan for Medicaid participation and seek approval of changes in it from the federal Health Care Financing Administration, which manages the Medicaid program for the federal government and pays the states the federal share.

Of course, procedural policies may have profound substantive effects. Oregon's request for a waiver of federal rules so that it could explicitly introduce the notion of rationing into its Medicaid plan was initially turned down by HCFA on grounds that came to be regarded as both substantive and political (too close to the election to endorse rationing), though initially the focus was on procedural inadequacies.

An even clearer example was the U.S. Ninth Circuit Court's 1994 order in *Beno v. Shalala* vacating a Section 1115 Social Security Act demonstration project waiver signed by the secretary of HHS. The waiver authorized California to conduct an AFDC work-incentive program, cutting benefits for most recipients except for 5,000 families assigned to a control group. The court noted that effects on human subjects had not been evaluated, as required by other statutes for all federally sponsored research. The federal statute requiring these reviews of human subjects delegated responsibility to the agency carrying out the study to perform the reviews, but California had not done so. Nor, the court added, had enough attention been paid to the merits of the study or its research design. Opponents of the study were successful in suing over a procedural infraction to stop a project that they did not like (on substantive grounds) and that they felt actually constituted a substantive policy change (a statewide cut in AFDC benefits) masquerading as a research project.

Environmental policy is fraught with opportunities for both sides to call in their attorneys to argue that proper procedures were not followed. Often the effect (and the intent) is to slow things down, delay, and wait for a better deal or make time for negotiation. Cynics have called the Administrative Procedures Act of 1946 "The Lawyers Relief Act."

Politics shapes policies, but policies also determine politics. Lowi (1964) delineated three types of policy, each with its own characteristic political structure, political process, leaders, and group interactions. The three are distributive, redistributive, and regulatory.

Distributive Policies

Distributive policies distribute benefits and produce mostly winners and few losers in a type of mutual noninterference pattern. Examples of distributive policies are hospital construction funds, research funding for the National Institutes of Health, Superfund cleanup dollars, and university capitation grants paid to medical and other health professions schools. Wilson (1989) added that distributive policies often concentrate benefits on the hospital corporations, medical schools, or others who win them, while costs are diffused among the taxpayers at large and concentrated on no specific group. So the winners have a big stake in the policy and actively support its passage, while the losers do not lose much and pay little attention.

A typical distributive program (described in more detail in Chapter 7) would be a program to set up federal scholarships for nurse-practitioners who agree to practice in medically underserved areas of the state. The witnesses before Congress would likely be nurse-practitioner groups, nursing school deans, and spokespersons from hospitals in rural areas that would benefit from the program. There would be few, if any, witnesses speaking against the program. The only possible opposition might come from physician assistants or other providers who might feel they should have similar programs. Overall, it would be a love-fest to be repeated in the other house and passed with little fanfare some weeks later. The only flaw in this seemingly idyllic situation is the relatively recent congressional concern for holding down federal spending. To the extent that the nurse-practitioner program is in competition with programs for physicians, pharmacists, or community housing advocates, the normally friendly politics of distributive programs become more turbulent and, sometimes, downright nasty. (The impact of the federal budgetary constraint on policymaking is described in Chapters 1 and 7.)

Regulatory Policies

Regulatory policies restrict the behavior of private or other governmental actors. In health policy this includes hospitals, physicians, nurses, graduates of foreign medical schools who want to practice in the United States, drug manufacturers, hospital janitors in charge of disposing of medical waste, dentists (who must wash their hands, change gloves, and wear masks to prevent infection), nuclear power plants, auto manufacturers, and the chief executive officers (CEOs) of hospitals who want to take over the competition. There are clear winners and losers in regulatory policies. Though the losses may be limited (nobody gets killed), they can also be substantial—the opportunity to earn millions or even billions of dollars may be lost.

Generally speaking, regulatory policies are more controversial than distributive policies, and they are often fought out on the congressional floor and in committee markup sessions. Many are salient and can easily arouse the ire of the group to be regulated. Regulatory policies have gained special notoriety in the health policy world as the subject of the debate over competition or regulation.

Many regulatory policies in health care are "self-regulatory." Physicians set the standards of practice for physicians, hospitals accredit one another as meeting the standards that their own Joint Commission on Accreditation of Hospitals has set, and schools of public health decide what courses will be required of graduating students to receive their association's imprimatur. Government often devolves authority to these self-regulating bodies, taking their seal of approval as evidence that minimal standards have been met and taking some of the political heat, and the cost of enforcement, off government actors themselves.

Redistributive Policies

Redistributive policies take money or power from some and give it to others. Lowi's taxonomy suggests that redistributive policies are the real battleground in political warfare. In health care policy, redistribution translates to taxing those with higher incomes to pay for health services to those with lower incomes. The U.S. income tax system is progressive—taking taxes at a higher rate as income rises—because those who have the ability to pay are believed to be the ones who should pay. Economists argue that extra or marginal units of any good are less valuable to the recipient than the first units. Following that logic, a little money to a poor person is worth a lot more social utility than a little more money to a rich person. Religious teachings make a similar point in parables of, for example, the poor widow whose small gift was valued more highly than the large gift of the rich man. Even some staunch conservatives tend to favor just enough free care to keep the work force healthy.

Medicaid is a redistributive program, taking tax dollars from the middle and upper classes to pay for health care for the very poor. Minority-hiring policies redistribute job opportunities from white middle-class males to females, African Americans, Hispanic Americans, Native Americans, and members of other minority groups.

Many expensive public programs are not very redistributive, and many of those that are redistributive are rather small. One exception is Medicaid. Once tiny, this program, which spends nearly three of every four dollars on people who were poor before they got the care, has grown to rival Medicare in size and has been dubbed the "PAC-Man" of state budgets (Weissert 1992).

Redistributive politics are fierce. They are combative, controversial, constantly under attack, hard to obtain, and hard to retain. When the Reagan administration ushered in its program of governmental spending cuts, which health care program was the first to be cut? Was it the (then) nearly $100-billion Medicare program serving all elderly Americans, most of whom are middle class—a group with a lower poverty rate than the population in general and roughly one-half the poverty rate of children? Or was it Medicaid, a program that requires recipients to spend all they own down to a few dollars a month of personal money before they can qualify? Of course, it was the latter. Because most people think that Medicaid is more or less exclusively a welfare program aimed at unwed mothers and their children, many of whom are members of a minority group, Medicaid is never a popular program with the voters.

After a fierce battle, led by the administration's Republican Senate majority on one side and opposed by such liberals in the House of Representatives as Henry Waxman, chair of the Health and Environment Subcommittee of the Energy and Commerce Committee, across-the-board cuts were instituted in Medicaid, with further cuts ready to go into effect if efficiencies were not produced. Though smaller than the Reagan administration wanted, the cuts were large in relation to the swelling demand for care among the poor and the states' concern over the growth of Medicaid spending as a share of their budgets. In his political novel *Facing the Lions* (1973), long-time political commentator for the *New York Times* James Reston made his leading character sagely observe that when all is said and done, it is redistributive policies that the establishment really fights against. That is all the government they really care about cutting, he said.

Tatalovich and Daynes (1988) identified an additional policy type to Lowi's categories, which they call social regulatory policy. These are instances in which government regulates social (not economic) relationships and where values, morals, or ideology bring people into conflict who might otherwise remain uninvolved. Abortion, gun control, assisted suicide, affirmative action, and school prayer are examples of social regulatory policy.

Extent of Policy Change

Not all policy changes are equal in their scope, range, and depth. Some changes are clearly monumental, generally reflecting a value change in society, often leading to institutional changes and pointing policy in a new direction. Welfare reform legislation in 1988, which redefined welfare from a "handout" to an opportunity for advancement through education and job training, was such a change. So was the enactment of Medicare in 1965, which was the first major federal health program guaranteeing health care for a large, targeted population.

Most public policies are not comprehensive. Rather, they build on earlier policies, are implemented by existing agencies and departments, and generally follow the policy direction of earlier policies. Such policies are called incremental, changing only slightly, or incrementally, from existing policies. Brown (1983) uses slightly different terminology. He refers to breakthrough policies, in which government is involved in a new activity, and rationalizing policies, in which attempts to solve problems are made through existing government programs.

The politics of the two types of policies are quite different. Comprehensive or breakthrough policies flow from major changes in public attitudes, often expressed through election results. They can be initiated by the public either with a positive image of enthusiasm or a negative image of criticism of the existing situation. Hayes (1992) argues that these nonincremental policies can only be adopted when values are agreed upon and when there is an adequate knowledge base. Even with these two predisposing criteria, the environment must be right for change, usually a turbulent environment characterized by a dramatic shift in the political world or public opinion. Public support is a crucial element to successful adoption of nonincremental change. Support by "elites" or those who are influential in the thinking of policymakers and the president is important as well. Finally, leaders who are willing to take a chance and opponents unable to defend their position can help as well. But as Hayes puts it, nonincremental change is simply impossible for many issues.

Incremental policies are most likely to emerge from situations where there is not much information and there is no national agreement on values. Incremental policies pit interests against interests in a situation where there is little public attention and where interest groups, federal agencies, congressional committees, and other interested parties grapple with the problems and the solutions best designed to solve them quietly and without public fanfare.

Some argue that the distinction between incremental and nonincremental change is extremely vague and may reside in the eyes of the beholder. The distinction is made more difficult because a series of incremental changes can have the combined power of major change, and seemingly nonincremental change may be simply an amalgamation of incremental steps. For example, changes in federal reimbursement systems encompassed in the prospective payment system in the 1980s have led to the redefining of health care delivery systems in hospitals and other providers. Yet the changes were accomplished across several years and several decisions and are hard to view as a single, comprehensive change.

The preference toward incrementalism is based at least in part on the number of actors involved and the knowledge available. The model advanced by Braybrooke and Lindblom (1963) called disjointed incrementalism embodies both aspects. The model notes that problems are identified in a disjointed manner by different affected groups. The participants are limited to consideration of a few familiar alternatives and only some possible consequences, and are not goal-directed. The process is characterized by trial and error and tends to intertwine policy goals and features of the problem itself. Far from being dismayed by the prevalence of disjointed incrementalism, Braybrooke and Lindblom note that "political democracy is often greatly endangered by nonincremental change," and such change can be accommodated only in certain limited circumstances (73).

Nonincremental change sometimes occurs first with an incremental step that provides knowledge to policymakers and mobilizes public or group support. In a second stage, convergence toward comprehensive reform occurs (Hayes 1992). Kingdon (1984) describes a situation of nonincremental steps perhaps leading to major changes. He quotes a Capitol Hill health staffer who observed that expansion of Medicare coverage to kidney dialysis in the mid-1970s might be viewed as an approach that focuses on procedures rather than population subgroups or care settings, calling it national health insurance "one organ at a time" (85).

This is not to say that nonincremental change is extremely rare or nonexistent. Kingdon (1984) notes that while incrementalism is one effective strategy for getting things done, it does not capture the tendency for ideas to catch on and suddenly gain momentum. "I analyzed all changes in my data and found that there were as many nonincremental as incremental changes," he said (85). Since Kingdon was tracking ideas, rather than policy enactments, he may have overstated the role of nonincremental policy change. However, Baumgartner and Jones (1993) agree that the policy world has a place for both types of policies. They argue that public policy is generally characterized by long periods of incrementalism, spiked or punctuated with change of a more comprehensive nature. They call this pattern punctuated equilibrium and describe it as a system of stability and change.

Aware of the higher likelihood of success with incremental versus nonincremental approaches, national health reformers have battled for forty years over which approach would produce more success: go for broke when the opportunity arises and try, as President Clinton did, to cover everything and everybody, or be satisfied with getting a little bit each year.

Despite the failures of most past presidents who had sought major change in health policy, President Clinton rejected a narrowly focused catastrophic-costs-only plan in favor of a broad plan that covered everyone, expanded benefits, reduced copayments, and mandated businesses to pay three-quarters of premiums. Political and health policy advisors urged him to focus on his vision of major change promised in the campaign and, they argued, demanded and expected by the American people. Economic advisors, sensing his preference for this visionary approach, swallowed their reservations and couched their support in conditional language that took advantage of the fact that the choice between broad and narrow reform was being made without the benefit of cost projections (Woodward 1994). Later postmortems would suggest that in addition to ignoring and then badly underguessing the costs, the boosters of major change had misread the voters. What the voters meant by major change was a guarantee of portability—a promise that insurance would not be lost or priced out of reach when a worker changed jobs or lost employment. To the Clinton administration and to their potentially most ardent supporters for reform—the American Association of Retired Persons, labor, and other beneficiary group lobbies—this type of piddling change was the worst kind of incrementalism.

Incrementalism is often an easier sell to the voting public and Congress because most people are risk averse. They are reluctant to make large and risky changes because the consequences and costs are hard to predict and unintended consequences can be costly. Kingdon (1984) observed that savvy politicians can and do use this understanding of the policy process to select a strategy for creating policy change. No one was a better master of it than House Health and Environment Subcommittee chair Henry Waxman. "He sets such ambitious policy aims that colleagues might consider him a pie-in-the-sky fool if they were not by now so familiar with his technique of taking a small slice at a time until years later he is holding the whole pie—even in the face of spending retrenchment. Persistence and patience are his strengths" (Duncan 1994, 188).

MODELS OF THE POLICY PROCESS

The policy process can be modeled in a variety of ways. Some models highlight the environment in which policy is made, others feature policy actors' perceptions, others the processes and institutions of government. Campbell (1992) found that he could not explain the development of aging policies in Japan with a model that assumed policy was either determined rationally by the dominance of an idea or by the conflicting power of interest groups. Standard operating procedures, the opening of an opportunity for making policy choices, and other factors also had to be considered. Many analysts highlight the steps most policy actors take most of the time in developing policy. Figure 6.1 is such a model, showing how issues progress from problem definition through criteria specification, generation of solution options, and their selection, implementation, and enactment. Feedback loops indicate that

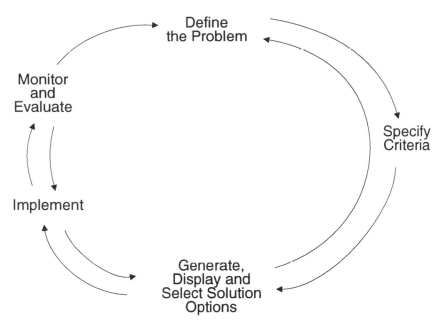

Figure 6.1 The Policy Process

sometimes the process of specifying criteria or selecting among solution options causes the analyst to rethink the problem definition. In actuality, the
process is much less well ordered than the figure suggests.

One of the most used "straw men" in public policy is what is known as the
rational-comprehensive model of policy, which generally follows the steps
shown in figure 6.1. A rational policymaker using this approach would clearly
define the problem, specify and prioritize the criteria, examine all the alternatives, compare the costs and benefits of the alternatives, and pick the one
that best meets the criteria. Since cost is generally a criterion, a cost-benefit
analysis is often a part of the ideal decision-making process. The idealized
model assumes that the policymaker has all the information needed to make
the choices and all the time needed to reach the most desirable solution (implied as well is that the solution is most clearly desirable to all "rational" observers). As we all know, and Simon (1945) was among the first to point out,
the model is not realistic. Policymakers do not have the time, resources, or
intellectual ability to go through the desired steps. Policy must be made in
consultation with others who may have different goals and objectives. Finally, successful policy must be forged considering its political and technical
feasibility in addition to its cost-benefit ratio. As House Ways and Means

Committee chair Dan Rostenkowski put it in April 1994, his three criteria for a health reform plan were universal coverage, cost containment, and the bill's ability to win 218 votes in the House ("Lawmakers Face Hectic Health Reform Timetable" 1994, 1).

Simon's solution was what he called "satisficing" or bounded rationality—policymakers and other decision makers must make the best feasible decision given the constrained information and alternatives available to them (Simon 1945). Nevertheless, as Light (1982) notes in his study of the presidency, sometimes decisions in the White House are made systematically in a way fairly close to the rational, comprehensive model. The somewhat simplistic display of the steps of policy development serves as a useful guide to understanding what goes on in policy development, even if it may be less easily modeled in real life.

The first and final steps of figure 6.1 need further elaboration. While disruptive or focusing events can catapult an idea to the top of an agenda, they are not the only way ideas arrive there. According to Kingdon (1984), the policy window can be opened with a new administration, a shift in congressional party control, a shift in national mood, or when a new problem captures the attention of governmental officials. Problems can come to the attention of policymakers in ordinary ways, such as routine monitoring of governmental agencies, and feedback or evaluation of existing programs.

The fact that the idea becomes a barrier to new ideas in the final stage is important, because even a new and daring idea will soon be the status quo, with its own supporters and implementors who will be threatened with the prospect of change. For Schon's model, as in Downs's model, most ideas do not successfully complete the stages but rather fall off at some point, often to return as "new" ideas slightly redefined or, more likely, renamed.

The Garbage Can Model

An eloquent criticism of the too-simplistic view of the policy process depicted in figure 6.1 was offered by Cohen, March, and Olsen (1972, 1), who described policymaking in universities as "collections of choices looking for problems, issues and feelings looking for decision situations in which they might be aired, solutions looking for issues to which they might be an answer, and decision makers looking for work." If nothing else, this characterization represents a profound indictment of the notion that policymaking proceeds in an orderly fashion. In their analogy, four separate streams flow into the "garbage can." The streams—problems, solutions, participants, and choice opportunities—flow independently. Policy outcomes result from the mix of garbage (the four streams) and often have more to do with the timing of someone's workload or the persuasiveness of a participant than the acuity of the problem being addressed.

Students taught the scientific method in eighth grade sometimes find this view of policymaking unreal. But consider the case of the Experimental Health Services Delivery Systems (EHSDS), a demonstration project mounted in the waning years of the era of health planning in the 1960s. It shows the effects of vague goals and the influence of actors who come and go, some with pet solutions they want to try, in a process definitely not rational in nature.

Planning groups had met without much success throughout the 1960s, trying to eliminate duplicate services. Critics charged that they had produced a million dollars' worth of planning and not a dime's worth of action. EHSDS was conceived on the rather vague notion that success could be achieved by putting "the movers and shakers" (CEOs from hospitals, insurance companies, public officials, and physicians) into the same room and letting them "work things out." Initial plans for the program were extraordinarily vague. As meetings were held to flesh out the idea and gain approval from agencies within HEW, participants came and went, in much the same way described by Cohen, March, and Olsen (1972). One prominent epidemiologic consultant who came to some early meetings insisted that no such effort should start without a household survey of needs. His strong personality and arguments prevailed. Though the consultant left the program after a number of meetings, his idea persisted and eventually became a major preoccupation of the project, though few understood why the survey was being done.

Twelve cities were funded to set up EHSDS organizations. They spent the first year arguing about bylaws and the wording of the household survey. In Southwestern sites the survey had to be translated into Spanish and, many argued, should also have been translated into languages used by various Native American tribes. Some cities refused to conduct the survey. Those that did had little time, energy, or resources for anything else. Few associated with the program ever figured out exactly what the organization was supposed to do or how it was supposed to do it. Some board members thought it was a health maintenance organization. Others thought it was a political action committee. Still others used the EHSDS funds to continue activities begun under an earlier grant, which had expired.

A project officer who took over after the first year decided that the most important product was a set of bylaws for the EHSDS board in each city. But he caused great furor when he rejected out of hand those produced by one site after months of local struggles and compromises. When a high-ranking bureaucrat associated with the project in its early days was asked how he could allow such a program to grow, he replied: "When you see something going wrong, you just want to get away from it" (Weissert 1972). Regrettably, this is not an altogether extreme example of how vaguely defined solutions can be put into motion with little clear sense of the problem they are intended to solve. The example typifies how the changing cast of characters brings different priorities and ideas to a policy. Individuals willing to invest the energy can move policy in a direction of their own choosing within the limits of other preferences and choice opportunities. Kingdon (1984) called these individuals "policy entrepreneurs."

Kingdon's Revised Garbage Can Model

Kingdon (1984) modified the garbage can model to fit health and transportation policymaking by the federal government. He reviewed case studies and conducted four sets of interviews with health policymakers and staff in Washington, D.C., to test his revised model.

From Cohen, March, and Olsen (1972) he adopted the notion that organized anarchy characterizes the federal government. He also adopted the "streams" notion, though his are slightly different: problems, policies, and politics. These streams develop and operate largely independently of one another. Problems are defined and moved to the governmental agenda; solutions are developed, whether or not they respond to a problem; the political stream may change suddenly with the election of a new administration, whether or not the policy community is ready or problems facing the country have changed. The separate streams come together at critical times: a problem is recognized, a solution is available, the political climate makes the time right for change. This critical time, or opening of the policy window, is an opportunity for advocates to push their pet proposals.

A policy window opens for a short time, then closes. Precipitating events may be enabling legislation that comes up for renewal or the influx of new members of Congress. The item suddenly gets "hot" because things come together at the same time: problems, solutions, and policymakers' attention and desire to act. Kingdon, like Cohen, March, and Olsen (1972), called this process "coupling." Typically this comes at the hands of a policy entrepreneur, a cabinet secretary, senator, member of the House, lobbyist, academic, lawyer, or career bureaucrat—inside or outside the formal policy circle— who does the brokering to make things happen. "Entrepreneurs do more than push, push, and push for their proposals or for their conception of problems. They also lie in wait for a window to open. In the process of leaping at their opportunity, they play a central role in coupling the streams at the window" (Kingdon 1984, 190). They bring to the debate several qualities that may afford them a hearing: they are experts or speak for others with a major stake in the problem, they are skilled negotiators, and they are tenacious. "When researching case studies, one can nearly always pinpoint a particular person, or at most a few persons, who were central in moving a subject up on agenda and into position for enactment" (Kingdon 1984, 189). While they wait for a policy window to open, they do the "softening up," giving speeches, chatting about, and otherwise working to make their ideas familiar to those who will be called on to adopt them when the timing is right.

Both Kingdon and the garbage can model suggest that the neat stages depicted in figure 6.1 miss some important qualities of the policy process. An important one is that solutions sometimes precede problems. The model also appears to omit exogenous factors, factors that make some problems more likely to be focused on than others. Finally, figure 6.1 captures only one cycle of the policy process. Sabatier and Jenkins-Smith (1993), among others, argue that policy change should be viewed over a long time-horizon—at least a decade. Problems are not "solved" and taken off the policy map. Rather as Wildavsky (1979) noted, once a solution is carried out, it creates whole new sets of issues, ensuring that no public problem ever really dies. They noted that figure 6.1 is not really a *causal* model because "it lacks identifiable forces to drive the policy process from one stage to another" (Sabatier and Jenkins-Smith 1993, 3). In our view, a final criticism of the heuristic model in figure 6.1 is that it fails to recognize that policymaking calls on two different sets of criteria for problem definition: criteria for deciding that a problem requires a public solution, followed by criteria for choosing among public solution options if the first set of criteria is met.

These are legitimate concerns that require that the policy process be viewed as more complicated than the simplified version depicted in figure 6.1. Yet this depiction of the policy process has been around a long time and has proved very useful, as even its most ardent critics concede: "[T]he stages heuristic [figure 6.1] has provided a useful conceptual disaggregation of the complex and varied policy process into manageable segments" (Sabatier and Jenkins-Smith 1993, 2).

DEFINING PROBLEMS IN HEALTH CARE POLICY

Problems are important, political, and transitory. Without a problem, there can be no policy action. Yet not all problems lead to public policies, and many problems fade from public concern well short of any type of solution. Simply put, a problem is a state of affairs that annoys, hinders, or injures a complaining group (Eyestone 1978, 5). Examples include little access to medical care, poor-quality care, costly care, insurance that may go away just when you need it or that locks you into your current job because your next job may require a physical exam that you cannot pass, unhealthy behaviors like killing ourselves with smoking or auto accidents, or killing others with guns and water pollution.

Baumgartner and Jones (1993) call problem definition the very engine of change because it is the essence of power. Problems are inherently political because they are not simply out there waiting to be solved. They must be formulated and defined, using political skill to mobilize support for the desired position. Definitions of problems are chosen strategically, "designed to call in reinforcements for one's own side in a conflict" (Stone 1988, 122). Is the transportation of disabled individuals to a health care facility a transportation problem with civil rights implications or a civil rights problem with a transportation solution? Is AIDS an epidemic with civil rights concerns or a civil rights problem of a group suffering an infectious disease? Is the health care of poor people a health or a welfare problem? The definition of a problem sets the parameters for discussion and lends legitimacy to an issue. The definition flows from the choice of values (Dery 1984) and can also determine whether the problem demands public policy action. Defined another way, a problem might be a market condition better left to the private sector or a personal attitude or preference not in the domain of public policy.

Not all problems are candidates for public policy. Some may be viewed as either intractable or not in the governmental domain. Eyestone (1978) provided three prerequisites for governmental recognition of a policy problem: governments must correctly identify a social problem or issue, governments must have the capacity to respond, and politicians must be persuaded that they should respond.

In health, the definition of a problem is crucial. Is the problem an unequal system of health care delivery, costs that are rising too rapidly, or the quality of the care provided? Is the problem with excessive paperwork or waste, profiteering insurance companies, greedy doctors, or a third-party payer system that encourages inefficiencies? Or is it all these things, as President Clinton proclaimed in his health address before Congress in September 1993. Part of his task as defined by Eyestone was accomplished: identifying the problem. But his harder task, convincing politicians and the country to respond, was only beginning.

Problems do not just emerge. Citizens, leaders, organizations, interest groups, and governmental agencies create them in the minds of their fellow citizens. Problems come to what Cobb and Elder (1972) called the systemic or public agenda. They may be brought by parties perceiving bias, a group seeking advancement or assistance, an unanticipated event, or a group seeking the public good. Triggering devices can be a natural catastrophe, an unanticipated human event, ecological change, or technological change. If sufficiently affecting many people, problems can go to the formal or institutional agenda, where policymakers will recognize and consider the matter. Problems can also reach the institutional agenda through interest group lobbying, congressional staff, bureaucrats, constituents, or the members of Congress themselves who discover a problem and wish to "solve" it with governmental action. In his study of how health care policy problems get on the public agenda, Kingdon (1984) found that no single source dominates the origination of problems across topics or issues. Surprisingly, he found that the press is rarely the source of problems, especially in fields like health care policy, which are complex and salient. The media merely serve to communicate problems among policymakers and constituents, and the specialized press helps policymakers communicate with one another.

Measuring Problems

Problems are usually ill defined and, more often than not, exaggerated. Advocates often approximate prevalence and severity in congressional testimony and press reports. Their goal is to dramatize the problem and create a sense of urgency. They want to make people feel the problem is so widespread that they could be its next victims. Advocates must "oversell" their positions to avoid losing their audience, Kingdon (1984, 137) contended. Some recent examples make his point. Estimates of the prevalence of battered women offered by the National Coalition against Domestic Violence were so large they included one-half of all married women. One-third, the group said, are battered multiple times each year. But when pressed for the source of the estimates by the *Washington Post* (Brott 1994), the coalition revealed that the numbers were actually guestimates. Eventually, on a major investigative news show the estimate was raised to 60 million women—a number that, the *Post* pointed out, exceeded the number of women living with men.

Somewhat more disciplined was the secretary of HHS, who, the *Post* reported, said that females were battered by their mates about as frequently as they bore children: 4 million victims. Though the number came from a Harris poll, it got so high by adding 1.1 million who said they had been "kicked, bit, hit with a fist or some other object" (a good working definition of battering) to 2.9 million who said they had been "pushed, grabbed, shoved, or slapped" (not desirable, but probably not battering). A more accurate estimate is one from the National Institute of Mental Health's National Family Violence Survey. It found violence in 16 percent of all American families, most of it slapping, shoving, and grabbing, while battering is limited to 3 or 4 percent of families, about 1.8 million families. Fewer than 200,000 women are actually harmed to the point that medical attention is required, according to the survey. This is far too many, to be sure, but not one-half of all of married women (Brott 1994).

Heterosexuals who contracted AIDS during its first decade were mostly intravenous drug users. Yet, many public education campaigns focused on heterosexuals. Some thought this was a deliberate effort to garner middle-class support for AIDS research (Furrento 1989). Others disagreed (Sherer 1990). Near-hysteria ensued when newspapers and the evening television news headlined the story that a small-town Texas high school had "discovered" six cases of AIDS in heterosexual young men with no homosexual experience (Suro 1992). The embarrassing follow-up story two weeks later, that the results could not be verified and the school nurse who had released the story could not be located, was given barely two inches near the bottom of an inside page (*New York Times* 1992; Associated Press 1992). Most papers simply ignored the follow-up.

Catastrophic health care cost problems were similarly exaggerated. Initial estimates dwarfed the available resources. Closer analysis showed that estimates of who experienced truly catastrophic costs were very sensitive to the definition used. Wyszewianski (1986) observed that thresholds for catastrophic expense varied widely, from $1,000 to 25 percent of income or 30 percent of wealth. The number of victims also varied: Did the patient actually bear the costs? Did the whole family's costs count? What if insurance paid the bill? Changing the definition changed the prevalence.

Bazzoli (1986) did similar work on uninsured persons. She showed that published estimates of their number ranged from 10 to 45 million. Each estimate carried the aura of science. They differed because a wide variety of techniques were used to vary the estimate, including:

—underreporting insurance among household survey respondents;

—overreporting insurance due to double-counting those with duplicate policies as separate people;

—including or excluding people sometimes uninsured or inadequately insured;

—failure to count Medicaid coverage as insurance or ignoring limits on Medicaid hospital days;

—overdramatizing the problem by including young people at low risk who were voluntarily uninsured.

Palumbo (1990) may have had such an example in mind when he observed that the interpretation of the facts drives policy, not just the facts themselves.

Another example of bad science shows how results can be exaggerated to promote a desired policy solution: public subsidy for home and community care for elderly people. The plethora of studies of inappropriate institutionalization of elderly people in nursing homes in the early and mid-1970s found too many people there. Up to three-fourths of them, some studies showed, were misplaced. They should have been in the community (U.S. Congressional Budget Office 1977). Later, controlled experiments replaced these subjective analyses. Surprisingly, only a very small fraction of would-be nursing home patients benefited. Despite the offer of community care, they went to nursing homes anyway (Weissert, Wan, Liveratos, and Katz 1980; Weissert, Wan, Liveratos, and Pelligrino 1980; Weissert, Cready, and Pawelak 1988; Weissert 1991).

Bad—or inexact—science can also lead to dramatic changes in the definition of a problem. Following decades of concern over an undersupply of physicians in this country and a number of high-level commission reports, culminating with an Institute of Medicine report in 1973, it became clear that the problem was an oversupply, not an undersupply, of physicians, and Congress in 1976 declared that the shortage was ended (and the battle "won"). While there were some extenuating circumstances affecting the estimates, such as an influx of foreign medical graduates and an increase in graduates from newly established medical schools, there were also problems of overestimation of the demand for services, underestimation of mounting health care costs, and unrealized assumptions about location choice and specialization. Regardless of the cause, the situation was no doubt confusing for national policymakers hearing a federal health official warn that the nation might soon be facing a physician surplus only a few months after receiving a prestigious report urging federal capitation for medical students to encourage the production of more young physicians (Ginzberg 1990).

Sometimes overestimation of the problem can get so out of hand that the only interpretation it produces is hopelessness. Public policy toward long-term care had been frozen for decades from fear that solving it would break the bank. The reason: most definitions equated having a long-term care problem with having a chronic illness. But most chronically ill people do not need human assistance in their daily functioning. What counts is whether or not one needs help bathing, dressing, using the toilet, eating, shopping, and doing household chores. Defined that way, estimates dropped from 30 million people to between 2 and 8 million (Weissert 1985).

Why the smoke screens? Lack of data, reliance on practitioners' anecdotes, and an absence of systematic analysis in the early stages of any problem's definition are some of the reasons.

The national Council on Wage and Price Stability's discovery in 1976 that Blue Cross/Blue Shield was a larger supplier to General Motors than U.S. Steel sent shock waves through the health policy field (U.S. Executive Office of the President 1976). Fears of deadening effects on international competitiveness galvanized policymakers into action on health care costs. Later analysis, however, has challenged the prevailing view of the dire consequences of the costs. Reinhardt (1989) noted that economists have long known that the costs of employee benefits are substantially shifted to employees through lower wages. Waste and rapidly rising costs are legitimate concerns, but not because they limit competitiveness, he argued. While not everyone agrees with Reinhardt, the lesson is clear: early characterizations of problems are rarely tempered by reasoned analysis and systematic evaluation of presumed consequences.

Political "Spins"

Sometimes the facts get bent on purpose. How an issue is framed can influence the type of politicking that will ensue, its chances of reaching the agenda of a particular institution, and the probability of a policy outcome favorable to the advocates of the issue (Petracca 1992b, 1).

Much of the framing of the problem involves linking the problem to its root cause. The solution then flows from the cause of the problem. In recent years, blame for smokers' deaths has shifted from individual smokers to cig-

arette manufacturers and (to a lesser extent) blame for highway traffic fatal-
ities from reckless drivers to faulty motor vehicles. When bartenders selling
drinks to obviously intoxicated drivers began to be recognized as part of the
problem of drunk driving, dram laws were passed in state after state. The
linkage is crucial to policy choice. In fact, Stone (1989) believes that people
choose causal linkages not only to shift blame but also to enable themselves
to appear to be able to remedy the problem. An example of this shift may be
the recent concern over identifying and extracting payment from teenaged
fathers and assigning parental responsibility for newborns to grandparents,
targets of policy opportunity perhaps more tractable, at least initially, than
teenaged mothers themselves.

Other linkages seem more loosely tied to specific policy solutions but rather
are designed to raise public concern or heighten sympathy. For example, the
aging lobbies initially described the homeless as "bag ladies" as a way of drawing attention to the needs of elderly women. It was only on closer examination of the homeless population that it became clear that most homeless
were nonelderly. Most are males, frequently Vietnam veterans and other young
and middle-aged men (Rosenheck, Gallup, and Leda 1991). An even more
blatant example was the Senate Aging Committee report in the 1980s that rising dog food sales must mean that the elderly were eating dog food, though
no evidence was ever offered to substantiate this claim.

A linkage was deliberately ignored when children's lobbies reported a massive outbreak of kidnapping. Pictures of missing children, presumably kidnapped, appeared on milk cartons. Only later did it emerge that most of
these claims involved divorces and child-custody disputes (Best 1988; Gelles
1984). A decade after its initial discovery, more systematic definition of the
stereotypical kidnapping as being a long-term, long-distance, or fatal episode
and analysis of the problem had reduced its incidence to roughly 150 to 300
cases per year involving an attack by a stranger (Hotaling 1988).

The elderly, kidnapped children, even hospitals, like to present themselves
as disadvantaged if it serves their policy interests. Many hospitals in the 1980s
complained that they were losing money on patients they wanted to discharge
but could not because there were not enough nursing home beds. Hospitals
said that states should pay for the wasted days (Dubay, Kenney, and Holahan
1989; Welch and Dubay 1989). However, in many states the problem barely existed. Further, there seemed to be other explanations for the delay, such as
slow Medicaid eligibility determination, which could be solved by more case-
workers or a presumptive payment system (Weissert and Cready 1989). Instead, the hospitals went to state legislatures for more money.

The point is that hospitals have a major stake in defining the problem, estimating its magnitude, and attributing its causes. They feel it is in their best interest to appear the victims, seeking legislative relief in the form of extra compensation for any stays they decide are unnecessarily long. Is this because hospitals are run by dishonest people always seeking a public handout? No, it is because hospitals are highly complex organizations facing urgent demands from many constituents. If they can solve one of their problems by shifting the load to public policy, they are likely to do it. The policymaking process must sort out the validity of the demands and decide whether a public policy solution is warranted, or the hospitals should be left to solve their own problems.

CRITERIA: THE LINK BETWEEN PROBLEMS AND SOLUTIONS

Much of the effort in problem definition goes into deciding when a condition is a public policy problem. Problems must meet certain criteria if they are not to be left to the market or private parties to solve. Once these public versus private criteria have been met, a second set of criteria comes into play. This second set is used to choose among solution options.

Public Problem Criteria

In health care, as in other areas, the lexicographic criterion involves the questions of public role. Is the problem one best settled by the public or private sector? Or put another way, should the government be involved in this area? While the government's role has been argued in health policy for decades (see Chapter 7), it is important to note that the issue is also important in policies as disparate as airline industry deregulation, sexual harassment, job training, international trade, and needle-exchange programs (Rochefort and Cobb 1994, 7–11). Bosso (1994) notes that the American culture is built around core beliefs of individual liberty—defined as freedom from government constraints—in a way that has a powerful effect on how people perceive the meaning of public problems.

People and policymakers differ in their views on the proper role of government. Many regard markets as the preferred solution. They take the view that the appropriate role of government should be limited to those instances in which flaws in the market preclude market-based solutions to the problem. Only under those circumstances should government enter the health care market. This opens a debate over when the market has failed. Those who want more governmental action argue that health care is not a well-functioning market because it has several distinctive characteristics. Patients as buyers and health care professionals as sellers are not equal players. Professionals have enormous amounts of technical knowledge needed to judge whether the care they are prescribing is needed by the patient. Most patients are completely or nearly completely ignorant of the science underlying clinical decision making. This information asymmetry distorts the principle of consumer sovereignty and, to many, justifies public action to at least license professionals to weed out unqualified providers. Others would go further, noting that the physician has the power to influence the patient's decisions concerning how much of a product to buy (Evans, Labelle, and Barer 1988; McCall and Rice 1983); they would regulate physicians' fees and review the appropriateness of prescribed care.

Externalities—costs or benefits falling on others—are also a concern in health care policy. Some health care problems affect more than the individual; infectious diseases are the principal case in point. The risks involved in the spread of diseases means that the government must take responsibility for ensuring that everyone is vaccinated and, under some circumstances, evaluated for the presence of disease. Public health and sanitation laws and enforcement are justified on this principle.

"Free riders" are another problem sometimes necessitating public action. Young healthy workers who decline to buy insurance are counting on the rest of us to pay for emergency rooms to care for them in the event that they get sick or are in an accident. They are free riders on an expensive health care system maintained by the insurance premiums paid by the rest of society.

These rationales for governmental involvement are intended to bypass issues of ideology and justify a limited role for government: correct the market failures, then get out. Disrupt the private sector as little as possible.

Yet these seemingly technical debates even among economists often turn into ideological arguments over whether or not the health care market functions well enough that further governmental intervention is unjustified. Advocates of limited government argue that government itself is the main source of market failure in the health care market. Licensing creates monopolies that allow providers to set prices without concern about competition from lower-priced suppliers. Those who believe these benefits will accrue through market reform assume that problems of information asymmetry will be overcome by consumers who take the trouble to inform themselves, through buying cooperatives or private information services, much as they do when buying other complex products about which they know little, including computers, universities, and foreign travel.

In health care, ideology plays an important role in determining what gets defined as a problem and what gets on the agenda for policymaking. Ideological differences about the role of governmental action help policymakers pick sides in the debate over whether or not governmental action is needed. Party affiliation helps make up their minds: Republicans tend to favor minimal government. They want the market to solve problems unless there is strong evidence that it is not working and cannot be fixed. Democrats, particularly liberal Democrats, are quicker to give up on the market and seek governmental intervention. Eyestone (1978) noted that most social questions are not neutral with respect to the governmental issue. For any two competing issues, he said, one will almost certainly call for more governmental involvement than the other, and the contrast will invoke the governmental role to some degree. Further, he noted, the appeal against bloated government is often a conscious political strategy—a charge made by Democrats when Republicans criticized President Clinton's proposed Health Insurance Purchasing Alliances.

Some have pointed out that the U.S. Constitution and the legal system both presume a capitalistic economic system based fundamentally and extensively on private property rights. For this reason, conditions are often presumed to be merely the product of a well-functioning market, meaning that governmental intervention is likely to be rejected. If the problem is defined as a market failure and conservatives can be convinced that this may be the case, intervention may be justified, even to conservatives. Convincing them is rarely easy. They point to past governmental failures (Weimer and Vining 1992) and worry that efforts to fix the current problem may produce future ones. Even if convinced that the market has failed, they will still argue for limited intervention, trying to leave as much of the problem's solution to the market as possible. In ideologically charged issues like health care policy, the political parties enter the fray, seeking further to shape the debate over the nature of the problem and the appropriateness of intervention (Baumgartner and Jones 1993). The public too is often skeptical of governmental intervention and evaluates a proposal by whether its extension of governmental power will affect the public directly or not (Eyestone 1978).

Public skepticism has a long history in health policy and has played a major role in stymieing the development of national health insurance. The arguments used in 1964 and 1994 regarding freedom to choose a physician, quality of treatment, and possibility of bureaucratic medicine were nearly identical. And both were effective. When poll respondents were asked to choose between a reliance on government and a private-oriented approach, large numbers identified the private approach (Jacobs 1993b). Further, while Democrats are more likely than Republicans to support a tax-financed national health plan, even liberal support is "tempered by concern over the problems of bureaucracy and the practical limits to what government can accomplish" (Jacobs 1993b, 634).

Donabedian (1973), a long-time student of and commentator on health care policymaking, called the two most extreme versions of the different views people hold toward health care "egalitarian" and "libertarian." The former want health care to go to everyone equally. The latter want only to prevent infections from spreading and keep workers healthy enough to keep a job. Egalitarians point to inequities between rich and poor patients in frequency of visits to physicians, waiting times, and variety of physicians and hospitals available to poor patients, and they demand the elimination of "two-tiered" care (better quality care to the rich than the poor). Libertarians want more aggressive screening to eliminate welfare cheaters, more oversight to eliminate fraud and abuse, and incentives to prevent unnecessary emergency room visits. Donabedian (1973) asserted that these ideologies play out in health care policymaking not merely as arguments over how much health care to provide but as manifestations of views of the kind of society we should live in. Libertarians, he argued, see governmental encroachment in health care as the first wave of attack on the very nature of American society.

Pooling Risk

Stone (1993) made a similar case on the issue of pooling risk. Arguing that the nation is a community, she rejected an insurance company's definition of actuarial fairness, which she quoted from a print ad. The ad defines actuarial fairness as "the lower your risk, the lower your premium" (288). On the contrary, she argued, each person paying for his or her own risk, when taken to its extreme, would mean that every person would have his or her own premium based on a perfect prediction of health care costs. The result would be the end of insurance, since all who could afford to would simply put the money in the bank to avoid insurance company profits and administrative costs. She called actuarial fairness "antiredistributive ideology" (294). In contrast, she argued, "social insurance operates by the logic of 'solidarity.' Its purpose is to guarantee that certain agreed-upon individual needs will be paid for by a community or group. . . . In the health area, the argument for financing medical care through social insurance rests on the prior assumption that medical care should be distributed according to medical need or the ability of the individual to benefit from medical care" (290).

Harvard philosopher John Rawls (1971) would most probably agree. Recognizing that most people are risk averse, in situations in which their future status is unpredictable (they wear a "veil of ignorance"), they tend to adopt policies that raise the position of the least advantaged. Fearing that they may become the minority, they adopt redistributive policies that lead to greater equality of outcomes.

In voluntary insurance plans, the sickest people buy insurance, well people (especially young people) wait until they get sick, and premiums rise over time, acerbating the problem. Insurance companies find it in their interest to try to sell insurance only to people who are not likely to use it, excluding those who are likely to get sick any way they can. Some of the ways they use are physical exams, exclusion for preexisting conditions, long waiting periods, and high and rising premiums for elevated risk, especially when "experience" shows that an individual has a tendency to use substantial care. Risk indicators and health care utilization experience are often detected at the time an individual applies for a new job that brings health insurance with it. The result is that people with elevated risk may be unable to change jobs without becoming uninsurable or facing prohibitive premiums. Sometimes the policies of an entire small firm face cancellation due to the risks or costs of one unlucky individual.

Mandatory national health insurance covering the young and old, sick and well, and those with no problems today but who may have them tomorrow is offered as one way to avoid such problems by increasing the size of the risk pool and sharing the costs of high-risk individuals among all policyholders. This raises the premiums of well people over what it would be in an experience-rated plan. It may also require expanding the benefits package provided to meet the needs of enrollees with special problems, including adaptive housing, transportation, special communications aids, and personal supervision needed by chronically ill patients. Since these are typically limited in the benefits package and premium calculations of private plans, they too may raise premiums over what private, experience-rated plans would cost. The result tends to be premiums that redistribute wealth from some premium payers to others and an expanding role of governmental control into vast new sectors of the economy as it referees disputes among beneficiary subgroups over what services should be covered.

Markets and Minorities

Reliance on the market to distribute income, wealth, and equity of access to health care may produce particular problems for minority groups. Any quick review of the data shows that the market has not worked very well to remove differences in health status between minority and nonminority Americans. Indeed, Winn concluded that advocates of market-oriented solutions to health care problems simply do not see racial barriers as a problem. African Americans are not regarded as a special group by free-market advocates, ignoring "the fact that blacks experience shorter life spans, a higher rate of chronic and debilitating illnesses, and lower protection against infectious diseases" (Winn 1987, 240).

Failure to confront the reality that poverty is highly correlated with minority racial status in society means that the special needs of minorities will not be met. Racially neutral policy therefore perpetuates the effects of racial discrimination and enhances its persistence. Likewise, policies that require poor individuals to pass through invasive and demeaning eligibility screening to prove that they are poor enough, and that also require them to accept care from providers willing to work for the invariably lower prices paid by government, are an affront to many champions of the poor because they produce two-tiered care, in which minority group members, often poor, face restricted access or lower quality care. Universal, equal access without regard to the ability to pay is for this reason considered one way to try to avoid aggravating the effects of past discrimination (McBride 1993).

CONCLUSION

These differences in perspectives between what are loosely referred to as liberal and conservative views reflect fundamental differences in social priorities and views about the efficacy of government as a solution to social problems. For these reasons, merely pointing out that a problem exists in no way ensures that there will be consensus on the need for governmental action. In defining health care problems for public policy intervention, technical arguments must take shape within an ideological context. Values are often at least as important as data.

The next chapter reviews some of the major health policy solutions attempted and in some cases adopted over the past several decades. During that period, policymakers' views of the problem of access to health care shifted from the shortage of facilities, personnel, and services to the lack of planning and coordination to concerns over distributional problems producing surpluses in some areas and shortages in others to the problems of inefficiency, wastefulness, ineffective care, and budgetary shortfalls. Solutions moved from supply subsidies to planning activities to incentives intended to alter the mix and geographic dispersion of services to utilization controls, price freezes, prospective budgets, fee schedules, and market-oriented solutions relying on competition to hold down prices. The criteria invoked to choose among these solution options are discussed in the next chapter.

7

Political Feasibility
and Policy Solutions

PROBLEMS ARE POLITICAL, and so are solutions. Though economists and others have done an excellent job of cataloging the generic types of solutions available to government, the actual choices and ways in which these options are combined is a political process. Like problems, solutions come to the decision-making agenda only if they have the right features to pass through ideological filters. They are adopted only if they meet certain criteria and interest in them peaks with the right timing and support. Gauging which solutions are likely to be chosen and shaping them to make them more acceptable to a majority requires an understanding of political feasibility.

Political feasibility has been critically important to the congeries of policy choices that make up what passes for national health care policy. National health insurance, for example, has failed to find acceptance as a solution to the problems of health care access for some fifty years. On the other hand, supply-and-demand subsidies have been a ready tool for policymakers, and cost-containment efforts have also been part of the health policy world since shortly after the passage of Medicare and Medicaid.

POLITICAL FEASIBILITY

In its most practical definition, political feasibility means being able to garner 218 votes in the House of Representatives and fifty-one in the Senate. But a large number of factors impinge upon the political feasibility of an issue. These include the appropriateness of the role of government proposed; the extent to which costs or benefits are concentrated on powerful interests; whether the proposal is means-tested and how much redistribution it involves; saliency and timing of the issue; its comprehensiveness, complexity, costliness, and prospects for solving the problem; and the amount of capital a president brings to his support of the issue or the savvy and effectiveness of another well-placed policy entrepreneur.

Appropriateness of the Government Role

A critical standard of acceptability for health care policies is whether they are viewed as an appropriate role for government. Advocates do their best to characterize problems in ways that make them public policy problems. During some periods that task is easier than at other times. During the Great Depression when the private market had clearly failed many Americans, they were willing to turn to the government for help. Again during the Johnson years, Americans seemed willing to experiment with public approaches to meeting a pent-up demand for solutions to a host of social concerns. Values seem to oscillate between relatively more liberal and relatively more conservative positions in cycles that are difficult to predict but seem at times to span perhaps three decades or so. During relatively more liberal times, a significant block of voters moves from serious distrust of the government's ability to solve problems to a willingness to suspend disbelief long enough to try out a new set of reforms. At such times it seems to be somewhat easier to successfully make the case for public intervention to solve a problem.

Yet even in such times a high level of distrust remains, making some proposals unacceptable. One such proposal has been mandatory participation in government health insurance programs. Little seems to enrage conservatives more than mandatory participation in a public program that they do not support. This is particularly true when the problem is, as Downs (1972) has suggested, one that is not affecting most members of society. National health insurance (NHI) proposals involve significant dislocations and costs for all who feel they are already well served in the private market. In health care, with premiums for nonelderly people substantially paid by employers and the elderly's care paid by Medicare, most people fall into that category when it comes to participation in a mandated federal program.

Calling a proposal "bureaucratic" is another rallying cry. Fear of bureaucratic red tape can bring a proposal under deep suspicion if opponents are successful in making a plausible case (often laced with exaggeration) that the proposal is likely to spawn bureaucratic growth and replace private decision making with decisions made by bureaucrats. This concern is paramount in health care. It puts proponents on the defensive and can greatly diminish the likelihood of adoption. Proposals that appear to replace physicians' clinical judgments with bureaucratic rules are strongly resisted, as are efforts to direct middle-class patients to specific providers.

Business, particularly small business, is viscerally fearful that any government-mandated compliance, however innocent at first, will eventually prove to be the nose of the camel under the tent as Congress, bureaucratic regulators, and the courts reinterpret the scope of their authority and the degree of compliance and reporting required. This fear has made business unwilling to accept federal subsidies intended to get them started on employee health insurance coverage, even when they could clearly benefit from the subsidies.

Other groups have been much more willing to accept optional subsidies. The subsidy has a long history in health care policy going back to merchant seamen, veterans, poor children, retarded children, and many other population subgroups, as well as hospitals and health professions schools. Though there was some initial Republican resistance to federally subsidizing health professions education beyond "bricks and mortar," a strong medical school lobby was willing to lay aside fears of government influence on their curriculum and continued to lobby for subsidies for many years. Republicans tend to remain skeptical of some subsidies, however, and are likely to cut them when they get the chance. They fear that federal subsidies bring federal control, for example over health professions education, and are likely to distort the relationship between supply and demand.

States have been very willing to accept subsidies and in the process have supported great expansion of the nation's idea of an acceptable role for the federal government. Though states sometimes jealously guard their autonomy and often see the federal government as the enemy of their individuality and discretion, frequently they use whatever discretion they can muster to increase the flow of federal dollars, often expanding the scope of federal influence and control. Federal budget deficits and a periodic resurgence of states' rights concerns have slowed the pace of such bargains from time to time.

Partisanship plays an important role in defining the appropriateness of government action. Republicans tend to favor market-oriented approaches, while Democrats have traditionally been more willing to use regulation to accomplish social objectives. Many solutions deemed appropriate under a Democratic administration or congressional majority are viewed as inappropriate options when Republicans are in control.

Over time, for some kinds of solutions, attitudes soften, and ideas that were once anathematic gain support and can be adopted. Seat belts were initially strongly opposed as government intrusion into private lives but later were grudgingly tolerated and eventually welcomed by many as a necessary safety device. Requisite for changed attitudes is the passage of time and accumulation of overwhelming evidence that benefits will justify the intrusion. Kingdon (1984) says that softening up occurs while time is passing: promoters are talking about their proposal and making people more familiar with it. They may also change it enough to make it more acceptable. The result is that ideas that fail the appropriateness test when first introduced tend to be introduced time and again, becoming better understood, more familiar, and easier to accept as time goes by. Prospective payments to hospitals are a case in point. Unfortunately, no set time is "enough," and for some proposals a half-century has not been sufficient. But there may be an interaction between the quality of the idea and its increasing likelihood of passage with time and familiarity. Kingdon (1984) concedes that there seems to be a compelling power to an idea whose time has come. Explicit rationing of health care to control costs is still unacceptable to most Americans, but the idea began creeping into public policy discourse in the 1990s (Lamm 1990) and was explicitly adopted for Oregon's poor early in the decade.

Conversely, some solutions grow less acceptable with time. Forced screening for various infectious or inherited diseases, particularly those affecting one minority group, is not a publicly acceptable method of solving the problem of controlling disease or costs and shows little sign of becoming acceptable, though quarantine for infection was more or less routine in the past.

Concentrated Costs and Benefits

Proposals that concentrate costs on powerful interests, such as business, are sure to be met by well-financed, well-organized resistance. Employer mandates fall on business, especially small businesses not offering coverage, often because an employed spouse can get coverage through the spouse's employer.

Likewise proposals that require members of Congress to set aside the interests of their districts are often doomed to failure. Sin taxes fall on a small number of industries usually represented by a block of important members of Congress, representing wineries in California and New York or tobacco interests in the South. Especially ill advised are proposals that offend an industry concentrated in the district of one or more key committee chairs (as graduate medical education reform did when the Senate Finance Committee was chaired by a New Yorker, a state with many teaching hospitals).

Proposals are likely to succeed—even well beyond the point they are needed—if they serve the interests of many members' districts and allow members to take credit for bringing projects and services to their districts, such as subsidies for hospitals.

Means Testing and Redistribution

Liberals and conservatives often part company over means testing as a way of limiting public subsidies and the scope of the public role. As discussed in Chapter 6, the parties subscribe to different philosophies of how best to improve the lot of the poor. Conservatives fear creating dependency among those given free care and worry that taxing the well-off will stifle investment. They prefer to restrict free care to only very poor people and count on a growing economy to provide more income for everyone. Physicians tend to side with the conservatives on this issue because they prefer to earn their incomes from middle-class, privately paying patients, restricting government health care programs to those who cannot pay on their own. Their fear is that with government subsidies will come fee schedules and other controls, eroding their income and freedom. Liberals prefer to use progressive taxation to raise revenues and provide the health care benefit free to all so there is no stigma attached to receiving "charity" care and the temptation to render poor care to poor people is mitigated (though it is still hard to avoid if the poor visit different providers than the middle class). Means testing is an approach to limiting the government's role and to making proposals more affordable.

The corollary of means testing is redistribution, however. Proposals that redistribute substantial fractions of income from the more affluent to the less well-to-do violate conservatives' sense of how to improve the nation's well-being and concentrate costs. The result: having favored means testing as a way of limiting the scope of government programs and their costs, conservatives then seek to limit funding for them. Highly redistributive programs are difficult to enact and support. Policies subsidizing middle-class voters are much easier to pass and very hard to cut. Tax deductibility of employee health insurance premiums is a prime example. Most of the revenue loss to the Treasury from this policy goes to higher rather than lower income earners. Efforts to end the subsidy have come to naught.

Comprehensiveness, Complexity, and Political Cost-Effectiveness

When policy analysts think of costs they think in terms of efficiency—the amount of output for each unit of input. Often they are concerned with cost-effectiveness or cost-benefit ratios: the relative benefit for a given expenditure. Politicians make a similar but slightly different calculation. They are worried about how to pay the political costs—dollars, disruption, and administrative burden—and whether the juice is worth the squeeze. Proposals that are very costly and of dubious effectiveness are dead letters.

Comprehensive proposals always face a tough road to enactment. Most people are risk averse, especially conservatives. Asking them not only to trust government but also to trust it to move on many fronts at once or a substantial distance from the status quo is threatening. Comprehensive proposals invariably offend many well-placed interest groups who are enjoying benefits from the way things are. Comprehensiveness also adds costs as well as complexity. The complexity of the proposal makes it more difficult to gauge potential effects and adds to perceived costs. Voters worry that complex systems will prove unreliable, that they contain hidden agendas, and that costs will exceed estimates while effectiveness will fall below expectations. Complex proposals make easy targets for critics who claim they simply will not work or will be highly burdensome because of reporting requirements to ensure compliance.

CBO estimates punctuated the Clinton administration debates over what percentage of the population would be insured under the various proposals competing for votes, each of which carried a different price tag. As the realization crept in that enormous additional spending would be required to produce small increases in the total population covered, zeal for reform waned: the juice no longer seemed worth the squeeze. Some call this the 20–80 or 90–10 rule: costs of solving the last 10 or 20 percent of a problem rival or even exceed the costs of solving the first 80 or 90 percent. Policymakers shy from such lopsided options.

Dollar costs have become much more important, especially in health care policy. For decades dollar costs were a secondary consideration in large, expensive projects costing billions of dollars and virtually of no concern at all in smaller ones of only a few million dollars. Mere thousands have long been rounded off in federal budgets. Certainly debate surrounding Medicare in 1965 addressed the cost issue, and even President Johnson's staff was concerned about the higher-than-expected rate at which costs of health care were rising after its passage. But those concerns were simply not given the weight that they are today. Nor were there so many sources of competing estimates. Computers, more number-crunchers, and deficit-reduction laws requiring that every piece of legislation coming to the Congress bring with it estimates of its costs and sources of the revenues to pay them have made costs a top concern. Since few politicians want to raise taxes, they must find other programs to cut or claim that their program will actually save money. An important aspect of the CBO staff's job is validating or, more likely, rejecting claims of expected savings (see Chapter 1).

Saliency and Timing

Saliency of an issue dictates the kind of politics that will accompany it. Salient issues draw heavy press attention, giving the opportunity for credit taking, which encourages individual grandstanding and partisanship. Compromise around a majority position becomes harder. Party discipline tends to break down because members know that voters will hold them accountable and may punish them for not protecting the district's interests. Salient issues involve big stakes for the president, making him vulnerable to demands for concessions by members willing to bargain with their vote.

An actual or perceived emergency—such as the Medicare Trust Fund going broke—can help proposals, giving legislators political cover from interest groups' pressures and allowing cuts to be made that would otherwise be impossible.

Timing can easily kill an issue, either because another issue pushes it off the agenda (foreign affairs events, for example) or because the issue has not been resolved as election time approaches. The policy debate becomes grist for campaign debate. Issues that had been the subject of negotiation and compromise become campaign slogans and sound bites, widening rather than narrowing the gap between the parties. Compromise becomes even harder if one party sees that it may gain enough seats in the election to change the lineup supporting or opposing a particular proposal.

Kingdon (1984) makes the point that the policy window opens but only briefly. Proposals ready to go when the opportunity arises have a better chance of being adopted than ones that have to be worked out. Downs's (1972) issue cycle characterizes the tenuous hold that problems have on the national agenda, especially if they are costly to solve. They enjoy saliency only as long as they are not replaced by another, more interesting, problem.

Policy Entrepreneurs

Proposals are much more likely to succeed if backed by a president with substantial political capital, including a large majority of his party controlling both houses. With two houses to get through, two parties, interest group opposition, a general distrust of government, affordability concerns, and issues as complex as health care policy, the default is policy failure. Any remaining hope must come from a policy entrepreneur, someone—often a member of Congress—pushing the solution forward, bargaining, and making persistent demands for progress (Kingdon, 1984). Success is affected by these individuals' legislative and policy prowess, how well placed they are on key committees, and their level of expertise and determination.

Not all these criteria of political feasibility get equally weighted. Weights on some criteria change based upon the issue, while others are always heavily weighted. Effectiveness is likely to be a less-important consideration in debates over subsidies than over mandates. Timing and comprehensiveness are less important if the issue is less salient. Concentrated costs and benefits are always important, however, because members of Congress place service to their districts at the top of their own priority lists. It is their job and their key to reelection, their proximate goal.

For many issues, the criteria for political feasibility are both additive and interactive in their effect on probability of success. Appropriateness of the government's role is especially worrisome if the costs of the proposal are high, its comprehensiveness concentrates costs on many powerful interests, its effectiveness is uncertain, and it remains unresolved as election time approaches and the parties are looking for issues useful for defining themselves. These additive and interactive effects highlight the difficulty of getting the "moon and the stars" in the right alignment for successful enactment of policy.

THE SOLUTION STREAM: A HALF-CENTURY
OF HEALTH POLICY CHOICES

Congress and the president have spent their time over the last several decades working on three major problems in health care policy: removing barriers to access, controlling rising expenditures, and trying to enact national health insurance. Against the goal of solving these problems, they have brought to bear many of the generic types of policy that governments use to accomplish their objectives (Weimer and Vining 1992), but they have strongly favored supply subsidies and a variety of caps and limits on capital investment, prices, and utilization. In choosing solutions, their preferences have clearly been influenced by ideological predilections that shape their views of good policy, including how they view the role of government (a paramount concern for their districts), sympathy toward hospitals and other provider interest groups, concerns over affordability, resistance to large changes, saliency of the problem, and efforts to position their party for the next election (see Chapter 1).

The remainder of this chapter will look at three classes of health policy solutions that have been proposed somewhat regularly over the past few decades: subsidies, cost-control efforts, and national health insurance. By looking at these in historical context, the persistence of solutions is illustrated, along with the political forces that determine their fate.

Subsidies

Supply subsidies have been a favorite policy approach for alleviating access problems. Congress wanted to eliminate supply shortages that made hospitals and physicians unavailable to many people. Programs subsidized hospital construction, personnel training, and services to disadvantaged populations. Subsidies are politically attractive. They allow members to be responsive to the many groups representing special populations' needs (for example, poor children, migrant workers and their children, and mentally ill people) or to focus on specific public health problems (for example, inadequate family-planning services). These programs also respond to constituents' pressure to expand facilities and services in members' districts.

If the major interest groups organizing the lobbying effort have done a good job, witnesses at hearings will include constituents of members on relevant committees and subcommittees. Authorizations, extensions, and budget increases are usually aired in hearings filled with like-minded witnesses and their supporters, each representing an affected subsidy recipient in the district of one of the members of the committee.

These are classic policy monopolies (Baumgartner and Jones 1993), in which everyone involved except OMB has a stake in continuing or expanding the program. The issues are not salient. Benefits are concentrated, costs diffuse. Usually only those affected show up for the hearings: interest groups, congressional staff and members supporting the programs, and bureaucratic agency staff implementing the program. The public at large has little interest, the populations served are typically unglamorous, and the content of the hearings tends to range from a presentation of deserving, often heart-wrenching cases being served by the program to arcane issues of administration. Frequently the hearings cast members in the role of fighting off an aggressive budget-cutting effort by the president and OMB. In the end, only OMB is likely to care that the program's worth was assessed in hearings in which only those with a self-interest in its continuation were called to testify.

A typical budget scenario for these types of program is for the president to propose phasing out the program or substantially reducing its budget over several years, only to be rebuffed by Congress, which is as likely as not to fund the program at a level substantially higher than the president requested. Programs are often continued long past the time when the president has told Congress that they are no longer needed, were never effective, or have been replaced by another program.

Points of contention over subsidies usually include:

—fights between Congress and the president over the need for the program and the size of the program's budget;

—bickering among members representing different types of constituents (urban versus rural, Northern versus Southern);

—professional group members' objections that additional personnel subsidies will produce excess supply, threatening their income;

—ideological battles over subsidies for abortion or family planning.

When the concern is excess supply, professional groups that feel threatened are likely to cast the argument in terms of an inability to control quality or an aversion to governmental interference into professional decision making, which they contend threatens quality. When the argument is over ideological differences, those with the strongest, best-organized opposition to governmental spending tend to prevail, in part because they are less willing to compromise than the other side and because it is relatively easy for a minority to stop a spending measure.

Subsidies have fallen on hard times in recent years. Compared to the early days, when budget deficits were rare and the major concern of Congress was whether a program was violating states' rights, the budget act requires that new subsidies must be accompanied by their own revenue sources: new or higher taxes or cuts in other programs. Members who want to see new services covered must turn to Medicare or Medicaid and hope that they can convince colleagues that offsetting cuts can be made in physician or hospital payments.

Hospital Supply Subsidies

More than three-quarters of a million beds had been built by the early 1920s, but consensus had grown that more were needed and construction standards should be imposed. The problem was well defined, and the solution easily quantified. Congress responded with the Hill-Burton Act of 1946. It provided one dollar of matching funds for every two dollars that states spent on nonprofit and public hospital construction, and it supported state surveys of bed needs. Members loved the idea of voting to put hospitals in their districts. In a spirit of bipartisanship, the act was introduced by and named for a Southern Democrat and a Republican. It was supported by both labor and the AMA.

Hospital subsidies moved through four phases:

1. construction subsidies, initially for hospitals but later expanded to embrace more types of facilities (including nursing homes and specialty hospitals), along with a larger federal government match;

2. efforts to shift from construction to modernizing facilities in urban areas (which failed when AHA supporters spurned the offer because they considered it too stingy to support their modernization plans and never really got it back);

3. the realization that too many beds had been built and efforts to end the subsidies (opposed by a coalition of Southern and rural members who felt they would not be allowed to catch up to Northern and urban areas);

4. efforts to obtain operating subsidies for financially troubled hospitals (especially those serving large numbers of poor people) to lessen the blow of Medicare PPS and continuing efforts to shore up the revenue stream of underutilized rural hospitals.

Throughout all these phases, support for hospitals remained popular with members of Congress. Most had one or more hospitals in their districts; benefits were concentrated on a few winners while costs were widely distributed.

The various solutions adopted represented incremental changes using familiar strategies. The budget deficit was not yet a problem. Hospital trustees and medical staff were highly regarded and presumed to be motivated only by public-spiritedness, and there were not many competing lobby groups in health care. Political campaigns were still cheap, the size of individual contributions was not yet limited, and a few large givers in a community could make a big difference to a member's reelection prospects.

Personnel Subsidies

Efforts to increase the supply of physicians began early with subsidies for the construction of medical and other health professions buildings. They moved into high gear in the 1960s with assistance for curriculum development and grants and loans to students. Some Republicans objected to expansion of subsidies to curriculum, seeing the specter of federal control.

This minority concern became the dominant policy attitude with the shift to a Republican president. The Nixon administration felt that physicians could pay their own way and would have preferred to see an end to subsidies for health professions. Failing that, his administration pressed for incentives and constraints that directed the subsidies to serving medically underserved areas, such as rural communities. The 1972 National Health Service Corps program allowed physicians to pay off federal loan obligations with service in underserved areas, exchanging a year for a year. Though later evaluation of the program would note that corps physicians saw fewer patients and worked fewer hours than other physicians, Congress would continue to extend the program despite presidential opposition. For some areas, corps physicians were the only option (*Congressional Quarterly Almanac* 1980).

The year 1980 brought a sea change to health personnel programs. HEW had been predicting future physician shortages for a decade. Now, both HEW and the Congressional Office of Technology Assessment changed their minds and predicted a slight surplus by the end of the decade (*CQA* 1980, 446). There would still be serious shortages in many areas, however, because physicians tended to concentrate in urban and suburban areas, leaving rural areas underserved.

The projected surplus coincided with a changed attitude toward support of physicians among some members of Congress. "Working people are taxed to finance the education of . . . people who are going to be rich," said a Texas House Democrat. It was time for the "free ride" to end, said Senator Richard Schweiker (D–Pa.), who as HHS secretary under the next president would help shape such policies (*CQA* 1980, 445).

Nurse training was similarly regarded as excessive as a shortage turned into a surplus. "We can't keep dumping funds into nurse education to train people to be administrative assistants and secretaries," said President Carter's HEW secretary, Patricia Harris (*CQA* 1980, 446). Schools of public health, on the other hand, argued that their graduates faced a market projected to need twice as many health administrators as were currently in place.

By the late 1980s most direct federal personnel-training subsidies had ended, following a stormy pathway marked by veto threats, vetoes, overrides, pocket vetoes (which could not be overridden because the session had ended), and congressional defiance by the repassage of parts of the same legislation in the new Congress, sometimes by large bipartisan margins.

Block Grants

Congress was highly supportive of new subsidy programs throughout the 1960s. Yet even President Johnson's advisors eventually became concerned about the lack of discipline reflected in the many narrow-purpose programs authorized. The federal government had been giving out money for a wide variety of programs with little attention to coordination or spending priorities. (Chapter 5 highlights the enormous growth in federal grants in aid and describes these grants.) Most federal grants had come in the form of categorical grants, which specified in detail how the money was to be spent. President Johnson, in his 1 March 1966 domestic health and education message, recognized the inflexibility of categorical grants as "an unnecessarily rigid and compartmentalized approach to health problems" (*CQA* 1966, 323). As part of a comprehensive health-planning act (see later sections of this chapter), the administration proposed the repeal of the formula and project grants and replacement with new funds with more general objectives, such as "providing services to meet health needs of limited geographic scope" and "stimulating new health services" (*CQA* 1966, 322). This was the first block grant, under which states are given money for broad areas of concerns and are allowed to spend as they see fit within a few federal guidelines. There were still some stipulations, however, such as a provision requiring that at least 15 percent of a state's allocation go to mental health.

In 1974 President Nixon proposed ending several existing health programs:

—the regional medical programs, which he said had not achieved regional health care systems;

—community mental health centers, which had been proved workable and had therefore accomplished their legislative goal;

—public health and allied health training programs, which he said had funds available from other sources;

—the Hill-Burton Act for hospital construction and modernization.

Congress refused.

President Nixon strongly supported the expansion of family planning. In addition, largely at congressional insistence, new initiatives were added to control lead poisoning, treat alcohol abuse, support and treat those with developmental disabilities, improve the quality of drinking water, and regulate medical devices and clinical laboratories.

President Reagan had more success in reducing health subsidies through the block grant mechanism. As part of a massive omnibus reconciliation bill in his first year of office, twenty-one categorical health programs were consolidated into four block grants funded at 75 percent of the categorical program spending level. "The federal government in Washington has no special wisdom in dealing with many of the social and educational issues faced at the state and local level," he said in his budget (*CQA* 1981, 464). The new president also succeeded where each of his predecessors since President Eisenhower had failed: he got Congress to agree to close the eight Public Health Service hospitals and twenty-seven clinics that had provided care to merchant sailors since 1798 (*CQA* 1981, 28).

His luck ran out in his efforts to turn community health center project grants into block grants. These had been one of the few programs substantially expanded during his predecessor's administration, largely at the behest of First Lady Rosalyn Carter. Overwhelmingly bipartisan support had sent to President Carter the Mental Health Systems Act, which pumped three-quarters of a billion dollars into the nation's mental health care system. The money was intended to continue the job of helping the nation build a new mental health care system. New drugs, altered therapeutic philosophies, and court rulings that patients had to be effectively treated (not just housed) or released had all but emptied the nation's mental institutions, dropping the resident population by one-half a million people in the past two-dozen years (*CQA* 1980, 432). The Community Mental Health Centers Act of 1963 had accelerated this trend with grants for centers that agreed to provide a specific list of services (*CQA* 1963, 222). Nearly 2.5 million clients were now served by 750 such centers, which formed a very strong and effective lobby against funding cuts.

Subsidies in Perspective

Subsidies in health represent the quiet politics of interests. Whether subsidies for medical schools, hospitals, or services to disadvantaged persons, the policies are often passed with little acrimony or public attention, with the subsidies continuing long after the problem has been solved. As budget constraints come down tighter and tighter on congressional decision making, the politics of subsidies may become more acrimonious as groups seek to maintain their "share" despite calls for reductions and phase outs. The strong ones will likely win (or lose in relatively small ways), while weaker interest groups will continue to see their funding diminish.

Cost-Control Initiatives

Presidents and the Congress have tended to shy away from direct regulation of health care delivery. They can be quite comfortable offering subsidies to encourage development in a particular direction, but they have tended to avoid specific orders to health care providers as to how to structure their industry or do their jobs. Yet subsidies create their own problems, encouraging disparate, uncoordinated growth and lack of planning. Worse, they do little or nothing to curb mounting expenditure rates.

Recognizing that something needed to be done and that the "market" was not doing it, the federal government began its foray into cost controls and restraint of delivery system growth by trying to encourage rational planning as a voluntary effort by the parties involved. When this failed, it added teeth by requiring planning decisions by the key actors involved. Later, when this too had produced little change in the upward spiral of spending, it turned directly to such cost-containment strategies as price controls, encouraging the growth of prepaid HMOs, review of medical bills to determine appropriateness, prospective reimbursement, and physicians' fee schedules. In the process, policy moved slowly but inexorably down a path that seemed to be leading to greater and greater federal control over provider delivery decisions or alternatively, by the mid-1990s, began moving aggressively toward steering public clients into tightly managed private delivery systems. These managed-care settings, resisted by the AMA in particular for decades, move the onus of cost control off federal regulators and on to private-plan managers by paying them a flat rate for most or all care received by an enrolled client.

Cost-control initiatives are a political anathema. They are a classic lose-lose situation because those likely to have their revenues or incomes curbed will fight hard to keep what they have. Those who potentially benefit—the public—usually do not see that they have gained. They perceive that they might not get the service they want, delivered when they want it, by their preferred provider. The politics of cost-control are brutal as interest groups muster membership ire over proposed cuts. It often comes down to "whose ox is gored" in cost-cutting, and the motto is "anyone's but mine."

Often it takes a perceived crisis or the structural imperative of deficit-reduction agreements to give legislators an excuse for making changes in payment policy. Under those relatively rare circumstances, interest groups' pressure is not enough to offset legislators' concern for good policy and fear of the electoral consequences of raising taxes, increasing premiums, or ballooning the deficit. A determined president can play an important leadership role in strengthening members' spines, but he can bring them along only so far and for so long. Even in response to a perceived crisis, initial victories are often eroded with subsequent delays and modifications to soften the blow of cost-cutting.

Yet Congress has gotten much tougher over the decades. In the early days after Medicare, public sentiment and legal restrictions against interference with the practice of medicine gave the federal government few options for controlling waste and duplication in the health care industry, even those parts that it subsidized, such as hospitals. Planning became the favored tool, a strategy that essentially counted on the public-spiritedness of providers to work together with community members to make more efficient allocation decisions. Failure of this strategy eventually brought policymakers to the realization that only payment policy would seriously alter provider behavior. States, in their Medicaid programs, began coming to that conclusion in the 1970s. It took the federal government considerably longer to adopt these ideas for Medicare.

Once begun, alterations of payment policy moved inexorably down a path of greater and greater control of some kinds of spending. Unfortunately, this often served only to spotlight the ability of providers to shift their activities to more lucrative procedures and less tightly controlled settings. Frustrated, policymakers turned to market-oriented strategies and tried to encourage competition among providers and insurance companies. A synthesis combining both strategies might impose global budgets on a competitive market—a one-two-punch approach offered initially by President Clinton in his ill-fated health reform plan. But global budgets for health care imply rationing, a policy that has not yet passed the appropriateness test of political feasibility and is strongly opposed by provider lobbies.

Supply Restrictions (Health Planning)

Building on the needs assessment and planning requirements for hospital construction under the Hill-Burton Act and citing that enterprise as a great success, the Johnson administration's 1966 Comprehensive Health Planning and Services Act provided funds for 75 percent of the cost of developing regional or local service coordination plans "to assure comprehensive, high quality health services for every person, but without interference with existing patterns of private practice of medicine and dentistry," which was code for no managed care.

The result was the spawning of state and local planning agencies throughout the country. Physicians, hospital administrators, government representatives, insurance company representatives, and many others formed discussion groups to try to bring rationality and order to the growth of the health care delivery system. Lacking any real authority over the private decisions of any of the major actors, however, these health-planning agencies were eventually charged with having done one million dollars' worth of planning while not changing the way one dollar was actually spent. That was an exaggeration, of course, but one reflecting a widespread sentiment that may have been substantially accurate in more than a few areas.

Seeing the flaw in the federal approach, state governments tried to put teeth into health planning. Nearly two-dozen states passed laws requiring hospitals to obtain certificates of need (CON) from state or local planning authorities before construction could begin. The Nixon administration decided to support a similar program at the federal level and proposed the 1974 Comprehensive Health Planning Act. Entities called health systems agencies—comprised of consumers, providers, and citizens incorporated into local planning boards similar to their predecessor planning agencies—would be given the power to withhold Medicare and Medicaid reimbursement of capital costs incurred in facilities not approved by them before construction as part of the agency's annual plan. There were more than 200 such agencies throughout the country. They would replace the regional medical programs and would shift the Hill-Burton program to hospital modernization only. Distrustful that county medical societies would find a way to have physicians selected to occupy too many slots on the boards by coming on as both provider and consumer representatives, Senator Kennedy inserted a requirement into the bill that 60 percent of the slots go to consumers. Governors opposed the bill until they were given authority to establish the size and shape of the planning areas. Senator Robert Dole (R–Kans.) opposed the bill as "further federalization, which goes hand in hand with increasing social-ization."

President Carter asked for a one-year extension of the 1974 Comprehensive Health Planning Act to enable his administration to review it. HEW wanted the breathing space to give it time to craft an important and controversial expansion of the law to reach outside the hospital to control technology, such as computerized axial tomography (CAT) scans in physicians' offices. Officials had grown weary of hospitals subverting the law's intent by arranging to have physicians purchase equipment and place it near the hospital. The AMA aggressively opposed the restriction but lost in committee. One Kennedy aide said it was the first time in a decade that the AMA had suffered a congressional defeat. A revised and expanded three-year extension passed both houses with bipartisan support and included the controversial provision. It extended CON requirements to major medical equipment even when bought and used in physicians' offices if those served were inpatients.

The legislation also supported the increasingly popular notion of competition among health care facilities as an approach to saving money. In this spirit, HMOs were largely exempted from CON requirements, and grants were provided for hospitals that closed or converted beds to other purposes.

A year and one-half later, the Reagan administration surprised few with a call to end health-planning programs. The Congress demurred, awarding a substantially reduced funding level for one year without addressing the termination issue (CQA 1981, 477). The president tried again in 1982 to kill the program. Existing authority was extended another year in the omnibus budget bill, setting funding at more than $4 million, compared to the $2 million suggested by the president. A reauthorization bill passed from Congressman Waxman's Energy and Commerce Committee's Health and Environment Subcommittee the following year but went no further, leaving the program to be continued for yet another year by continuing resolution.

Eventually, the program and the era of federal support for health planning were allowed to die a quiet death, starved of both dollars and supporters. Some states dropped their own programs immediately or shortly thereafter, while others kept them in place.

Freeing Markets

Health maintenance organizations began as an experimental program in 1971. Their appeal to President Nixon was largely due to their great potential as a cost-saving mechanism—an idea he got from HMO promoter Paul Ellwood. The president pitched the idea of bringing federal support to their expansion in his 18 February 1971 message to Congress: "The most important advantage of health maintenance organizations is that they increase the value of the services for each health dollar. This happens, first, because such organizations provide a strong financial incentive for better preventive care and for greater efficiency" (*CQA* 1972, 769). He proposed mandating all insurance plans—public and private—to offer an HMO option and $23 million in planning grants plus loan guarantees to HMO start-up sponsors. Different versions of an earlier bill that would have provided Medicare beneficiaries with an HMO option had passed both houses in 1970 but died with the ninety-first Congress before it ever got to conference committee.

Senator Kennedy opened hearings in his Labor and Public Welfare Health Subcommittee in late February 1972, focusing on both the administration bill and an HMO bill of his own. Administration spokespersons praised their own bill and criticized Kennedy's. The AFL-CIO criticized both, saying the administration's bill did not go far enough, while Kennedy's went too far. The full committee, by a vote of seventeen to zero, reported the Kennedy version in late July. It authorized planning grants, development grants, construction grants and loans, and interest subsidies. It also took the all-important step of preempting restrictive state legislation, which had retarded HMO growth. Furthermore, it provided per-capita grants to support HMOs that cared for indigents, offered malpractice reinsurance, and encouraged the development of quality-control mechanisms through incentive awards and a national commission. Clearly the committee sought to fan the sparks of HMO growth.

By late September the bill had passed the Senate sixty to fourteen with strong bipartisan support. Liberal Jacob Javits (R–N.Y.) said that "in full committee, on the whole, there was no dissent with the fundamental purpose" (*CQA* 1972, 773). But Peter Dominick (R–Colo.), a member of the full committee, called it "unrealistic both in terms of cost and scope" saying that he would nonetheless vote for it because "it addresses some important health care problems" (*CQA* 1972, 773).

In the House the AMA opposed the bill in subcommittee testimony. "Believing in a pluralistic approach, we feel that HMOs should be given a trial. But the basis should be limited, experimental. . . . What disturbs us is the prospect of a heading rush into a large-scale HMO program without hard evidence that it would fulfill the anticipated hopes" (*CQA* 1972, 774). The Optometric Association asked that its members' services be included in the list of basic services.

September passage by the House Interstate and Foreign Commerce Committee was not soon enough for action before the end of the Ninety-second Congress, and Nixon's enthusiasm seemed to die with the Congress (many believe because of pressure from the AMA; see Chapter 3).

The legislation passed the next Congress (in 1973) despite the AMA's opposition. The physicians' group was successful in convincing the Republicans to produce a scaled-down version. In the end, the bill that passed was budgeted at $375 million, down substantially from the $5.2 billion version passed a year earlier by the Senate. The legislation required HMOs to provide a wide variety of social responsibility roles, such as community rating, and a wide range of patient benefits. HMO managers would in coming years complain that these provisions made their costs prohibitively high and made it impossible for them to compete with regular insurance plans.

Still the window had opened for development of an idea that had been popular for many years but kept off the public agenda by the concerted efforts of the AMA. Strong interest group opposition and partisan differences had come together in a way damaging to a proposal that had begun with bipartisan support. President Nixon liked its inherent market-oriented, cost-control incentives. Kennedy, Congressman Paul Rogers, and other Democratic liberals saw it as a chance to alter the health care delivery system while at the same time moving to limit its benefit-cutting potential by legislating a large package of benefits. The AMA saw it as a threat to their markets and eventually their independence. Delays produced by these differences allowed events in the political stream to close the policy window. The president lost political capital with the expanding Watergate scandal. He needed strong support wherever he could get it. The AMA offered such support but used the opportunity to bargain for a less-expansive public role in support of HMOs.

HMO legislation passed again in 1976, acceding to industry demands to lighten the burdens placed on it by the 1973 act. Success reflected the organizational and lobbying efforts of Group Health Association of America and other HMO supporters to repeal the demanding benefit list Congress had included in the earlier legislation.

President Reagan did not share his Republican predecessor's faith in HMOs' potential to bring market discipline to health care. He argued that they had been given enough subsidies to make it on their own and asked Congress to cut them off. Congress was not convinced. Viewing them as money savers compared to fee-for-service arrangements, members voted to continue subsidies and relaxed community rating requirements, permitting classification of patients so that higher-cost groups would pay a higher premium (*CQA* 1981, 480). The president appeared to win the war, however. No new funds were provided under the program, and in 1986 a three-year phaseout and re-peal of the program's legislative authority were approved as part of the an-nual omnibus budget act (*CQA* 1986, 244). A year later, over White House ob-jections, the House passed legislation making it easier for HMOs to obtain federal certification.

Cost Controls in Medicare and Medicaid

With the implementation of Medicare and Medicaid in 1966, the federal government had moved squarely into the policy strategy of contracting for health care services. The participation of physicians and hospitals in the pro-gram, which had initially been far from certain, was quickly won by gener-ously reimbursing them at their costs or, in the case of hospitals, their costs plus 2 percent (Feder 1977). With both supply and patient demand subsi-dized, both costs and expenditures rose. By the time the Nixon administra-tion took office, that rise had become substantial. He had been in office only six months when he told Congress that action had to be taken soon to avoid a "massive crisis" in health care (*CQA* 1969, 867). His administration capped physician payments (which HEW showed had increased faster than projected) and eliminated as inherently inflationary the 2-percent-over-cost bonus pay-ments to hospitals. This payment methodology gave providers an incentive to spend more, but so did simple cost reimbursement, even without the 2-percent bonus.

The following year, HEW Undersecretary John G. Veneman was back to suggest that Congress make further changes to improve efficiency incentives and impose some budget control. Medical care costs had risen faster than general inflation since the enactment of Medicare and Medicaid. Use rates were said to be about 20 percent higher than expected, and physicians and hospital workers had substantially increased their rates of pay, according to testimony. He summed up the problem (retrospective cost reimbursement) and prescribed a solution: prospective payment (which would finally be adopted more than a decade later), under which "a provider would be chal-lenged to stay within the limits of known reimbursement and would share in any savings achieved through effective management. . . . Reimbursement to physicians should be tied to an index. . . . In the future the level would move up only in proportion to wage-price indices" (*CQA* 1970, 580).

Though the idea gained widespread support within the health policy com-munity, including hospital comptrollers, clinical lab directors, drug manu-facturers, and the Ohio Nursing Home Association, it quietly slipped from the national policy agenda for reasons not at all clear. Noteworthy, however, was the omission of the AMA from the list of supporters. The issue would return again to the agenda, but much later.

Meanwhile, Senate Finance Committee chair Russell Long (D–La.) wanted to make sure that somebody was minding the store. Long said he wanted "to get a responsible, hard-headed businessman's attitude into the administration of these important health programs" (*CQA* 1970, 577).

Long wanted to focus on fraud and abuse, and with this characterization of the problem ushered in a specific cost-containment solution that would wax and wane in saliency but continue as an active federal policy through at least the remainder of the century. His committee's staff report had charged "laxity" and said "physicians sometimes took advantage of poor administration through abuse and sometimes outright fraud" (*CQA* 1970, 578). Blamed were inadequate staffing and lack of loyalty to the program's interests among the private insurance companies that administered the program for the federal government. The federal government itself was inadequately staffed to provide oversight, according to agency heads. And if all this was bad, state administration of the Medicaid program was worse, according to HEW's Veneman: "Federal officials have been lax in not seeing to it that states establish and employ effective controls on utilization and costs, and states have been unwilling to assume the responsibility on their own" (*CQA* 1970, 578).

Health spending continued to rise in double digits. The short-lived Ford administration tried a variety of regulatory approaches to holding down costs, including demands for preadmission review of Medicare patients seeking hospitalization. A 1976 proposal to bundle Medicaid and fifteen other health programs into a budget-capped state grant program was ignored by Congress. The president vetoed the 1977 health appropriations bill as too expensive and because it ignored his administration's requests for various cost-saving measures in Medicare and Medicaid, but Congress overrode him. Not related but not unnoticed by those called upon to cut provider payments, California physicians struck to protest their rising malpractice premiums.

Hospital Prospective Budgeting

The real money was in hospital payments. As long as hospitals were paid on a cost-reimbursement basis, they had little incentive to stop spending. President Carter made hospital cost control his cause célèbre, asking Congress on 25 April 1977 to cap inpatient acute care—regardless of payer source—at a 9-percent increase in the coming year and at lower rates of increase in the next three years. The proposal trended forward 1976 spending and permitted small increases in the volume of patients. HEW would work to devise a better method of paying for hospital care, but in the meanwhile, the proposal also called for an end to new beds in areas with a surplus, estimated to be more than three-fourths of the nation.

Carter's HEW Secretary Joseph Califano set about pushing the plan with vigor. Calling American hospitals "fat," he went before Congress to urge immediate adoption of hospital cost controls. His proposal would avoid "massive bureaucracy" by drawing the information it needed from current Medicare and Medicaid cost reports, he said (*CQA* 1977, 502). Hospitals retorted that the president's assessment of their role in the cost problem was wrong, would ruin the quality of care, and usher in rationing of technology, beds, and quality. They were being blamed for the rising costs of medical care when in fact prices were rising on all fronts, they said. Labor worried that charity patients would be dumped.

Congress delayed. By October only Senator Kennedy's committee had reported a bill. Three more committees were still working on other items in a heavily loaded agenda. The hospital lobby and its allies continued to argue that the proposed controls were unworkable and threatened good-quality care. Members were concerned about the plan's technical feasibility and concluded that more performance incentives should be built in. The year ended with the legislation stalled in committees.

President Carter renewed his push the following year. Hospital costs were rising at $1 million a day, two-and-one-half times the rate of inflation in other products. But Congress had already concluded that the president's plan for controlling costs—a cap on annual inflation from a hospital-specific base, plus a $2.5-billion cap on overall capital spending—was too complicated. It also had political problems in its lineup of powerful opponents: the AMA, two hospital groups, and labor (which feared that savings would come from wages). Labor wanted costs controlled, but not on the backs of health care workers. Worse, almost nobody supported the bill. Lobbies for the insurance industry and the elderly were supposed to be supporters, but they did not work very hard. The public was not actively engaged. To the extent they supported any position, many consumers were concerned about the specter of rationed hospital admissions, services, and technology. Few seemed to understand the ramifications of high health costs, perhaps because they did not pay them directly. To top it off, some complained that the administration had not done "the basic educational job for members of Congress and staff," as one lobbyist for the elderly put it (*CQA* 1978, 620).

The hospital industry stepped into the breach, announcing the creation of a national steering committee and a network of state medical and hospital committees that would engage in a "voluntary effort" to cut hospital spending by 2 percent in each of the coming two years. Ways and Means Subcommittee chair Rostenkowski, whose committee still faced a full legislative agenda and a very tough sell on the president's bill, responded favorably, giving the hospitals a year to prove they could deliver, after which mandatory controls would kick in if spending had not dropped by 2 percent. Labor and the hospitals would have none of it and continued to battle against the bill in committee.

Compromises began to surface. The administration responded to labor's demand for its support of a pass-through provision for labor costs of blue-collar workers. Labor was still not satisfied and joined with the hospital lobby to stall action in key House committees.

Senate action was only slightly more favorable. After months of committee struggle, the Senate passed a bill that applied prospective payment to all hospital charges, regardless of who was the payer. The era of prospective payment had crept in on cats' feet, under cover of the larger Carter cost-containment initiative. One reason for success in the Senate may have been senators' awareness that the version on which the House was working was going nowhere. The president claimed victory in the Senate, but three days later, Congress adjourned sine die with the bill stuck in the House Ways and Means Committee with too few votes. When the dust settled, the president, who had made controlling hospital costs a top priority, was the big loser.

He tried again the following April. His new proposal asked for mandatory controls that would trigger if industry revenues rose by more than 9.7 percent in real dollars. An additional rise of nearly 2 percent could be justified by changes in the population or product, and the controls would apply to fewer than one-half the hospitals in the nation. The president used his awareness that the nation's high and rising overall inflation rate was becoming a major concern among both Congress and the people. He challenged Congress to stand up to the hospital lobby in a move to do something about inflation. This time, administration lobbying for the bill was coordinated in the White House rather than in HEW (perhaps a precursor to the president's decision to fire his HEW secretary in midyear, many said, because he showed too much support for Senator Kennedy, who was increasingly becoming the president's nemesis on national health insurance reform and a likely primary election rival).

Though the president sought to muster support from big business, it demurred, leaving the job of supporting cost controls to a congeries of state and local governmental officials, labor (now supportive because the new proposal included a wage pass-through), elderly people, and the health insurance industry. Hospital associations lined up on the other side, charging that they had been unfairly singled out to control inflation. They feared rationing of care, undue reporting and paperwork burdens, and a "regulatory nightmare" (*CQA* 1979, 513). Their voluntary effort would do just as well, they said, and, indeed, rates of hospital cost inflation had slowed by 2 or 3 percent since the president started his effort.

Senator Kennedy's Labor and Human Resources Committee reported the president's bill in June, largely intact. The Senate Finance Committee, which shared jurisdiction, was much less supportive, flatly rejecting the president's plan. The vote was eleven to nine to substitute a bill limited to Medicare and Medicaid payments, and the split was largely partisan: all but one Republican voted against the administration, as did three Democrats.

House action was little better. After accepting more than thirty damaging and weakening compromises, many of which the administration offered itself to win votes, the House Ways and Means Committee reported the bill with no Republican support. The Commerce Committee came excruciatingly close to losing the bill altogether, voting once to table it in subcommittee and defeating a gutting amendment by a tie vote in full committee. The final vote to report a further weakened bill was close and garnered little Republican support while losing nearly one-quarter of the Democrats on the committee. Representatives from rural and Sunbelt states feared that the bill would hold back needed expansion of new hospital services in their areas, preventing them from catching up with more developed areas (*CQA* 1979, 515).

Cognizant of slender hope for victory on the bill, the House Rules Committee held off providing a rule until the administration demanded it. An earlier vote by the committee had been delayed by its chair when it became clear the votes were not there to pass a no-amendments rule.

The administration should have listened to its congressional advisors. Two major arguments by lobbyists were credited with the bill's 234–166 trouncing on the House floor. Members were persuaded that new medical technology would be denied. "The American people demand the best," Tim Lee Carter (R–Ky.), a physician (and one-time supporter of cost containment) told the House (*CQA* 1979, 518). "It's doubtful we would now have intensive care units and recovery rooms and cardiac care units" had the bill been in effect, argued Willis Gradison (R–Ohio) (*CQA* 1979, 518). Members also abhorred it as new governmental regulation. Efforts to picture hospitals as "fat cats" had not been successful. Speaker of the House O'Neill's pitch to help "bill-paying Americans" ignored the fact that most Americans never saw their hospital bill. Lined up against the bill in what was described as "single-minded opposition" were the hospital industry and big business (*CQA* 1979, 518). Pressuring calls from the White House to wavering Democrats were no match, and Monday-morning quarterbacks wondered why the president had pressed forward with such a losing cause.

The legislation finally accepted—a product of the open-rule debate—was a substitute plan offered by Dick Gephardt (who ironically would be Speaker of the House under President Clinton and a key player in that health reform debacle). The Gephardt proposal set up a national commission to study hospital costs.

A year later President Carter tried one more time with a more incremental approach limited to Medicare hospital costs. The package was included in the first-ever omnibus reconciliation act, a bill with so many provisions that a lobbyist called it the largest health bill of the Ninety-sixth Congress (*CQA* 1980, 459). It included a provision long sponsored by Senator Herman Talmadge (D–Ga.) limiting Medicare and Medicaid hospital payments to average rates for various categories of hospitals. Other provisions paid hospitals for closing unused beds, limited Medicaid patients' use of expensive hospitals, and cracked down on hospital practices of transferring overhead charges from outpatient departments to other departments (*CQA* 1980, 460). All were deleted from the final product.

Cost containment, it appeared, simply could not be gotten past the provider lobby. The issue had been put on the front burner, however, and in the process had subjected a number of solution options to what Kingdon (1984) called softening up. The next administration would not start from zero even if the last one had seemed to casual observers to have ended there.

Medicaid Cuts

President Reagan's decisive 1980 election victory on a platform of major reductions in government's scope and cost put him in a strong position to demand cuts in health care spending. But he did not start with hospitals. Instead, he demanded a cap on federal Medicaid payments to states: for the current year, they would be held to just 5 percent more than last year, and in future years to no more than the increase in the gross national product. This inflexibility, his new OMB director, former Congressman David Stockman, called the only way to arrest the 15-percent annual increase in Medicaid outlays (*CQA* 1981, 479).

The National Governors' Association was apoplectic, lamenting that their budgets were already being consumed by Medicaid spending. The Reagan proposal would merely shift more costs to them. Neither house fully supported the president's approach, though both felt they had to achieve his target level of spending cuts from Medicaid as part of their effort to meet Gramm-Rudman-Hollings spending targets. The Senate Finance Committee changed the cap on growth from 5 to 9 percent. But falling short of his billion-dollar savings target from Medicaid, they voted to cut the federal share of Medicaid in the wealthiest states from 50 to 40 percent. The dozen states that would be affected begged their colleagues for relief, but for the present got none.

Meanwhile, the House did its best to accommodate all parties. Calling the growth cap "too simplistic," House members cut federal Medicaid support by 3, 2, and 1 percent in each of the coming fiscal years, thus meeting the billion-dollar goal.

Members of the House-Senate conference committee settled on the House approach but changed the annual figures to 3, 4, and 4.5 percent. They dropped the federal matching reduction, and in a quid pro quo to governors in exchange for the cuts, they granted the HHS secretary authority to give them waivers of "freedom of choice" requirements in Medicaid, thus allowing states to lock Medicaid patients out of expensive hospitals, as had been proposed under Carter. No longer would states be required to permit welfare mothers to make a normal delivery at an expensive university research and teaching hospital. Conferees also gave states a stronger defense against lawsuits from providers dissatisfied with payment rates and methods by changing the provider payment clause in Medicaid from requiring payment based on "reasonable cost" to payment that would ensure "reasonable access to services of adequate quality" (CQA 1981, 478).

They also granted additional waiver authority, allowing states to pay for home- and community-based care as an alternative to nursing home care. The House version allowed overall Medicaid spending to rise to cover new patients who might use home care. The Senate allowed more home-care spending only if nursing-home spending went down dollar for dollar. Unable to choose between the House and Senate language on that provision, conferees adopted both, despite their obvious conflict (CQA 1981, 479). HCFA, favoring the budget implications of the Senate version, would later write its regulations to conform to the Senate paragraph, ignoring the House paragraph in the law in a classic example of bureaucratic power in regulation writing.

Medicare Cuts

Hospital costs had continued to soar, rising more than 20 percent in two years, convincing Senate Finance Committee chair Dole (in the now Republican-controlled Senate) that he and Congress might have made a mistake in rejecting President Carter's mandatory hospital cost-containment plan (*CQA* 1982, 471).

President Reagan also called for cuts in Medicare, but got only phantom cuts achieved by moving costs back into the previous fiscal year that had been artificially moved forward the year before to show savings in that year (*CQA* 1981, 479). He fared better in 1982, signing Medicare changes that cut more than $14 billion from the program over the coming three years (*CQA* 1982, 471). Savings were achieved primarily by adopting former Senator Talmadge's long-supported notion of setting Medicare hospital payment rates for bed, board, and routine nursing at or near the average for a group of similar hospitals rather than the individual hospital's own experience. But Congress took two more important steps:

—It adopted the notion that hospitals should be paid a fixed amount per case based on a recent prior year's costs. If the current year's costs fell below that amount, the hospital could keep one-fourth of payments as a bonus. On the other hand, only one-fourth of costs above the fixed amount would be reimbursed.

—It required HHS to come back within five months with a prospective payment system for hospitals and nursing homes (*CQA* 1982, 471). This would put an end to the perverse incentive system that paid hospitals more for spending more.

Because federal policy analysts had been working on a prospective payment plan as a demonstration project for the state of New Jersey, HHS was able to comply with the tight deadline, submitting a Medicare hospital PPS in late December of the same year (Morone and Dunham 1985). The approach would pay hospitals flat rates for each of over 400 diagnostic groupings with similar lengths of stay and complexity of treatment. The diagnostic groups had been developed by health services researchers at Yale University. Though the New Jersey demonstration had been operating too short a time to produce results, Congress quickly adopted it anyway, stampeded by predictions that the Medicare trust fund would run out of money within the next few years if hospital payments were not reduced. Much as the garbage can model predicts, events in the political stream caused a problem to move to the top of the agenda, a window opened, the problem was well quantified, a solution was ready to go, and it was adopted.

The legislation also established an advisory group of experts who would meet annually after 1986 to review the need for rate adjustments (the Prospective Payment Assessment Commission). In the meantime, the new system would be budget neutral, allowing payments to rise with costs plus 1 percent for three years. During the three-year phase-in period, costs were to be increasingly set at regional and national averages, with declining adjustments for hospitals' individual costs. Hospitals serving an especially large number of poor beneficiaries were designated "disproportionate share" institutions and provided with exceptions or exclusions. Teaching and capital costs were excluded from the program in the short run but were to be collapsed into the overall rate later until, by the end of four years, 100 percent of hospital costs were paid in one rate. To protect patients against the new incentives for hospitals to skimp on care or increase admissions, Congress added to the president's package creation of peer review organizations (PROs).

Proving that Congress can act quickly and decisively when it wants to, the House Ways and Means Health Subcommittee reported the plan before the end of February, attaching it to a major Social Security bill. The full committee approved the plan a week later, and the full House passed it in less than a week. The Senate followed a similar schedule, and on 20 April 1983 the president signed into law the most significant change in Medicare policy since the program's enactment: case-by-case prospective payment for hospitals based on diagnostic groupings. Additional payments were permitted for exceptionally long-staying cases (later called outliers).

This extraordinary legislative feat—almost revolutionary given the stakes for interest groups—was possible for several reasons:

—Congress was panicked over the prospect of bankrupting the Medicare hospital trust fund;
—the proposal had in other forms been considered many times by Congress and was in its basic incentive approach familiar to members;
—legislatively, it was "ready to go" and already drafted;
—major party differences had dissipated when Republican Senate Finance Committee chair Dole became convinced by continuously rising hospital costs that the change was needed;
—the change was an incremental movement from the steps taken the year before;
—the leadership attached the payment plan to Social Security legislation

reforming that system to avoid bankruptcy of the Social Security trust fund.

The bill was brought to the House floor with a rule permitting no amendments to its Medicare provisions (*CQA* 1983, 393).

In contrast, other Medicare cost-saving strategies proposed by the president and considered through the normal legislative process were not reported during the session. These included higher premiums for beneficiaries, a one-year freeze on physicians' fees, and vouchers for beneficiaries who wanted to leave the Medicare program and buy care on their own.

On the heels of the controls on hospitals, physicians seemed the next likely target. As the *Congressional Quarterly Almanac* of 1983 put it, "there was a general sense that it was the doctors' 'turn' to accept some new limitations" (394).

By 1985 medical inflation in general had slowed. Hospital admissions also dropped as more care shifted to newer ambulatory settings, such as surgery centers. Though later research would question whether Medicare's new payment system (PPS) actually helped create the trend or merely benefitted from it, the shift from inpatient care raised alarms in the minds of some, who saw it as a threat to the quality of care. A brief investigation by the advocacy-oriented Senate Aging Committee concluded that "seriously ill Medicare patients are inappropriately and prematurely discharged from hospitals" (*CQA* 1985, 285). Hospital representatives responded that such charges were anecdotal and provided no evidence that the quality of care was falling or that prospective payment was creating a problem with quality (*CQA* 1985, 285). Despite news stories from time to time indicating that "quicker and sicker" discharges were occurring, Congress chose not to respond.

With yet another round of budget cuts required by the deficit reduction act, coupled with the imposition of both PPS and caps on physicians' fees, Congress now found itself squarely in the middle of deciding how much should be paid for various health care services. Some $3 billion had to be cut from Medicare and Medicaid for the coming fiscal year (*CQA* 1986, 256).

Nonetheless, both houses agreed to delay the implementation of the full brunt of PPS for another year, making myriad changes in the way hospitals were paid, inflation rates, special help for disproportionate share hospitals, and ordering HHS to go easier on home health, hospice, and other regulations (*CQA* 1986, 253). In a display of personal legislative prowess, Senate Finance Committee chair Robert Packwood (R–Ore.) persuaded his colleagues to exempt his state from the PPS extensions, because hospitals there had found PPS to their benefit and wanted to get on with its implementation.

While spending cuts were widely agreed to be necessary, they were often hard to support, with hometown providers and hospitals making personal appeals for leniency. Even House Republicans who demanded the elimination of the new spending proposals declined (with a few exceptions) to vote for them when given the chance (*CQA* 1986, 256). To raise revenues, the legislation cut supplemental payments to teaching hospitals for the next two fiscal years and set a per-capita payment rate for graduate medical education costs, rather than simply agreeing to pay costs, as had been past policy.

The president asked for further cuts in both Medicare and Medicaid in 1987. Weary of such thankless labor, House members balked before realizing that they really had few options, thanks to deficit-reduction targets. Of their work in the Ways and Means Committee, ranking Republican Willis Gradison from Ohio said after his committee agreed to cut hospital and physicians' payments in the coming year: "It was a budget-driven exercise pure and simple. . . . We did what we had to. I'd be the last one to try to justify each of these actions as being the right way to run Medicare" (*CQA* 1987, 562).

His comment did not describe the reality of how the cuts had pitted members who would normally support new spending against one another in a fight to protect their own district's interest. Ways and Means Health Subcommittee chair Stark had put his own state's interests aside to help craft a provision giving rural hospitals relief from what they felt was an unfair PPS effect: equipment and other nonlabor costs were set at rates that presumed steady, heavy use typical of only urban areas. Rural hospitals argued that they needed the same equipment but did not have the volume of patients to produce economies of scale. Stark gave rural hospitals special relief in his subcommittee bill.

Urban state representatives from Illinois, Michigan, California, and Massachusetts who sat on the full committee were not buying. Fuel and malpractice insurance were more expensive for urban hospitals, they argued (*CQA* 1987, 562). Compromises gave both types of districts a break on PPS rates and infused higher spending levels into urban disproportionate share hospitals and rural "swing-bed hospitals" (*CQA* 1987, 559). Swing beds are certified for both acute and long-term care, used as demand dictates. To offset the new costs, the committee cut special subsidies for teaching hospitals and increased the number of days physicians and hospitals had to wait to be paid their claims.

Stark scorned the compromises, saying they were crafted in ways designed simply to get votes and had nothing to do with good health policy. "Proponents were looking for ways to direct money into a few states. All hospitals get soaked a little to provide the transfers," he said (*CQA* 1987, 563). Three Congresses later, the game had not changed, only the players. Newly installed Senate Finance Committee chair Moynihan announced that the new protected class would be his state's teaching hospitals.

Physician Fee Controls

Both the House and Senate considered a six-month freeze on physicians' fees as part of the 1984 round of cuts. But no further action was taken on these recommendations, in large part because they would have increased beneficiary costs as physicians billed patients for the difference between what Medicare paid and their charges. Members had agreed earlier in their budget resolution not to do that. With this impediment removed the following year, both houses agreed to increased patient copayments, a freeze on physicians' payments to extend through October 1985, financial penalties for physicians who raised beneficiaries' copays, and a slowed rate of hospital cost increases (*CQA* 1984, 480). These measures were regarded as not fully adequate to save the trust fund, but it was an election year. Further cuts were unattractive (*CQA* 1984, 449).

The cap on physicians' fees was due to expire the next year. Unless Congress acted to stop them, payment rates would rise more than 3 percent with general medical inflation. Both House Ways and Means and Commerce Committees had hoped to take some savings from holding down increases when the caps expired, but members also wanted to encourage physicians to go easier on their patients' out-of-pocket expenses. Resolving substantial differences among the committees and between the houses, the caps were extended until the end of the year for physicians who did not "accept assignment" (that is, they charged patients above the Medicare-assigned rate), but the fee caps were removed on May 1 for those who accepted the Medicare payment as full payment (*CQA* 1986, 255).

While both houses debated Medicare catastrophic insurance reform in 1988, a report quietly came into HCFA in compliance with a study Congress had demanded four years earlier on the feasibility of using a relative value method to pay Medicare physicians (*CQA* 1988, 328). Though HCFA had funded the study, its current administrator, Bill Roper, did not support the idea that it endorsed. The report computed the input costs of physicians' education, office expenses, and other expenses within specialty groups and compared these specialty-to-specialty differences with Medicare payment differences. Its conclusion was that Medicare paid much more for technology-based medicine than for diagnosing and spending time with patients, even though input costs were not much different for specialists compared with internists and pediatricians. The study proposed adjusting payments to more evenly reflect input costs by lowering specialists' pay and raising generalists' pay. Roper opposed it because it had no volume controls and did not purport to cut expenditures, just redistribute them (*CQA* 1988, 329).

Congress decided to ignore the HCFA administrator. It moved quickly to hearings on a bill with three major features:

—a relative value-based fee schedule;

—a cap on utilization to prevent physicians from making up for lost revenue by delivering more services;

—limits on how much physicians who did not accept assignment could charge their patients.

Some physicians would be winners under RBRVS, while others would be losers, but all of them hated one aspect: volume controls. Several studies had suggested and others seemed to show rather conclusively that when physicians' fees were fixed, they found ways to pump up the volume. One approach was by "unbundling" services and charging separately for each. Another was to "induce" demand by suggesting that the patient needed to come back for something else (Rice and Labelle 1989). Physicians hated this interpretation. In their view, if they gave more than was needed, it was either because the patient demanded it or because they feared lawyers would sue them for malpractice if they did not do every test and give every treatment regardless of their own medical judgment.

House Ways and Means Health Subcommittee chair Stark had a simple view: "There is no control over what we pay physicians, and they are basically charging what the traffic will bear and getting away with it. That's not a good system" (*CQA* 1989, 158).

Volume controls would prevent a surge in use that could otherwise offset some or all of any reduction in prices. Volume controls meant that physicians who provided care beyond the limits would not be paid for it, or overall payments to all physicians would be cut by a like amount the following year. Members felt it was time to do something. Six years earlier they had adopted a revolution in hospital payment; now it was the physicians' turn—indeed, many felt it was quite late for their turn. The Ways and Means Health Subcommittee adopted (eleven to three) a package drafted by its chair, adding only a provision to intensify research into the effectiveness of various physician practices, later to be known as "medical outcomes research." The package included volume controls: next year's physicians' payments would drop to offset any amount by which aggregate targets were exceeded (*CQA* 1989, 161–62).

After two more weeks of closed-door sessions by the Ways and Means Committee, its contribution to the year's reconciliation bill included the physicians' fee package, a $3-billion cut in physicians' inflation adjustments, and a provision restricting their ability to refer patients to labs or other providers (except hospitals) in which they held a financial interest.

But Ways and Means was not the only player. While Congressman Waxman's Energy and Commerce Subcommittee agreed to most of the same provisions, members would not agree to expenditure targets. They would penalize the just as well as the unjust, Waxman said: physicians who had worked hard to meet patients' needs as well as those who had abused the system.

The Senate Finance Committee agreed that a fee schedule was needed and sought a compromise position between the two House committees on the volume control issue. Senate Finance Medicare and Long-Term Care Subcommittee chair John Rockefeller (D–W.Va.) pitched in with ranking Republican Dave Durenberger to forge a proposal. Their solution: phase the program in between 1991 and 1995. Both the AMA and the Bush administration agreed (*CQA* 1989, 166). The compromise also eased the limits on balance-billing (charges to the patient over what Medicare would pay), and most important for the AMA, the Finance Committee's compromise took discretion in fee setting away from HCFA. In the future, either Congress would adjust the increases in physicians' payment rates allowed under the fee schedule or a formula would automatically adjust them. Cynics would later note that one effect of keeping Congress in the loop would be to ensure AMA contributions to key members. The package also included relief for small hospitals.

While many health reforms of the 1980s were contained in the reconciliation acts, it appeared initially that the fee schedule would be an important exception to the trend. It was removed from the reconciliation bill in the Senate by a decision to strip nonsavings provisions from the bill. Because it was budget neutral, the RBRVS plan had to be removed because it saved no money—at least not in the near term. Left on its own, it seemed destined to die for lack of action on a compromise. Members credited Senator John Rockefeller with salvaging it. "He wouldn't take 'no' for an answer," Durenberger recalled (*CQA* 1989, 167). Rockefeller was told by his committee chair, Lloyd Bentsen, that the plan was "dead" and that he should "lay off it." "But I wasn't going to stand for it. It was ridiculous," Rockefeller said (*CQA* 1989, 167). Taking the bull by the horns, he called together a powerful rump group of conferees, staff, and the HCFA administrator and kept them there through the day and into the night and again three more times until they found a way to agree, eloquent testimony to the power of the determined policy entre preneur.

Waxman's Medicaid Mandates

Meanwhile, a historical first had occurred: the 1982 Medicaid rate of spend-ing increase fell as states used their new discretionary authority to limit eli-gibility and select lower-cost hospital providers (*CQA* 1982, 470). Some thought the 1981 cuts might have helped. Congress used the news to spurn President Reagan's request for more cuts.

Indeed, the House Energy and Commerce Health Subcommittee chair, Henry Waxman, had quite different ideas. Others could cut; he would ex-pand. Weary of watching comprehensive reform fail, he opted for an incre-mental approach using the tools at hand: the Medicaid program over which his subcommittee had jurisdiction. His first proposal was to expand cover-age to pregnant women and needy children. His subcommittee and commit-tee quickly complied, as did the Senate Finance Committee. But action stalled and died before reaching either floor (*CQA* 1983, 419).

He was not one to give up easily. The next year he prevailed in what would be the first of many eligibility expansions he would offer, first as an option, then, a year later, as a mandate, to state Medicaid programs before the states were able to stop his incremental approach to national health insurance. One of his greatest accomplishments was breaking the traditional link between Medicaid and welfare eligibility. By the early 1980s some states covered fewer than one-half of their residents who fell below the federal poverty line. Wax-man set a deliberate course toward a solution to this problem: mandating el-igibility for deserving groups that met or modestly exceeded federal poverty standards, thus subsidizing health care without adding to state welfare cash-assistance rolls. Because of the tie between welfare eligibility and Medicaid, states could expand Medicaid eligibility only with the undesired result of making more people eligible for welfare cash assistance. Waxman's efforts were intended to break that link.

Undeterred by President Reagan's requests for cuts, Waxman pressed on. His next proposal offered further expansion of coverage to children and mothers higher on the near-poverty scale as well as to older children. Sub-stantial changes were also made to extend the period during which individ-uals whose incomes rose above welfare limits could continue to receive Med-icaid. Waxman wanted it extended from six to eighteen months, plus another eighteen months at state option, and he wanted the income ceiling raised to

185 percent of poverty before these extended benefits would be lost. Additional discretion was granted to states to provide home- and community-based care services, further permitting them to incur new total spending, which had previously been severely limited by HCFA's interpretation of earlier versions of the provision.

In Medicare Part B, Waxman offered redefinitions intended to subtly expand the eligibility for various services, such as the Medicare definition of homebound. In the 1987 Omnibus Budget Reconciliation Act, he added language to allow home health coverage to beneficiaries who could leave the home for short periods. Previously, such individuals would have been ineligible. These improvements—add-ons in terms of cost—were in addition to the full package of nursing home quality-assurance provisions that he included in the same bill. The full Energy and Commerce Committee approved the subcommittee's proposals largely intact, as did the House after differences with Ways and Means were resolved (CQA 1987, 563).

Senators balked, however, over the cost. One staffer said that the Congress "looked silly" spending money it did not have (CQA 1987, 558). In conference negotiations with the White House, the Democratic Senators sided with the Republican administration to contain Waxman. Senate Finance Committee chair Bentsen said "we have to meet the realities of the budget" (CQA 1987, 558).

The situation highlights some key differences in partisanship and ideology of the House and Senate members. House members, notably Democrats Waxman, Stark, and Dingell, fought long and hard for their programs and accused the Senate Democrats of selling out to the Republican White House and OMB. The House members distrusted the OMB budget numbers, best expressed by Representative John Dingell, who said "no one around here with any brains at all trusts OMB, because they lie and cook figures" (CQA 1987, 566). Senators felt bound to abide by recent budget summit agreements to cut $2 billion from Medicare and Medicaid. Waxman disagreed, saying that he had not been party to the budget summit and could therefore ignore it (CQA 1987, 567). He was the last to relent, managing in the final days to retain the provisions relating to pregnant women and to children, a shorter extension of coverage during periods of ineligibility, liberalization of home- and community-based services, and a few other provisions. He was also able to keep a number of Medicare add-ons, while Stark and other House members were able to exclude a Senate provision raising the Part B deductible by $10 annually.

Stark was not gracious in this small victory, however. "Those dim bulbs in the Senate won't accept that rising Part B costs are due to greedy doctors," he said. "They think they're due to greedy beneficiaries" (CQA 1987, 567).

When the dust settled, the conference had cut $500 million more than had been promised at the budget summit. Most of it came from cuts in physicians' and hospitals' payments and the extension of a temporary requirement that one-quarter of Part B costs be borne by beneficiaries (*CQA* 1987, 563, 567). A GAO report summed up the cuts with an almost confirming conclusion: "Reagan-inspired Medicare cuts made by Congress between 1981 and 1985 avoided new Medicare spending of $13 billion from the $81 billion program. But beneficiary costs went up by 49 percent for hospitals and 31 percent for physicians during the same period" (*CQA* 1987, 558).

Despite tremendous pressures to cut spending, Waxman again succeeded in including in the 1989 reconciliation package more Medicaid mandates, making this the fifth straight year that he had succeeded in slipping into reconciliation bills important expansions of Medicaid coverage of poor and near-poor mothers and children.

His success reflected his persistence and knowledge of the technical details of the programs under his committee's jurisdiction. In expertise, he found power. But there was no denying that part of his success was because other key members agreed with him. Allies in his effort included Bentsen, Senator Bill Bradley (D–N.J.), conservative, antiabortionist Representative Henry Hyde (R–Ill.), and others (*CQA* 1989, 172). Several problems seemed to be focusing their efforts:

—the persistently high infant mortality rate, making this country rank near some underdeveloped nations in infant survival rate;

—equity concerns: the feeling that near-poor people who worked were worse off than welfare recipients because the welfare recipient could qualify for Medicaid while the working poor mother was disenfranchised;

—state-to-state differences in Medicaid coverage of poor people;

—declining rates of Medicaid eligibility among the nation's poor people because states chose not to raise their welfare income eligibility standards to keep up with inflation;

—a view of Medicaid expansion as a feasible strategy for moving toward greater access for some children even if it could not be accomplished for all through national health insurance;

—the fact that the Medicaid program is means tested and limited to the very poor;

—until this point, opposition from only one interest group, the nation's governors, which had been rather tardy in turning to the effort and not yet effective.

In short, the problem met the criteria for success (Kingdon 1984):

—it was well defined, with numbers and good examples;
—it was widespread and severe but not so widespread or severe that it was a budget buster;
—the problem, but not the solution, offended many members' sense of fairness;
—it was a salient problem but using Medicaid as the solution made the debate complex and not at all salient;
—the solution was clearly technically feasible and ready to go legislatively;
—it had limited opposition from interest groups;
—it had a powerful, persistent, savvy, well-placed, and determined entrepreneur pushing it who happened to be chair of a key health subcommittee and was well supported in the effort by the other key committee and subcommittee chairs.

Furthermore, members of both parties could claim, and they did, that Republican presidential candidate George Bush had endorsed the expansion of Medicaid (*CQA* 1989, 172). No need to mention that his endorsement was offered as an alternative to broader health care reform.

The party finally ended the next year. What had become known as the "Waxman wedge" was finally blunted as the governors were able to marshal their power and present intense opposition. "There was literally an eruption of concern from governors from every part of the country and every place on the political spectrum," said Ohio Governor Richard Celeste, a Democrat (*CQA* 1989, 174).

Flexing their political muscle (combined with the increased budget consciousness on the Hill), governors garnered the support of Republicans, budget committee members, and the Senate Finance Committee, including its chair, Lloyd Bentsen, who abandoned his earlier support for higher income eligibility levels in favor of 133 percent of the federal poverty line. "I think the states deserve time to catch-up," he said (*CQA* 1989, 175). The catch-up period would stretch on indefinitely as the Clinton reform plan displaced other health reform efforts, died, and moved off the national policy agenda as the Republicans' budget-cutting "Contract with America" took center stage.

Cost Control in Perspective

Cost control first became a federal concern in the late 1960s, only a few years after the enactment of Medicare and Medicaid. Health planning, regulation, and incentive strategies were all tried and most continue in some form. Global budgets to control overall spending, such as those used by Japan and other countries with national health care systems, have only recently been introduced as a policy solution here. They were quickly rejected from the initial version of the Clinton national health reform plan. Reminiscent of PPS and RBRVS, their gestation period is likely to be quite long and to require major developments in the political stream to overcome opposition by interest groups.

Politically, cost-control policies are difficult to enact. The public (as President Carter found, to his dismay) is simply not engaged on the issue. In contrast, interest groups representing those whose "ox will be gored" are highly energized and well organized to fight the proposal.

In health, Gramm-Rudman-Hollings and other budget targets have become a major factor in cost cutting—forcing the Congress to look at where the money is, mainly Medicare and Medicaid—often forcing them to come up with new ideas and approaches that might have been ignored without the budget constraint. Under Gramm-Rudman-Hollings, spending had to be cut to avoid triggering automatic cuts in spending. Under later budget agreements, new spending had to be offset by new cuts or new taxes, while deficit-reduction targets and new definitions of baseline spending levels adopted by Republicans who took over the House caused reluctant Democrats to cut Medicaid and increase Medicare beneficiary out-of-pocket spending. Usually those actions were aimed at cutting hospitals' and physicians' payments. In lean years, when cuts were required, they came first as fee and rate limitations and next as major reforms directed at changing the incentive structure of hospital payments and the specialty preference in physicians' payments. When budget developments permitted, reduction targets were relaxed and delayed.

Opposition by provider interest groups has been generally ineffective in avoiding cuts when spending-cut targets demanded them, but they have been quite successful in delaying implementation. Constituents' interests have dictated which provider subgroup cuts would be treated as worthy of special protection. High-volume urban and low-volume rural hospitals for many years enjoyed protection of powerful committee chairs, pressing the interests of their districts during conference committee negotiations. Teaching hospitals in New York were protected for as long as their powerful senator could fend off critics.

National Health Insurance

Ideological concerns are a big part of the reason the national health insurance problem remains unresolved. Though every president of the past five decades has wanted to pass one form or another of national health insurance, more often than not, they have had to ask for less than they wanted, accept defeat, or accept major compromises to try to pass something, or all three. Many of the same proposals prominently featured in any current debate have formed the essence of offerings going back five decades or more. Table 7.1 highlights how many of the same solutions have been debated (and discarded) with some regularity since the 1970s, and some much earlier.

Democrats tend to favor comprehensive change. Their proposals typically include universal coverage; mandatory participation; a full range of benefits, including mental health, prescription drugs, and long-term care; publicly formed insurance risk pools and public administration through a national board or regional boards that set budgets, pool risks, and purchase insurance; community rating to equalize premiums; no means testing; portability; noncancelability; very limited waiting periods; small business incentives; employer mandates and payroll and sin-tax financing; fee schedules; spending caps; and quality-assurance monitoring agencies.

Republicans prefer incremental proposals typically offering voluntary participation, voluntary risk pools with subsidies to states to form pools for those at high risk, means testing, substantial copayments or catastrophic coverage, and a limited range of benefits.

Provider and other interest groups play a major role in shaping the debate. The AMA wants public coverage limited to the poor. Insurance companies want their industry preserved. Business, especially small business, opposes employer mandates. Labor opposes copayments, larger premium shares, taxation of benefits, and other measures intended to raise price consciousness and encourage prudent buying. Hospitals oppose budget caps or limits on rate of expenditure growth. HMOs oppose global budgets limiting growth of health spending as a percentage of the gross domestic product (GDP).

NHI proposals typically violate one or more aspects of political feasibility. Proponents often argue for a large role for government by demanding mandatory participation, taking over the insurance function, and failing to means test. They invoke interest groups' ire by saddling business with premiums and paperwork and providers with prospects of lowered income and reduced discretion in their caregiving operations. NHI proposals are very expensive while promising only limited improvement in the breadth of cov-

Table 7.1. Features of Major NHI Proposal, 1940s–90s

	'40s	'50s	'60s	'70s	'80s	'90s
Eligibility						
Means tested	x	x	x	x	x	x
Elderly only		x	x	x	x	x
All ages	x			x	x	x
Coverage						
Hospital surgical costs of the aged	x	x	x	x	x	x
Long-term care		x	x	x	x	x
Mental health			x	x	x	x
Physician's fees	x	x	x	x	x	x
Prescription drugs				x	x	x
Mammograms						x
Preventive primary care				x	x	x
Catastrophic care			x	x	x	x
Lab	x				x	x
Dental	x					
Alcohol treatment and drug abuse treatment				x	x	x
Ambulatory				x	x	x
Medical equipment			x	x	x	x
Outpatient drugs			x	x	x	x
X-rays	x	x	x	x	x	x
Immunization			x	x	x	x
Pre/post natal care			x	x	x	x
Well child exams			x	x	x	x
Obstetrics and gynecology			x	x	x	x
Family planning			x	x	x	x
Hospice care				x	x	x
Financing						
Payroll tax			x	x	x	x
General revenues			x	x	x	x
Sin taxes						x
Employee mandate				x		x
Beneficiary cross-subsidies					x	
Expand Medicare, Medicaid eligibility						x
Mandate employers to cover laid-off workers and families					x	
Mandate employers to provide coverage to workers				x	x	x
Individual mandate with subsidies for poor						x
Social Security system	x	x	x	x		
States with federal help	x	x	x	x	x	x
Increased payroll taxes	x	x	x	x	x	x
Joint employee-employer contributions			x	x	x	x

Table 7.1. *(cont.)*

	'40s	'50s	'60s	'70s	'80s	'90s
Risk pooling						
Relax antitrust to encourage pools			x		x	
Subsidize voluntary pools			x		x	
Require insurance companies to join			x		x	
Mandate community rating			x		x	
Prohibit refusals, cancellations			x		x	
Sponsor state insurance pools			x		x	
Cost controls						
25 to 50 percent employee premium contribution					x	x
Higher copays for "fee-for-service" care					x	x
Purchasing cooperatives						x
Global budgets					x	x
Health individual retirement savings accounts						x
Managed competition						x
HMOs				x	x	x
National health care board						x
Administration						
Federal SSA, independent SSA	x	x	x	x	x	x
Private insurance		x	x	x	x	x
State				x	x	x
National advisory board				x	x	x
New public agency				x		
Incentives to possible financing sources						
Big business: government responsible for retirees, copays					x	x
Small business: phase-in, subsidize copays					x	x
States: Medicaid flexibility				x	x	x

Source: Compiled from proposal descriptions and debates chronicled in *Congressional Quarterly Almanac,* 1945–95.

erage of most Americans and a less-than-complete solution to the problems of the poor and uninsured. Because the many features of the health care system are interactive, proposals are complex and tend to involve major change and high downside risks if cost estimates or behavioral impacts are wrong. Many of the mechanisms included are untested and, to all but those schooled in health policy, unfamiliar. The issue is salient, but most reporters and television commentators have no clue about it and must pass through a bewilderment stage before catching on to the issues well enough to inform the public.

The longer the debate drags on, the more interest groups figure out the changes they need made in the proposal to avoid losses or gain benefits. Interests without Washington, D.C., representation scramble to hire somebody or reassign someone to head an office. Old hands at the AMA, the insurance lobbies, and the hospital associations share information and point out problems to newcomers to broaden the base of opposition. Members start hearing from constituent groups that will be hurt. Ad campaigns are mounted to scare the public. Naive presidential staff who slaved over the details of the proposal, often thinking they had figured out ways to win supporters, are shocked at the high level of intensity. They call for members to stand up to the lobbies and are surprised when the nature of the debate turns to personal criticism of presidential political ineptitude. Compromises spurned earlier now cannot be struck. The next election looms, PAC money flows, the parties stake out their differences and lay aside hopes of compromise.

All this ugliness is reasonable if one considers some underlying truths: the parties have real differences over how they view the role of government in health care; powerful interests have much to lose; the system is so complex that there is no real agreement on what will work; the stakes are so high that norms of expertise and reciprocity break down; though many of the ideas are old, they are new to most members; and the public has little sustained interest in expensive, comprehensive reform. They tend to equally value fairer health care and lower taxes.

The nature of an NHI debate can be understood by answering the following questions:

—What will the role of government be in insurance risk pooling and participation requirements, bureaucratic administration, and provider price and practice controls?
—Who will pay the costs?
—Will there be means testing?
—How comprehensive and expensive will the plan be?
—How close is the next election?
—How large is the president's political capital?

These questions serve as the organizing framework for analyzing the roughly six decades of NHI history in the United States.

What Will the Role of Government Be?

The Roosevelt-Truman Era. Liberals started a half-century ago with their most expensive proposal: Social Security would collect money from payroll taxes, pool risks equally by charging no premium regardless of health status, set payment rates, and pay the bills—in today's argot, a single-payer system with community rating. These were the plans of early reformer groups as well as Presidents Roosevelt and Truman, though Roosevelt's was never actually introduced. These proposals offended conservative ideologies on every possible front.

Conservatives, appalled at the prospect of that much governmental control, quickly dubbed it socialism. When President Truman offered his Social Security–based plan, an organization said to be funded by the American Medical Association distributed 25 million propaganda leaflets, some featuring a copy of the classic painting of a devoted physician sitting at the bedside of a sick child with the caption "Do you want the Government in this picture?" (Anderson 1990, 118). Though fear of governmental interference in their business and possible loss of income were probably paramount concerns of the AMA, it is also clear from the debate that this largely conservative group had strong ideological opposition to an expanded federal role in health care.

Conservatives, tending to rely on the private sector, felt in Truman's time that the private sector would handle the job. Blue Cross plans reported, perhaps with some exaggeration, that they had enrolled 20 million members in forty-three states by 1946 (Anderson 1990; Harris 1966). Other plans gained footholds in some states, and some believe that 40 percent of the population was covered by hospital insurance by 1948 (Anderson 1990), though some are now skeptical of the numbers (Harris 1966). While Congress sat on pending health insurance legislation, voluntary health insurance became the "backbone of health services funding" (Anderson 1990, 139).

The Eisenhower and Nixon Administrations. Republican President Dwight Eisenhower tried to solve the problem of insuring high-risk enrollees with government-run risk-pooling schemes. Government would sell "reinsurance" protection against catastrophic claims to private insurance companies. House members rejected his plan by a vote approaching two to one in a debate that teamed conservatives, who opposed it as creeping socialism, with liberals, who charged that it was not enough. Two years after the reinsurance plan was rejected, a more humble effort aimed at the same problem was also unsuccessful. It would have legislated permission for small businesses to enter into risk pools without fear of antitrust prosecution (Anderson 1990). It too was defeated.

Under President Nixon's 1971 plan, states would administer risk pools and private insurance companies would sell insurance with federal supervision. PSROs would review claims and quality. Providers would be paid "reasonable charges" but physicians could bill patients extra. Medicare would be continued (*CQA* 1971).

A competing proposal offered by Massachusetts Democratic Senator Edward Kennedy and Michigan Democratic Representative Martha Griffiths proposed a single-payer system. Private insurance companies would have no role. A national board would administer the plan through regional offices, which would review records for quality. Medicare would be abolished, and Medicaid would pay for only services not included in the national plan (*CQA* 1971).

The debate surrounding the two proposals brought into focus the ideological difference between the parties over the role of government versus the private sector when it came to the administration of the insurance function. Of his plan, President Nixon said, "There simply is no need to eliminate an entire segment of our private economy and at the same time add a multibillion-dollar responsibility to the federal budget" (*CQA* 1971, 543). Kennedy disagreed: "I do not believe we can afford the health insurance industry in this country—nor do I believe we have any responsibility to maintain it at the public's expense now that its failure is apparent" (*CQA* 1971, 543).

In revisions over the next several years, Senator Kennedy substantially curtailed the role of the federal government in his national health insurance plans, though still not enough for conservatives. His 1978 bill would have established a public authority in charge of a mixed public, highly regulated private system. State agencies would implement the system as contractors to the public authority. A benefits package would be mandated and employers would pay most of the cost for employees and dependents. His bill related premiums to wages rather than health history, thereby inherently mandating community rating. Enrollment would be open and without regard to preexisting conditions. Industry risk pooling for reinsurance would be encouraged to protect against catastrophic costs of some patients. The federal government would pay for unemployed or elderly persons. Budgets would be fixed annually through negotiation among the major players (1978).

The AMA complimented Kennedy on the features of his revised plan, including the preservation of a role for private insurance, but said nonetheless that it would still mean rationed care, poor quality, and bureaucratic waste.

The Carter Administration. The Democratic Carter administration followed a more conservative line, offering only catastrophic coverage. Full-time employees and their families would be covered by employer-provided health plans meeting federal standards. Private insurers would market an employer's plan and a public plan for elderly, disabled, or poor people under federal regulations. The federal government would administer only the public plan. To raise price consciousness and control costs, tax deductions for insurance premiums would be dramatically cut.

The Reagan and Bush Administrations. A much more ambitious plan somewhat reminiscent of Eisenhower's efforts to form reinsurance risk pools passed the House after an effort led by Ways and Means Health Subcommittee chair Stark in 1986. It required states to set up risk pools to offer insurance to chronically ill and other "uninsurable" individuals. Six states already had such pools, and four others had put legislation on the books but had not yet implemented it. The plans would be allowed to charge premiums no more than 50 percent over the average premium for similar insurable clients in the state. Employers of twenty or more would be mandated to make up any deficits suffered by the risk pool or pay a 5-percent excise tax. Opposition by the business community defeated the proposal in the Senate and in conference, including a compromise offered by conferee Stark merely to form the pools.

Republican President Bush expressly sought to minimize public administration by relying on a voucher system for low-income people based on tax credits and tax deductions for middle-income earners. States would be encouraged to design innovative delivery systems and establish networks of small business groups to reduce the cost of administration (1992).

The Clinton Administration. Despite the continued lack of success of public or quasi-public administration of the insurance function, President Clinton's plan took many of the features of Kennedy's plan, including its name, a national board to set global budgets to be administered by the states, and health alliances to collect premiums, risk adjust the premiums, and purchase health insurance from private insurers on consumers' behalf.

His plan made community rating its central selling point: health alliances would collect equal premiums from all enrollees but would pay risk-adjusted premiums to insurance companies on their enrollees' behalf. The realization that young enrollees would pay more than their expected costs while older, higher-risk enrollees would pay less led some to ask how young people could be induced to enroll once the mandatory aspect of the proposal was dropped as negotiators sought compromise on the major sticking points. If young and healthy people dropped out, reaching the target of 95-percent coverage by early in the next century would seem to defy technical feasibility. Moreover, experience in New York State showed that voluntary plans actually performed according to theory: sick people enrolled, well people departed, and the percentage of the eligible population enrolled actually declined (Clymer 1994).

Negative reaction to President Clinton's proposed health alliances was swift and fierce. Conservative critics charged that there would be fifty or more new bureaucracies wielding unlimited power. Clinton officials responding to these criticisms quickly modified the scope of the alliances' responsibilities to essentially a clearinghouse function and greatly expanded the number of firms for which participation would be voluntary. It had initially been mandatory for firms with 5,000 or more employees. Congressional modifications made it voluntary for firms of only 100 or more employees. The insurance industry led the charge against the Clinton plan in part because it expected adverse effects on small insurers. Because they could not exclude high-risk clients, they would need the protection of very large numbers of enrollees, a situation that seemed to favor large companies.

Republican proposals in the next Congress emphasized self-paid health savings funds involving no risk sharing at all.

Who Will Pay the Costs?

Paying for national health insurance invariably falls to one of two groups: businesses (through a governmental mandate or another form of taxation) and taxpayers in general (usually through a payroll tax, such as Medicare supplemented by sin taxes, or taxation of health insurance premiums). In the 1980s a catastrophic health insurance plan for elderly people tried a third approach: it taxed wealthy beneficiaries of the program to pay some of the costs of poorer beneficiaries. The law was repealed the following year as those who were targeted to pay complained of the cost for the value received.

Employer Mandates. When business is targeted, the mechanism is employer mandates. President Nixon, a Republican, was the first president to propose an employer-employee mandate: he suggested employers pay 75 percent, employees 25 percent. Though voluntary for employees, it was mandatory for employers. Federal subsidies would be provided for firms with up to ten workers. The National Association of Manufacturers opposed the plan, saying that health insurance coverage should be left to the collective bargaining process.

When Ways and Means Committee chair Wilbur Mills tried to pass a compromise version of the Nixon bill through his committee, he worked the members through the first dozen provisions, which drew most heavily from the administration bill but took bits and pieces from other bills. Things seemed to be going well. Then he got to the employer mandate, and the committee began to splinter. An AMA means-tested plan with no employer mandate failed, twelve to twelve. Finally, a committee-staff-designed, employer-employee financed, compulsory plan passed by one vote. But Mills would have no part of it, refusing to take to the floor anything that had passed by such a narrow margin.

As the 1970s closed, long-time Senate Finance Committee chair Russell Long also tried his hand at legislating employer-based financing. He first proposed a plan that gave small employers a 50-percent rebate on their premiums, fined employers who did not provide coverage, and required that coverage extend to dependents and workers up to six months after employment. By the following year, he was forced to scale back his proposal to only tax credits for small businesses that voluntarily provided catastrophic coverage, expansion of the existing Medicaid program, and reduction of cost-sharing for Medicare skilled-nursing care. Even that scaled-down bill failed.

Employer-mandate provisions passed Senator Kennedy's committee again in 1988 and 1989. Votes during the committee's consideration of the 1988 bill were instructive for future efforts to use employer mandates to finance national health insurance. The sixteen-member committee split: nine Democrats in favor to seven Republicans against reporting the bill. President Reagan's HHS secretary, Otis Bowen, opposed the idea, saying it would "open the door to broad new federal regulation of the private health-care sector, exacerbate health-care inflation, and upset settled wage and benefit arrangements" (1988, 314).

The proposal, strongly opposed by small business and the U.S. Chamber of Commerce, died without going to the Senate floor. "A majority of our members would oppose mandated minimum benefits on philosophical grounds," a Chamber of Commerce spokesperson commented (CQA 1988, 317), even though, he agreed, it would probably benefit them. Liberal Republican Senator Lowell Weicker said small business "doesn't want a bill. Period. Over and out" (CQA 1988, 317). Kennedy argued that his current bill was very similar to Republican President Nixon's proposal (which Kennedy had rejected as too little), but Republicans would have no part in supporting the mandate provision. It was too fiercely hated by the business community.

President Clinton boldly ignored the sullied history of the employer mandate, calling in his 1993 proposal for employers to cover 75 percent of the cost of a standard health policy. While some provider groups, such as hospitals and physicians, welcomed the employer mandate, others, especially small businesses, targeted the mandate as something akin to the devil himself taking control of their businesses. They worked to defeat it in the House Commerce Committee, succeeding so well that the bill died there without even the dignity of a vote. (Not surprisingly, the states too have had difficulty encouraging business to provide health insurance. See Chapter 5.)

Tax Increases. In August 1974 Gerald Ford, newly installed as president after Richard Nixon's resignation, said in a congressional address, "Why don't we write . . . a good health bill on the statute books before Congress adjourns?" (*CQA* 1974, 391). But he quickly changed his mind. Worried about inflation and the newly discovered federal deficit, and reluctant to raise taxes, President Ford asked that no new federal programs be enacted, officially abandoning support for health insurance legislation.

A year later (1975), faced with high unemployment, the House Ways and Means Committee passed legislation to insure unemployed workers by mandating companies to provide extended coverage to ex-employees. This too soon died. The Ways and Means Committee funded its 1979 proposal for insurance coverage of the unemployed with a 1-percent payroll tax. It was not popular in the Senate, however, where Finance Committee chair Russell Long eliminated it, preferring to tap savings in Medicare and Medicaid. Long would later propose revenues from liquor or cigarette taxes to pay for his own program for the unemployed.

Another way taxpayers can be forced to contribute is through taxing the value of health insurance premiums provided by employers, either in full or over some threshold premium value. This form of financing is appealing economically because in addition to raising money, it can make consumers more aware of their health care costs in a way that might help restrain spending. President Carter's 1979 proposal would have eliminated most of the middle class's tax deduction for health insurance, and proposals floated by President Bush would have similarly taxed some portion of the health insurance premium for many Americans.

The initial version of President Clinton's plan would have taxed as income employer-paid health benefits above a standard benefits package, but labor objected. The proposal was then modified to phase in the tax on only benefits won under new labor agreements, but labor again objected, and this major source of financing (not to mention strategy for creating consumer awareness of price) was dropped.

Another financing scheme considered in the late 1980s was targeted at a special group of taxpayers—those who would benefit from the program and who could afford to pay. But that plan did not work so well either.

It began at the urging of HHS Secretary Bowen. President Reagan agreed to support his idea for insurance to cover the catastrophic costs of hospital and nursing home care for elderly people—costs above Medicare's lifetime limits for hospitals and those beyond the 100 days of skilled nursing home care covered by Medicare. President Reagan endorsed the idea in two State of the Union addresses. Long-term care costs quickly proved to be too expensive, however, and were dropped from the proposal, except for an education effort to make seniors realize that their Medigap insurance did not cover it. When junior members tried to add more extensive long-term care coverage during committee markup, Democratic subcommittee chair Pete Stark and ranking Republican Willis Gradison said such benefits would make the proposal unaffordable. There was simply no money for such costly coverage. "Let's not ruin the good with the perfect," Stark said (*CQA* 1987, 495). The bill left committee with only minimal long-term care changes, including the removal of the three-day hospital stay required for nursing home coverage and an increase in covered nursing home days from 100 to 150 per episode.

Administration estimates for nursing home and home-care services sought by elderly or disabled people were $60 billion for the first five years (*CQA* 1988). While support among the public ran high in the polls, so did support for cutting the deficit. "It's going to take time to put together a program that will satisfy not only those it will benefit, but those who will have to pay the bill," said a Democratic senator's aide (*CQA* 1988, 295). "Any big spending program is going to be hard to sell, even if it's self-financed. These guys may find themselves all dressed up with no place to go," Ways and Means Committee chair Dan Rostenkowski said (*CQA* 1988, 295).

When catastrophic coverage finally passed, without the long-term care provision, it was financed by beneficiary premiums and increased taxes on those elderly whose income was high enough to incur taxes. This blatant redistribution from well-to-do elderly to less-well-off elderly persons was complex enough to pass unnoticed for a time, but eventually seniors took notice. The new 101st Congress had barely begun when in January 1989 members started making it known that they were seriously rethinking passage of catastrophic health insurance. House Republicans, in particular, had gotten enough flak from constituents to feel they had made a mistake. Grass-roots organizers pushed elderly people to demand relief from what they were told were onerous, $800 increases in their Medicare premiums, though in reality only the highest-income elderly people would pay those top premiums. Many of those misled by the anticatastrophic campaign would, in fact, have paid none of the "supplemental" premium, since it was estimated to fall on only 40 percent of beneficiaries (*CQA* 1989, 149).

As the year wore on, members were besieged by complaints about the new law. A peak event was network news coverage of Chairman Rostenkowski surrounded in his car by angry senior citizens, one of whom flung herself over the windshield. Though later, more sober analysis showed that she was almost certainly among the 60 percent who would get new benefits while paying very little extra, she had been told otherwise and believed it.

Monday-morning quarterbacks gave a variety of explanations for the sorry fix in which members found themselves. "Seniors . . . resent paying twice for the same benefits, or paying for benefits they don't want or need," said one (*CQA* 1989, 149–50). "We did too much all at once, and we decided we were going to charge them for it," said another (*CQA* 1989, 150). "The most prevalent misconception about the bill is that everyone was going to pay the $800," said another (*CQA* 1989, 150).

A fifteen-hour meeting among some of the major power brokers on the conference found no way out. "I tell you with some sadness that we should vote for repeal," a subdued Waxman conceded (*CQA* 1989, 156). Senate Finance Committee chair Bentsen agreed and eventually recommended outright repeal of all but the Waxman Medicaid provisions. Both Houses quickly signed on in an overwhelming repeal vote.

Politicians and reporters began to talk about health care reform as "the third rail: touch it and you die."

Will the Proposal Be Means Tested?

The Kennedy-Johnson Era. Liberals have tended to favor health reform that does not charge premiums to the beneficiaries but instead relies on a broadly financed system that provides health care as if it were a right citizens should be able to expect from their society. Conservatives have felt that those who could pay should pay, reserving full subsidy for only very poor people; as a corollary, government should target its involvement in the financing and management of health care to only those groups that could not fend for themselves through the private market.

The American Medical Association is a case in point. After its initial 1940s revulsion against any kind of governmental role in paying for health care, a decade later the AMA joined with the American Hospital Association to put forward a recommendation for a limited role for government. In a 1959 joint resolution, the two groups pledged that they would "mobilize their full resources to accelerate the development of adequately financed health care programs for needy persons, especially the aged needy" (Anderson 1990, 163). True to their word, when just such a program was introduced by Ways and Means Committee chair Wilbur Mills and in the Senate by Robert Kerr (D–Okla.), it was supported by the AMA and other conservatives and was signed into law by President Eisenhower without controversy. It came to be known as the Kerr-Mills program and was later modified to become Medicaid. As Kerr-Mills, it offered block grants to the states to help them pay for health care for poor people.

As hearings began on Medicare in 1964, the AMA, AHA, U.S. Chamber of Commerce, Blue Cross/Blue Shield, the major for-profit nursing home association, and others all testified against Medicare, citing in particular its lack of means testing. AMA President Dr. Edward R. Annis strongly supported means testing, saying that there is "no justification for the use of tax dollars collected from workers at the low end of the income scale to pay these expenses for the entire elderly population, including the self-supporting and the wealthy" (*CQA* 1964, 233). He, with most other conservative groups, supported instead the expansion of the state-federal Kerr-Mills program, noting that it had provided one-half billion dollars in benefits in 1962 and would soon be operational in forty states and territories.

Medicare did eventually pass without means testing over fierce Republican objection, emerging from the House by a comfortable 313–115 vote but only after a narrower victory (191–236) over a means-tested Republican version of the AMA plan. Had not the Democrats held an extraordinary majority, the bill would have been means tested or died.

The Kerr-Mills program was expanded to permit near-poor individuals to subtract from their income what they spent on health care to help them meet the poverty definition, and it was renamed Medicaid. It was a means-tested program, even for elderly people, paying Medicare premiums, deductibles, and copayments for poor elderly who could not afford them.

The Nixon and Carter Administrations. When the national health insurance debate heated up again a decade later under President Nixon, the AMA still wanted a targeted, means-tested program but had expanded its perspective to support coverage of those who incurred catastrophic costs of health care: "The AMA strongly favors a system of private, medical insurance for everyone—for the poor at no cost, for others at a cost related to income. The organization supports insurance for everyone against the financially catastrophic cost of a protracted illness" (*CQA* 1971, 549).

President Nixon's 1971 proposal required beneficiaries to pay one-quarter of their premiums and a $100 annual deductible per person. Low-income families would pay less, and poor people would pay nothing. Physicians could bill patients extra. The rival Kennedy-Griffiths bill required no cost sharing and no means testing. Kennedy's 1978 version also made few demands on patients' pockets. Nothing passed.

President Carter tried to strike a compromise. His 1979 plan began its coverage only after a deductible of $2,500 plus part of premiums. Poor people, disabled people, and workers who received comprehensive coverage from their employers would have the deductible or most of it met for them.

Senator Kennedy criticized the Carter administration plan's deductible as "too harsh" and his subsidies for poor people as supporting "separate but unequal" care for those privately versus publicly insured. Yet he too showed substantial movement toward the conservative position on means testing. His revised 1979 plan would charge wage-adjusted premiums with employees paying up to 35 percent. President Carter's spokespeople called Kennedy's plan "a potential $200 billion-a-year pork barrel" that would raise employer costs by 80 percent (*CQA* 1979, 540).

The Clinton Administration. President Clinton tried to pick a middle ground on the means-testing issue by charging employees 25 percent of premiums, copayments if they used a fee-for-service plan, and reduced tax deductibility of premiums. Low-income individuals would be subsidized. As prospects for the president's bill looked dimmer and dimmer, Senator Kennedy—a supporter of the Clinton plan and from whose earlier bills the 25-percent employee premium contribution had come—suggested that the employee's share be raised to 50 percent, with employers providing the remainder.

Over the course of fifty years, the Democratic position, now personified by Senator Kennedy, had moved from no premiums or copays to subsidies for poor people only and 50-percent premiums for employees along with nontrivial copayments. This was twice the employee premium suggested by Republican President Nixon two decades earlier. Meanwhile, however, many Republicans had moved not only to means testing but also to medical savings accounts or self-financed savings plans for employees. Compromise proved out of the question.

How Comprehensive and Expensive Is the Proposal?

National health insurance reform proposals of the past fifty years have been both incremental and comprehensive, although, of the two, the incremental changes are clearly the more successful. The only major comprehensive health insurance proposal to pass was Medicare in 1965, possible only with strong political will and a large number of Democrats. Other proposals sponsored by key health legislators and presidents have tended to be scaled back and finally abandoned.

Following President Ford's change of heart on national health insurance, Democrats pinned their hopes on President Carter, but he surprised them by advocating incrementalism. It is time to give up "rigid" demands, he called them, for "all or nothing at all" and "rise above differences that have created . . . stalemate" for thirty years "and act now" (*CQA* 1979, 537). His efforts to pass a catastrophic-coverage-only bill were stymied by Senator Kennedy, who insisted on a comprehensive bill.

Expanding the scope of benefits helped lead to repeal of catastrophic coverage when it did pass ten years later under President Reagan. For a time, ideological differences appeared to have been set aside as the Democratically controlled Ways and Means Health Subcommittee moved to pass a catastrophic costs bill offered by President Reagan. The bill's most prominent feature was its innovative, progressive financing strategy—charging well-to-do beneficiaries more than those less well off (1986). The full committee made it even more explicitly progressive. Efforts to add a variety of new types of coverage had been mostly battled off, though a few items had been added. A major ideological hurdle had been surmounted as the proposal went through conference. Democrats and Republicans were making common cause to pass a means-tested, targeted, catastrophic version of national health insurance that would be self-financed and limited in scope.

The Democrats could not stand it. Speaker of the House Jim Wright (D–Tex.) told his House Democratic caucus colleagues that adding a drug benefit would "put a Democratic stamp" on the legislation (*CQA* 1987, 495). In a last-minute twenty-four to twelve partisan split, Democrats on the committee added a prescription drug benefit to the bill, over near-unanimous Republican objection.

But the drug benefit was expensive. It could be afforded only by phasing in its implementation while beginning the collection of the new premium immediately. Seniors saw their premiums and taxes going up with little to show for it. They were outraged and ultimately killed the program. The Democratic stamp added at the last minute had turned out to be one straw too many on an overloaded camel. "If you really want to make a difference in the short term, you have to accept the incremental way policy is actually made," a Durenberger aide said after the repeal (*CQA* 1988, 295).

Though President Clinton claimed that his plan would lower the deficit by reducing health care spending, the CBO estimated the plan would increase deficits by $74 billion between 1995 and 2000. It would start saving money only by 2004. By the time of his second State of the Union Address, it had become clear that President Clinton would get much less than he had asked for. Strategically, he retreated to a single nonnegotiable demand, universal coverage: everybody would have to be covered or he would veto the bill. By midyear, he began looking for new definitions of "universal"; clearly it meant something less than 100 percent, since even Social Security got only 97- or 98-percent participation. And phasing in would be entirely acceptable—indeed, welcomed—even if it took until 2002.

How Close Is the Next Election?

Timing has generally been unkind to NHI proposals. They tend to be submitted early in the legislative session, but their complexity often holds up serious battles over the most important features—the role of government and financing—until well into the first year or early in the second year. By then, the congressional midterm elections are looming. What had been differences of agreement over policy issues become the focus of ideological tirades. One or the other party or both begin looking to the election and thinking about either how to use the health care debate to embarrass the other party or how to delay a vote on the legislation. If things go as hoped, they will come back with additional seats, thereby improving their bargaining power on the health bill. This political maneuvering has been the death knell of health reform proposals for decades.

The Nixon administration's second-term experience is a case in point for the importance of timing—or strategically waiting for a Congress or president more amenable to health reform. By 1974 prospects for historic action on national health insurance could not have looked brighter. President Nixon introduced his revised plan, called for speedy action, designated national health insurance his number-one domestic priority, and expressed willingness to compromise with Congress (*CQA* 1974, 387). Senator Kennedy sounded a similarly compromising note, while labor continued to support the very liberal bill now carrying only the name of Democrat Martha Griffiths (originally the Kennedy-Griffiths bill). Kennedy had taken his name off and joined with Ways and Means Committee chair Mills on a bill shorn of some of the ideological red flags of the Griffiths bill.

But labor would not compromise. They called the Kennedy-Mills bill a Kennedy sellout and decided to wait for the 1974 elections, in which the Watergate-weakened Republicans were expected to lose big. Labor let it be known that they hoped to elect a "veto-proof" (heavily Democratic) Congress (*CQA* 1974, 387).

Election results were just as labor had hoped. With the Democrats' victorious return after the election, Speaker of the House Carl Albert predicted that NHI would be the first order of business in January 1975 (*CQA* 1974, 394). Inflation worries changed all that, causing President Ford and many members to abandon their enthusiasm for health insurance legislation. Democrats then decided to wait until pronational health insurance candidate Jimmy Carter won the presidency in 1976. Even then, things did not turn out as planned.

Similarly, in the late summer of 1994, the looming midterm elections had a major effect on the health care debate. Although the Democrats had initially thought the failure to pass a national health reform proposal would hurt the Republicans, by the summer they realized that the public was ambivalent at best. Worse, many feared the specter of large governmental interference in their own health relationships, a situation portrayed by many Republicans and interest groups alike. The president's ratings continued to tumble, if not nosedive.

Finally, majority party leaders of both houses met with the president to tell him that the best they would get would be something "less comprehensive, less bureaucratic, and more phased-in." In fact, that was putting it in the best possible light. What they really hoped for was anything at all. As the president's approval ratings slumped even further and Republicans became bolder, Clinton lost a crucial vote on a major crime bill—by eight votes. The vote reflected a split within his party over the death penalty, testifying eloquently that his power to persuade the recalcitrant liberal and conservative wings of his heterogeneous party was all but nonexistent. It seemed clear that the price of winning the one group was losing the other. Sensing disarray, Republicans converged to deliver the block of opposition needed to ensure defeat.

On 26 September 1994 Senate Majority Leader Mitchell, who had passed up a Supreme Court seat to shepherd national health reform, finally admitted that national health insurance was dead for the year. Correspondent Bob Schieffer had broadcast an obituary two days earlier on the CBS Evening News. Others had been even less decorous, doing postmortems a week or more earlier. Finally the First Lady, who had been the administration's visible leader on health reform, told reporters that the fight for national health insurance was not something that ended after fifteen rounds. It would begin again next year, she said. She did not mention the virtually certain additional barrier of a lower ratio of Democrats to Republicans in both houses. Election results were much worse for the Democrats than expected, and health care reform was quietly, if unceremoniously, off the agenda. Though the president mentioned health reform a time or two following his party's electoral trouncing, by the end of the celebrated first 100 days of the newly Republican Congress, the topic had fallen off the list of top priorities he then articulated in an effort to regain control of the policy agenda.

Electoral maneuvering is not always limited to interparty differences. In the 1970s health care reform became the primary policy fulcrum for a sitting Democratic president and the most likely presidential rival. When he did not like President Carter's bill, Senator Kennedy pressed his own version, which, many said, seemed to be functioning as a campaign tool for a primary fight. When the battle finally ended with the passage of nothing more than a national commission to look into the problem, Carter had clearly lost, but Kennedy had not really won. The biggest loser was national health insurance reform. Fifteen years later, a still-bitter Jimmy Carter would say in plain English on a national news show that the country would now have national health insurance if it had not been for Senator Kennedy—in spite of the fact that no name in Congress is more associated with national health insurance reform than Kennedy.

How Large Is the President's Political Capital?

Big plans require big majorities and a powerful policy entrepreneur. For NHI, this means a president who must be popular and whose party commands a large majority in both houses. Medicare slipped through by the size of the 1964 lopsided Democratic victory. Votes can be lost by the traditional disagreements between the parties, but also by the inevitable tension between liberals who favor comprehensive change and other liberals who want something more scaled down. Carter and Kennedy and labor and then Carter and labor split their support for national health reform over the issue of comprehensive cradle-to-grave coverage versus catastrophic-only coverage. Single-payer Democrats versus managed-care Democrats did the same thing during the Clinton proposal debates.

Presidents with small majorities are simply not able to muster the votes for large, comprehensive proposals. As criticism of their proposal heats up, it tends to cost them support in the polls as well, further depleting their reserve of capital.

National Health Insurance in Perspective

Ideological differences continue to plague the national health insurance debate and translate into major disagreements over risk-pooling strategies, means testing, and financing. Though the Democrats have moved nearly completely to what was for many years the prevailing Republican position, agreement seems further away than ever.

The specter of rationing likely to result if use and costs are actually controlled makes governmental interference in health care decisions a convincing case for those who distrust government anyway and are especially repelled by the massive complexities of major system reform. A long record of bad estimates of utilization effects and costs, and a track record of consistent inability to control provider behavior makes confidence in public solutions to the health care cost problem even harder to sell. Large-scale proposals challenge believability in our ability to predict what will happen a few years down the road. Interest groups have much to lose if reform comes too suddenly or changes too many settled arrangements.

Whatever approach future reformers use, they will have to come to grips with the realities of serious ideological differences that cannot be overcome without a very large majority and a new funding source. Incremental approaches may be the only feasible option, yet they must be carefully structured so that they eventually build to controls on use and costs and do not encourage adverse selection. Other countries effect the necessary controls through global budgets set by national or regional boards. Eventually, the United States is likely to have to resort to those tools too if the growth of the share of the GDP devoted to health care costs is to be arrested. More time must pass and more Americans made uncomfortable by their health care costs or lack of coverage before such strategies will pass the acceptability test.

CONCLUSION

The saga of post–World War II health care policy outlined here in three areas—subsidies, cost control, and national health insurance—illustrates the institutional roles, power of interest groups, political motivations, and serendipity discussed in earlier chapters. Reading Chapters 1 through 6, one might wonder how any bill can ever make it through the process to become law. Reading this chapter, one knows: many times bills fail, especially the first time. They rarely pass in their "purest" form or in the most rational manner. Many arguments for and against are exaggerated or misguided, and the final vote may hinge on a member's party, district, relationship to an interest group, or proximity to an election. But many good (and some bad) health policies are enacted and revised (and sometimes repealed). The solutions for health problems facing the country come from members, interest groups, the bureaucracy, and academia. Sometimes bills pass long after sponsors have retired or have been defeated and after administrations have changed. Many solutions are recycled until they become familiar enough to gain acceptability (prospective budgeting, physicians' fee schedules). Some are still "not yet ready for prime time" (global budgets).

This chapter belies those who think that because we have no national health insurance program, we have no national health policy. We have had many policies—subsidies to improve access to care and upgrade its quality, planning, reimbursement controls, competition, and probably global budgeting eventually. Lacking are national health insurance and any real commitment to force Americans to ration their consumption of health care. Our national health policy is eclectic, dynamic, and evolving, but it also has an inexorable quality. Eventually it will get there—cost-effective, prioritized, and constrained. If it moves slowly, and it does, its hesitancy seems to be responsive to both vested interests who benefit from the insuring and delivery of care and a public who is generally satisfied with the care it receives. Ideological differences, especially over the appropriate scope of national health insurance, have stymied past efforts at comprehensive reform. Budget constraints are likely to do so in the future. But policy will continue to be made. Few solutions are adopted if they move too quickly or too far. Yet with time, despite their overwhelming initial and subsequent successes, provider interests have been forced to accept hospital prospective payment, a physicians' fee schedule with volume controls, and support for expansion of HMOs. Kingdon's notion of the force of ideas whose time has come seems to be borne out in health care policy more often than not. Getting the timing and content right just takes persistence and a lot of time.

8

Conclusion

OVER MANY DECADES, a variety of ideological, institutional, and political factors have served to stymie, if not obliterate, dozens of proposals for comprehensive health care reform. But failure to enact a national health insurance system does not mean that health care reform in this country has not occurred. On the contrary, as this book has illustrated, health reform in Washington and the states has blossomed since 1965, often in ways unrecognized by much of the country's population.

Health care policy changes range from small to large and differ in the politics they engender and their rates of success. It is the proposals for large, comprehensive change that attract the most attention. Indeed, when most people think of health care politics, they think of the big, ideological fights over comprehensive reform: Truman and the AMA, Clinton versus the insurance companies, Nixon and the Democrats, Carter and the hospitals, or Congress and the senior citizens outraged over the costs and financing of Medicare catastrophic coverage. These are the battles royal with major stakes and high public interest. Each begins in similar ways: struck either by the madness of what public spending for health care is doing to the domestic discretionary budget or by compassion, a presidential candidate will often feel compelled to push for major health reform. Briefly, the public's interest quickens. Health care policy becomes salient; reform is in the wind, and reporters scramble to understand the issue. Big, ideological battles over the role of government in health care ensue between White House policy advocates and insurance, providers, and business titan coalitions. Reform advocates seek to expand governmental control over health care practice and spending and to make access to insurance coverage more available to poor people and special populations through various risk-pooling arrangements.

Though a variety of sources of financing are explored, the real choices invariably come down to employer mandates, a payroll tax, or both. (Taxing the beneficiaries à la Medicare catastrophic blew up so badly that it probably will not be tried again for some time.) Interest groups with much to lose and little to gain by disrupting the status quo resist. They mount grass-roots campaigns, appealing to core values by threatening that reform plans will restrict the choice of physicians and bring governmental interference into the doctor-patient relationship. They point to the plan's complexity and the inevitability of rationing and queuing if spending is capped. And they raise the specter of massive growth of the federal bureaucracy. Patient cost-sharing and means testing further aggravate differences. Providers, hoping to restrict any broadened governmental involvement in health care to those who cannot afford to pay privately anyway, favor it. Liberals want the program to cover all equally, because programs for only poor people are regarded as welfare and are poorly funded.

The debate lasts until, as Downs (1972) characterized it, "reality sets in," when middle-class voters realize that the costs of reform will be high. Though the plan's promoters try to emphasize features that protect freedom of choice and quality, doubt is sown. Voters and policymakers understand that governmental agencies serve multiple missions, favor equity over efficiency, are constrained by cumbersome procedures designed to ensure compliance with law, and employ managers who exercise little control over an agency's financing and personnel. Small businesses see initial subsidies and risk-pooling arrangements included in most reform bills as the nose of the camel under the tent: voluntary participation and subsidies likely to be followed by regulatory demands and mandatory spending. Few believe official cost and utilization estimates and are easily persuaded that projected financing obligations should be increased several-fold before calculating what reform is likely to cost them.

In a climate of skepticism over government's ability to fulfill its promises, the public becomes confused over whom to believe and withdraws its support. Reform zeal abates. Promoters are accused of overreaching.

Why is comprehensive change in health care so difficult? Major reasons include:

1. ideological differences over the role of government;

2. the massive expense of expanding access before costs are under control, especially in the light of the large effort required to make small improvements in access;

3. the reality that the middle class, which will pay the bill, does not have much problem with health care coverage;

4. the fact that major changes concentrate costs on many powerful groups who will pay for or otherwise suffer the costs of reform, while benefits accrue to the public in general or the poor and other disenfranchisees with little political clout.

Few presidents enjoy sufficient political capital (congressional votes, electoral margin, and sustained popularity) to ignore minority views and overcome well-funded opposition media campaigns. The balkanization of policymaking into the hands of subcommittee staffs and micro-interest pressure groups aggravates the situation. The congressional enterprise favors staking out single issues rather than participating in comprehensive reforms. With little party discipline especially among Democrats and the ability and willingness of subcommittee chairs and even individual members to go their own way, introducing bills as substitutes for their president's or party leaders' bills, majorities are hard to form around compromise proposals.

On top of all this, features inherent in the way health care is marketed, consumed, and paid for make it especially hard to tackle comprehensively. Politically speaking, there is something special about health care. Everyone's fear that he or she will fall victim to heart disease, cancer, or a disabling condition puts stories from each issue of the *New England Journal of Medicine* at the top of the evening news. Researchers on breast cancer, heart attack, and mental disease have become regulars on the morning television news shows. Medical breakthroughs keep the outputs of the health care system—though not the rest of it—highly salient.

Health care is special. Leaving aside traditional economists' concerns with information asymmetry, entrance barriers, and other characteristics of the noncompetitive market that is health care, the health care market is politically unique. It combines fear of disease and death, third-party payment, and publicly supported biomedical research continuously fueling demand for new forms of care. Everyone is a consumer of health care and, in the usual course of events, cares only that new cures are being discovered and physicians are aware of them. This makes medical breakthroughs highly salient and helps fuel their demand.

Other aspects of health policy are much less salient. Except for periods of high unemployment when employee coverage lapses for some laid-off workers, it is primarily the uninsured who face financial barriers to care. In some rural areas and most inner-city poor neighborhoods, supply shortages present problems. But most access problems afflict few middle-class Americans in ways that they understand. During 1993, when it appeared that national health care reform was imminent, virtually everyone knew someone who was unemployed and without health insurance and feared he might soon be next. When things changed—fewer people were out of work or fearful of losing their jobs—the issue began to decline in public saliency. Most people believe that emergency care is available to uninsured persons so that extreme hardships will be avoided and need not weigh on the national conscience. Other public programs are presumed ready to intervene to control the spread of infection.

Third-party payment means that most Americans feel few of the costs of their unbridled consumption of health care. The RAND Health Insurance Experiment saw a one-fourth reduction in health care consumption when patients had to pay a substantial amount for their own care. Health status did not decline as a result of using less care, so prone to health care overconsumption are most Americans. Yet first-dollar coverage or coverage without any copayment continues to be the norm. Few middle-class Americans appreciate the reality that costs of delayed, inappropriate, unneeded, and inefficiently delivered care—their own or others, including uninsured persons—actually erodes their wages. The route is indirect: unpaid bills are shifted to insurance companies, which pay the (already-too-high) bills of middle-class patients. The insurers then raise the premiums of employers, and employers reduce the wages they might have paid had health care costs not raised their fringe-benefit contributions.

This makes escalating costs the least salient of all health reform motivations. The result is a policy issue bifurcated into salient and nonsalient aspects. The public cares deeply about those aspects of policy that might reduce their access to treatments and cures. It cares little about the costs of producing them or about those who are disenfranchised from insurance coverage.

As long as government stays out of the picture, it is a safe assumption that insurance will cover most care demanded by most people most of the time and that the quest for new forms of care will continue. Portability and cancelability, problems that do affect middle-class wage earners, are relatively easy to fix without comprehensive reform. Preexisting conditions present a much more difficult challenge, but can be somewhat mitigated with limited intervention, and affect a minority of voters.

Moreover, the shift toward managed-care arrangements, which accelerated in the early 1990s (greatly escalated in response to the Clinton administration proposal), promise more market-driven accountability among the parts of the system. A million market conflicts will produce hundreds of thousands of compromises over drugs and dosages, appropriate services, reasonable payment, treatment effectiveness, adequate quality, short- and long-term efficiencies, scope of practice, mix of skills, and a multitude of decisions to be worked out between providers, payers, and consumers. Self-interests and consumer power will obviate the need for public intervention in many aspects of the health care market. Concentrated power and information asymmetry will point more clearly to situations where intervention is needed.

Why then should Americans support comprehensive reform? It is opposed by powerful provider, insurance, and business interests; it employs roughly one-seventh of the work force, which has a stake in keeping things as profligate as they are now; the average citizen cares greatly that the quest for new cures continue at its present rate but is uninformed and indifferent concerning items on the reform agenda that relate to cost controls and access for the underprivileged—unless controls are suggested that might put them into a queue for care. Americans have been told through mass-media campaigns that reform will be expensive to them, may limit their choices of providers and types of care, will adversely affect quality, and even if it works is likely to make only very small improvements in access over the status quo, changing from 85 percent insured to perhaps 95 percent. In short, the system works pretty well for many Americans. Why risk mucking it up and possibly making things worse? These realities make it hard to convince a majority of either policymakers or the public that the juice will be worth the squeeze.

While attempts at comprehensive health reform in this country have come up woefully short, they have served an important role in focusing policymakers' attention on health care issues, moving the policy analysis process forward, broadening and deepening policymakers' understanding of the problem and its solution options, sometimes adding new options to the solution list, and perhaps defining the agenda for incremental reform. But such efforts stand little chance of wholesale adoption. Budget constraints have made any change involving substantial new revenues even harder to pull off today.

At the other extreme of the continuum of health care politics is normal, incremental client and interest group politics of the kind that goes on day in and day out, year in and year out. In ordinary health politics, those who make their living from health care—the caring professions, insurance carriers, facility management and support staff, university training program faculty, drug and equipment suppliers, and a host of others—have learned to get what they want quietly, away from the glare of news coverage and intense public scrutiny. What they want is usually a small change in the status quo: changes in reimbursement policies, for example, that benefit the nebulizer industry or rural hospitals or optometrists. They go after policies that support these changes with both guns blazing.

These incremental changes are often predicated on well-defined, quantified problems and are familiar to policymakers who have debated and voted on these or similar issues in previous sessions. Proposals that raise few problems of technical feasibility, are not too expensive, broadly diffuse costs, offend no one's sense of the appropriate limits on the role of the federal government, garner little press and public attention, are complex enough to discourage interlopers, and seem to promise benefits that make them worth their cost are likely to be easiest to pass. A student of health policy who watched only these ordinary day-to-day client and interest group politics would capture much of what happens in health care policy and over time might witness considerable change.

Yet incremental successes and comprehensive failures provide an incomplete story of health politics and mask much of the dynamics of policy change. Somewhere in between massive and small changes are moderate-sized bursts of reform that offer a kind of "punctuation" (Baumgartner and Jones 1993) to the normal equilibrium of incremental change.

An important aspect of this type of politics may be problem redefinition, as noted by Baumgartner and Jones. Health planning had to die a lingering death while policymakers came slowly, grudgingly to the realization that the problem with the health care system was not just access, fragmentation, and duplicate facilities. It was more fundamental: under the existing payment systems' incentives, nobody cared about costs and prices. Planning was not going to change those incentives. The shift to reimbursement-based reform waited patiently in the wings until the evidence accumulated that the problem needed to be redefined and a different type of solution tried.

Usually—but not always—Kingdon's (1984) focusing event occurs, a crisis has been declared, or a congressionally appointed commission has refined and worked on a proposal, honing it to the point that it is ready to go.

It passes quickly, with little fanfare. Some recent examples are Medicare PPS, Medicare RBRVS, outcomes research, and nursing home quality reform. These reforms were very important turning points in health care policy. They were not comprehensive, but they were not business as usual either.

The idea of prospective reimbursement was first introduced by President Nixon's health staff: hospitals should be paid on a prospective basis, and physicians should be paid on a fee schedule. Georgia Senator Talmadge pushed it for years, doing what Kingdon (1984) called "softening up," compromising and bargaining on its behalf. President Carter tried to pass it as the keystone of a comprehensive reform, and though he failed, he further contributed to redefining the problem from fragmentation and duplication to perverse incentives in the payment system.

Hospital CEOs saw it coming, and the smart ones began to position themselves to deal with it, perhaps mitigating their opposition when it finally came. Ultimately, events in both the problem and the political stream changed: projections showed that the Medicare trust fund would go bankrupt if costs were not controlled; a Republican president and Senate majority were elected; and Senate Majority Leader Robert Dole, who had opposed hospital fee caps when proposed by a Democratic president, became convinced that rising prices were indeed a problem inherent in the payment system. A decade had elapsed since the idea was first introduced.

Six more years lapsed between the time Congress reformed hospital costs and when a Harvard researcher's report showed that a reasonable-looking fee schedule could be designed. Though the plan was nearly sidetracked as part of a larger problem with the year's reconciliation bill, when it did pass it went through Congress remarkably intact in the form it was proffered by the PPRC.

This kind of politics has two key features:

—it involves big change but gets little notice (only the most ardent watchers of health policy knew that PPS had passed; fewer still knew that RBRVS had passed or that funding for outcomes research was included in it; still few know today that major nursing home reform passed in the late 1980s);
—the interest groups that would normally be effective in warding off such incursions are rendered essentially ineffective.

Nonsaliency and the inexorable process of problem redefinition may be important parts of the explanation. These kinds of policy are highly complex. Few reporters understand or care about them when they pass. Policies of this type represent the quintessence of the Weberian notion of the bureaucratic role: highly technical, rational, essentially apolitical responses to a problem that everyone agrees has to be solved but few politicians understand well enough to tackle without major bureaucratic support. One bureaucrat who had been detailed to the Senate to help refine the RBRVS draft claimed to have been the only person on the Hill who knew what was in the bill at the time it passed. Nursing home reform passed into legislation in approximately the same form as it was reported from the Institute of Medicine's reform commission.

Baumgartner and Jones (1993) used the term "punctuated equilibrium" to characterize policy change that departs from the usual incrementalism in response to a change in the problem definition. Kingdon (1984) too probably had such change in mind when he noted the overwhelming power of an idea whose time has come and the usefulness of the "softening up" process. PPS, RBRVS, outcomes research, and nursing home reform all represented overdue corrections for long-acknowledged policy distortions. Arguments against the proposed reforms had been persuasive for a long time, but lost their appeal as the data contradicted them over time. Interest groups appeared in each case to have come to the conclusion that passage was inevitable and not worth spending further chits on a frontal defiance. Instead, in the case of PPS and RBRVS, they chose to work at the margins, redefining, delaying, and altering in small but important ways after passage of the initial legislation.

Awareness of these moderate bursts of reform may be helpful in anticipating future policy direction for one very important reason: their evolutionary process means that changes in the next ten years are probably already on the table for all to see. Some of these include:

—taxing health insurance premiums, at least initially above an average cost (perhaps coupled with health IRAs as a sweetener);

—means testing Medicare so that well-off elderly people pay more of the program's costs;

—adding the actuarial insurance value of Medicare, Medicaid, and other safety net programs to the incomes of some or all taxpayers;

—altering statutes and regulations to allow greatly expanded reliance on non-physician personnel to augment the supply of primary care practitioners;

—refocusing GME payments to produce more primary care clerkships and residencies;

—malpractice tort reform and limits on awards;

—reduction of federal Medicaid-matching payments to the largest states;

—modification of ERISA so that it no longer applies to health insurance;

—shifting more of the health care reform effort to the states;

—capping overall health spending as a percentage of the gross domestic product and the public budget;

—heavier reliance on outcomes research studies to guide clinical and coverage decisions, public and private.

Each of these proposals addresses an important aspect of the health care cost problem. Over time, research and analysis on them will accumulate, and as the budget binds, answers are likely to be seriously sought and variations on these themes are likely to be among those that pass many tests of political feasibility. The softening-up process for them has already begun.

Politics too evolve and change, reflecting the public's ongoing response to economic, social, and political forces. As this book has illustrated, America's institutions are far from moribund, but are as dynamic and changing as the people they represent and the policies they initiate, adopt, and implement. Governing health in this country is a major undertaking—one accomplished with care and caution befitting both the country's long-standing distrust of strong government and the tremendous economic impact that health spending has on the nation as a whole. Those who fail to understand how the governing process works are likely to find themselves paying the bill for those who do.

Acronyms

AARP	American Association of Retired Persons
AFDC	Aid to Families with Dependent Children
AHA	American Hospital Association
AHCCCS	Arizona Health Care Cost Containment System
AHCPR	Agency for Health Care Policy and Research
AIDS	Acquired immune deficiency syndrome
AMA	American Medical Association
BB	Bureau of the Budget (became OMB)
CAT	Computerized axial tomography
CBO	Congressional Budget Office
CDC	Centers for Disease Control
CEO	Chief executive officer
CON	Certificate of need
DRGs	Diagnostic related groups
EHSDS	Experimental Health Services Delivery System
EPA	Environmental Protection Agency
EPSDT	Early Periodic Screening, Diagnosis, and Treatment
ERISA	Employee Retirement and Income Security Act
FDA	Food and Drug Administration
GAO	General Accounting Office
GDP	Gross domestic product
GME	Graduate medical education
GSA	General Services Administration

HCFA	Health Care Financing Administration
HEW	(U.S. Department of) Health, Education, and Welfare (became HHS)
HHS	(U.S. Department of) Health and Human Services
HMO	Health maintenance organization
IPA	Individual practice association
NCHCT	National Center for Health Care Technology
NCHSR	National Center for Health Services Research (became AHCPR)
NHI	National health insurance
NIH	National Institutes of Health
OBRA	Omnibus Budget Reconcilation Act
OMB	Office of Management and Budget
OSHA	Occupational Safety and Health Administration
PAC	Political action committee
PHS	Public Health Service
PPRC	Physician Payment Review Commission
PPS	(Medicare) Prospective Payment System
PRO	Peer review organization
ProPAC	Prospective Payment Assessment Commission
PSRO	Professional Standards Review Organization
RBRVS	Resource-based relative value scale
SOP	Standard operating procedure

References

Abramson, Jill, and Daniel Pearl. 1993. Congressman's Sojourn in Washington Teaches Bitter Political Lesson. *Wall Street Journal*, Dec. 15:A1, A4.

Advisory Commission on Intergovernmental Relations. 1985. *The Question of State Government Capability.* Washington: Government Printing Office.

"AHA Launches Massive Grassroots Effort." 1994. *Medicine and Health* 48 (Mar. 7):2.

Allen, E. 1992. The Crisis of Family Abductions in America. *FBI Law Enforcement Bulletin* 61 (Aug.):18–19.

Allison, Graham. 1971. *Essence of Decision: Explaining the Cuban Missile Crisis.* Boston: Little, Brown.

Alston, Chuck. 1989. Belt-Tightening in Medicare Pits Doctor vs. Doctor. *Congressional Quarterly,* Oct. 7:2605–9.

Altman, Drew, and Harvey M. Sapolsky. 1976. Writing the Regulations for Health. *Policy Sciences* 7:417–37.

Anderson, J. E. 1994. *Public Policymaking: An Introduction.* 2d ed. Boston: Houghton Mifflin.

Anderson, Odin W. 1990. *Health Services as a Growth Enterprise in the United States since 1875.* 2d ed. Ann Arbor: Health Administration Press.

Anton, Thomas. 1989. *American Federalism and Public Policy.* New York: Random House.

Appleby, Paul H. 1945. *Big Democracy.* New York: Knopf.

Arnold, R. Douglas. 1990. *The Logic of Congressional Action.* New Haven: Yale University Press.

Arrandale, Tom. 1994. A Guide to Environmental Mandates. *Governing,* Mar.: 73–86.

Associated Press. 1992. Inquiry Discounts Texas H.I.V. Cases. *New York Times,* Aug. 2:C6.

Austen-Smith, David, and John Wright. 1994. Counteractive Lobbying. *American Journal of Political Science* 38:25–44.

Babcock, Charles. 1993. Health Care Fears Open Up the Pocketbooks. *Washington Post National Weekly Edition,* June 7–14:14.

———. 1994. The Overrated Power of PACs. *Washington Post National Weekly Edition,* June 20–26:15.

Bailey, Stephen K. 1970. *Congress in the Seventies.* New York: St. Martin's.

Balla, Steven J. 1995. Participation and Physician Payments: The Decisions of Interest Groups and Citizens to Oversee Bureaucrats. Paper presented at the annual meeting of the Midwest Political Science Association, Chicago, Apr. 6–8.

Barber, James David. 1985. *The Presidential Character: Predicting Performance in the White House.* Englewood Cliffs, N.J.: Prentice-Hall.

Barnes, Fred. 1985. On the Hill, Raging Representatives. *New Republic,* June 3:9.

Baumgartner, Frank R., and Bryan D. Jones. 1993. *Agendas and Instability in American Politics.* Chicago: University of Chicago Press.

Baumgartner, Frank R., and Jeffery C. Talbert. 1995. From Setting a National Agenda on Health Care to Making Decisions in Congress. *Journal of Health Politics, Policy and Law* 20:437–45.

Bazzoli, G. J. 1986. Health Care for the Indigent: Overview of Critical Issues. *Health Services Research* 21:353–93.

Behn, Robert D., and Kim Sperduto. 1979. Medical Schools and the "Entitlement Ethic." *The Public Interest* 57:48–68.

Benda, Peter, and Charles Levine. 1986. OMB and the Central Management Problem: Is Another Reorganization the Answer? *Public Administration Review* 46:379–91.

Bendavid, Naftali, T. R. Goldman, and Sheila Kaplan. 1993. Handicapping Health Care's Major Players. *Legal Times,* Oct. 11: S28–45.

Benenson, Bob. 1987. Savvy "Stars" Making Local TV a Potent Tool. *Congressional Quarterly Weekly Report,* July 18:1551–55.

Berry, Jeffrey M. 1984. *The Interest Group Society.* Boston: Little, Brown.

Best, J. 1988. Missing Children, Misleading Statistics. *The Public Interest* 92:84–92.

Beyle, Thad. 1989. From Governor to Governors. In *The State of the States,* edited by Carl Van Horn, 33–68. Washington: Congressional Quarterly Press.

Bicentini, J. S., and M. A. Anzick. 1990. Employee Benefits in Total Competition. EBRI Issue Brief 111:4. Cited in Dogmatic Slumbers: American Business and Health Policy by Lawrence D. Brown, 1993. *Journal of Health Politics, Policy and Law* 18:339–57.

Blumenthal, Sidney. 1994. The Education of a President. *New Yorker,* Jan. 24: 31–43.

Bolling, Richard. 1964. *House Out of Order.* New York: E. P. Dutton.

Bond, Jon R., and Richard Fleisher. 1990. *The President in the Legislative Arena.* Chicago: University of Chicago Press.

Boodman, Sandra G. 1994. Health Care's Power Player. *Washington Post National Weekly Edition,* Feb. 14–20:6–7.

Bosso, Christopher. 1994. The Contextual Bases of Problem Definition. In *The Politics of Problem Definition,* edited by David Rochefort and Roger Cobb, 182–203. Lawrence: University Press of Kansas.

Bowler, M. Kenneth. 1987. Changing Politics of Federal Health Insurance Programs. *PS* 20:202–11.

Braybrooke, David, and Charles Lindblom. 1963. *Strategy of Decision.* New York: Free Press.

Brinkley, Joel. 1993. Cultivating the Grass Roots to Reap Legislative Benefits. *New York Times,* Nov. 11:A1, A14.

Broder, David. 1993a. Clinton Finds His Voice. *Washington Post National Weekly Edition,* Dec. 20–26:4.

———. 1993b. Who Does the Senate Represent? *Washington Post National Weekly Edition,* Aug. 23–29:4.

———. 1994a. Can We Govern? *Washington Post National Weekly Edition,* Jan. 31–Feb. 6:23.

———. 1994b. Congress Cranks Up Its Health Reform Sausage-Maker. *Washington Post National Weekly Edition,* Apr. 25–May 1:10.

———. 1994c. Congressional Staffers Wield Power in Health Care Reform. *Ann Arbor News,* July 13:A9.

Broder, David S., and Stephen Barr. 1993. Going Over the Top on Oversight? *Washington Post National Weekly Edition,* Aug. 2–8:31.

Brooks, Phil, and Bob Gassaway. 1990. Statehouse News Coverage: A Question of Efficiency. *News Computing Journal* 6:51–55.

Brott, Armin A. 1994. Battered-Truth Syndrome. *Washington Post,* July 31:C1.

Brown, Lawrence D. 1983. *Politics and Health Care Organization: HMOs as Federal Policy.* Washington: Brookings Institution.

———. 1993. Commissions, Clubs and Consensus: Reform in Florida. *Health Affairs* 12 (summer):7–26.

Browne, William. 1985. Variations in the Behavior and Style of State Lobbyists and Interest Groups. *Journal of Politics* 47:450–68.

————. 1991. Issue Niches and the Limits of Interest Group Influence. In *Interest Group Politics*, edited by Allan J. Cigler and Burdett A. Loomis, 3d ed., 345–70. Washington: Congressional Quarterly Press.

————. 1993. Group Leaders, Grassroots Confidants, and Congressional Responses. Paper presented at the annual meeting of the Midwest Political Science Association, Chicago, Apr. 6–8.

Brownlow, Louis. 1949. *The President and the Presidency.* Chicago: University of Chicago Press.

Burns, James MacGregor. 1984. *The Power to Lead.* New York: Simon and Schuster.

Butler, Patricia. 1994. *Roadblock to Reform: ERISA Implications for State Health Care Initiatives.* Washington: National Governors' Association.

Califano, J. A. 1994. Imperial Congress. *New York Times Magazine,* Jan. 23:40–41.

Calvert, Randall L., Mark J. Moran, and Barry R. Weingast. 1987. Congressional Influence over Policymaking: The Case of the FTC. In *Congress: Structure and Policy,* edited by Mathew D. McCubbins and Terry Sullivan, 493–522. New York: Cambridge University Press.

Campbell, John C. 1992. *How Policies Change: The Japanese Government and the Aging Society.* Princeton, N.J.: Princeton University Press.

Campion, Frank D. 1984. *The AMA and U.S. Health Policy.* Chicago: Chicago Review Press.

Carney, Eliza Newlin. 1994. Pesky Critters. *National Journal,* Oct. 29: 2507–11.

Carter, Jimmy. 1981. President Jimmy Carter's Farewell Address. *Congressional Quarterly Weekly Report* 39 (Jan. 17):196.

————. 1982. *Keeping the Faith: Memoirs of a President.* New York: Bantam Books.

Cater, Douglass. 1964. *Power in Washington.* New York: Random House.

Ceaser, James. 1988. The Reagan Presidency and American Public Opinion. In *The Reagan Legacy: Promise and Performance,* edited by Charles O. Jones, 172–210. Chatham, N.J.: Chatham House.

Center for Responsive Politics. 1994. Health Contributions Up. Soft Money Switches Parties. Oct. 19, press release.

Centers for Disease Control. 1991. *Profile of State and Territorial Public Health Systems: United States, 1990.* Atlanta: U.S. Department of Health and Human Services.

Chirba-Martin, Mary Ann, and Troyen Brennan. 1994. The Critical Role of ERISA in State Health Reform. *Health Affairs* 13 (spring):142–56.

Cigler, Allan. 1991. Interest Groups: A Subfield in Search of an Identity. In *Political Science Looking to the Future. Vol. 4 of American Institutions,* edited by William Crotty, 99–135. Evanston: Northwestern University Press.

Cigler, Allan J., and Burdett A. Loomis. 1991. Organized Interests and the Search for Certainty. In *Interest Group Politics*, edited by Allan J. Cigler and Burdett A. Loomis, 3d ed., 385–98. Washington: Congressional Quarterly Press.

———. 1995. Contemporary Interest Group Politics: More Than "More of the Same." In *Interest Group Politics*, edited by Allan J. Cigler and Burdett A. Loomis, 4th ed., 393–406. Washington: Congressional Quarterly Press.

Clapp, Charles L. 1963. *The Congressman: His Work as He Sees It.* Garden City, N.Y.: Anchor Books.

Clark, Peter B., and James Q. Wilson. 1961. Incentive Systems: A Theory of Organizations. *Administrative Science Quarterly* 6:129–66.

Clarke, Gary J. 1981. The Role of the States in the Delivery of Health Services. *American Journal of Public Health* 71:59–69.

Clausen, Aage R. 1973. *How Congressmen Decide.* New York: St. Martin's.

Clawson, Dan, Alan Neustadtl, and Denise Scott. 1992. *Money Talks: Corporate PACs and Political Influence.* New York: Basic Books.

Clymer, Adam. 1994. With Health Overhaul Dead, a Search for Minor Repairs. *New York Times*, Aug. 28:A1, 11.

Clymer, Adam, Robert Pear, and Robin Toner. 1994. For Health Care, Time Was a Killer. *New York Times*, Aug. 29:A1, A8–9.

"Coalition Starts Reform Campaign." 1993. *Medicine and Health* 47 (Sept. 20):2.

Cobb, Roger W., and Charles D. Elder. 1972. *Participation in American Politics: The Dynamics of Agenda-Building.* Boston: Allyn and Bacon.

Cohen, M. D., J. G. March, and J. P. Olsen. 1972. The Garbage Can Model of Organizational Choice. *Administrative Science Quarterly* 17:1–25.

Cohodas, Nadine. 1987. Press Coverage: It's What You Do That Counts. *Congressional Quarterly Weekly Report*, Jan. 3:29–33.

Colamosca, Anne. 1979. The Trade Association Hustle. *New Republic*, Nov. 3: 16–19.

Common Cause. 1992. The Medical-Industry Complex and Its Pac Contributions to Congressional Candidates. *Journal of Public Health Policy* 13 (summer): 224–41.

Congressional Quarterly Almanac. 1945–95. Washington, D.C.: Congressional Quarterly Press.

Cooper, Joseph, and William F. West. 1988. Presidential Power and Republican Government: The Theory and Practice of OMB Review of Agency Rules. *Journal of Politics* 50:864–95.

Council of State Governments. 1992. *Book of the States* 1992–93. Lexington: Council of State Governments.

Cronin, Thomas. 1970. Everybody Believes in Democracy Until He Gets to the

White House: An Examination of White House Departmental Relations. *Law and Contemporary Problems.* Duke University School of Law.

Davidson, Roger H. 1981. Subcommittee Government: New Channels for Policy Making. In *The New Congress,* edited by Thomas E. Mann and Norman J. Ornstein, 99–133. Washington: American Enterprise Institute.

———. 1984. The Presidency and the Congress. In *The Presidency and the Political System,* edited by Michael Nelson, 363–91. Washington: Congressional Quarterly Press.

Davidson, Roger H., and Walter J. Oleszek. 1994. *Congress and Its Members.* Washington: Congressional Quarterly Press.

Dearborn, Philip M. 1994. The State-Local Fiscal Outlook from a Federal Perspective. *Intergovernmental Perspective* 20:20–23.

Demkovich, Linda. 1994. Breakthrough or Blackmail?: Emotions on TennCare Run High. *State Health Notes* 15:1,2,8.

Denzau, Arthur, and Michael Munger. 1986. Legislators and Interest Groups: How Unorganized Interests Get Represented. *American Political Science Review* 80:89–106.

Derthick, Martha. 1970. *The Influence of Federal Grants.* Cambridge: Harvard University Press.

———. 1975. *Uncontrollable Spending for Social Services Grants.* Washington: Brookings Institution.

———. 1990. *Agency under Stress.* Washington: Brookings Institution.

Dery, David. 1984. *Problem Definition in Policy Analysis.* Lawrence: University Press of Kansas.

De Tocqueville, Alexis. 1956. *Democracy in America,* edited by Richard D. Heffner. New York: Mentor Books.

Diamond, Martin. 1985. What the Framers Meant by Federalism. In *American Intergovernmental Relations: Foundations, Perspectives and Issues,* edited by Laurence O'Toole, Jr., 28–35. Washington: Congressional Quarterly Press.

Dolbeare, Kenneth M., and Murray Edelman. 1985. *American Politics, Policies, Power and Change.* 5th ed. Lexington, Mass.: D. C. Heath.

Donabedian, A. 1973. *Aspects of Medical Care Administration.* Cambridge: Harvard University Press.

Downs, Anthony. 1967. *Inside Bureaucracy.* Boston: Little, Brown.

———. 1972. Up and Down with Ecology: The "Issue-Attention Cycle." *The Public Interest* 28:38–50.

Dubay, L. C., G. G. Kenney, and J. Holahan. 1989. Should Medicare Compensate Hospitals for Administratively Necessary Days? *Milbank Quarterly* 67: 137–67.

Dubnick, Melvin J., and Barbara Romzek. 1991. *American Public Administration: Politics and Management of Expectations.* New York: Macmillan.

Duncan, Phil, ed. 1993. *Politics in America.* Washington: Congressional Quarterly Press.

———. 1994. *Politics in America, 1994: The 103rd Congress.* Washington: Congressional Quarterly Press.

Dye, T. R. 1984. *Understanding Public Policy.* 5th ed. Englewood Cliffs, N.J.: Prentice-Hall.

Eckl, Corina L., Karen C. Hayes, and Arturo Perez. 1993. *State Budget Actions, 1993.* Denver: National Conference of State Legislatures.

Edelman, Murray. 1964. *The Symbolic Uses of Politics.* Urbana: University of Illinois Press.

Edwards, George C. 1980. *Presidential Influence in Congress.* San Francisco: W. II. Freeman.

———. 1989. *At the Margins: The Presidential Leadership of Congress.* New Haven: Yale University Press.

Elazar, Daniel. 1984. *American Federalism: A View from the States.* 3d ed. New York: Harper and Row.

Ellwood, John, and James Thurber. 1977. The New Congressional Budget Process. In *Congress Reconsidered,* edited by Lawrence Dodd and Bruce Oppenheimer, 163–92. New York: Praeger.

Epstein, David, and Sharyn O'Halloran. 1994. Administrative Procedures, Information and Agency Discretion. *American Journal of Political Science* 38:697–722.

Epstein, Samuel. 1979. *Politics of Cancer.* Garden City, N.Y.: Anchor Press.

Evans, Robert G., Roberta J. Labelle, and Morris L. Barer. 1988. Fee Controls as Cost Control: Tales from the Frozen North. *Milbank Quarterly* 66, 1:1–64.

Eyestone, R. 1978. *From Social Issues to Public Policy.* New York: John Wiley.

Falkson, Joseph. 1980. *HMOs and the Politics of Health Systems Reform.* Chicago: American Hospital Association.

Feder, Barnaby. 1993. Medical Group Battles to Be Heard over Others on Health-Care Changes. *New York Times,* June 11:A12.

Feder, Judith M. 1977. *Medicare: The Politics of Federal Hospital Insurance.* Lexington, Mass.: D. C. Heath.

Feder, Judith, John Holahan, Randall Bovbjerg, and Jack Hadley. 1982. Health. In *The Reagan Experiment,* edited by John L. Palmer and Isabel V. Sawhill, 271–305. Washington: Urban Institute Press.

Feingold, Eugene, and George Greenberg. 1984. Health Policy and the Federal

Executive. In *Health Politics and Policy,* edited by Theodor Litman and Leonard Robins, 99–113. New York: John Wiley.

Feldstein, Paul J. 1977. *Health Associations and the Demand for Legislation.* Cambridge: Ballinger.

Fenno, Richard. 1973. *Congressmen in Committees.* Boston: Little, Brown.

———. 1978. *Home Style: House Members in Their Districts.* Boston: Little, Brown.

Fiorina, Morris. 1977. *Congress: Keystone of the Washington Establishment.* New Haven: Yale University Press.

———. 1981. Congressional Control of the Bureaucracy: A Mismatch of Incentives and Capabilities. In *Congress Reconsidered,* edited by Lawrence C. Dodd and Bruce Oppenheimer, 2d ed., 332–48. Washington: Congressional Quarterly Press.

Flemming, Arthur S., and Ray Marshall. 1994. Tyranny of the Minority. *New York Times,* May 30:17.

Foltz, Anne-Marie. 1975. The Development of Ambiguous Federal Policy: Early and Periodic Screening, Diagnosis and Treatment (EPSDT). *Health and Society* (winter): 35–64.

Foreman, Christopher. 1995. Grassroots Victim Organizations: Mobilizing for Personal and Public Health. In *Interest Group Politics,* edited by Allan J. Cigler and Burdett A. Loomis, 4th ed., 33–53. Washington: Congressional Quarterly Press.

Fossett, James W. 1993. Medicaid and Health Reform: The Case of New York. *Health Affairs* 12 (fall):81–94.

Fox, Daniel, and Daniel Schaffer. 1989. Health Policy and ERISA: Interest Groups and Semipreemption. *Journal of Health Politics, Policy and Law* 14:239–60.

Friedman, Sally, and Robert T. Nakamura. 1991. The Representation of Women on U.S. Senate Committee Staffs. *Legislative Studies Quarterly* 16:407–28.

Fritschler, A. Lee. 1989. *Smoking and Politics.* 4th ed. Englewood Cliffs: Prentice-Hall.

Fuchs, Beth, and John Hoadley. 1987. Reflections from Inside the Beltway: How Congress and the President Grapple with Health Policy. *PS* 20 (spring): 212–20.

Furrento, M. 1989. *The Myth of Heterosexual AIDS.* New York: New Republic Books.

Gelles, R. J. 1984. Parental Child Snatching. *Journal of Marriage and the Family* 46:735–39.

Georges, Christopher, and Katherine Boo. 1992. Capitol Hill 21510. *Washington Monthly,* Oct.:36–43.

Gilmour, John B. 1990. *Reconcilable Differences: Congress, the Budget Process and the Deficit.* Berkeley: University of California Press.

Ginzberg, Eli. 1990. *The Medical Triangle: Physicians, Politicians and the Public.* Cambridge: Harvard University Press.

Glazer, Nathan. 1975. Towards an Imperial Judiciary? *Public Choice* 41 (fall): 104–23.

Gold, Stephen. 1992. One Approach to Tracking State and Local Health Spending. *Health Affairs* 11 (winter):135–44.

Goodsell, Charles T. 1994. *The Case for Bureaucracy.* 3d ed. Chatham, N.J.: Chatham House.

Gore, Al. 1994. *From Red Tape to Results: Creating a Government That Works Better and Costs Less.* New York: Times Books.

Gormley, William. 1982. Alternative Models of the Regulatory Process: Public Utility Regulation in the States. *Western Politics Quarterly* 25:297–317.

Grant, Daniel, and Lloyd Omdahl. 1993. *State and Local Government in America.* 6th ed. Madison, Wisc.: WCG Brown and Benchmark.

Gray, Bradford H. 1992. The Legislative Battle over Health Services Research. *Health Affairs* 11 (winter):38–66.

Green, Mark. 1982. Political PAC-Man. *New Republic* 188 (Dec. 13):18–24.

Greenberg, George. 1975. Reorganization Reconsidered: The U.S. Public Health Service 1960–1973. *Public Policy* 23:483–522.

Grenzke, Janet. 1990. Money and Congressional Behavior. In *Money, Elections and Democracy,* edited by Margaret Nugent and John Johannes, 4–44. Boulder, Colo.: Westview Press.

Grier, Kevin B., and Michael Munger. 1993. Comparing Interest Group Contributions to House and Senate Incumbents, 1980–86. *Journal of Politics* 55: 615–43.

Grover, William F. 1993. Outside In: Bernie Sanders in the U.S. Congress. Paper presented at the annual meeting of the American Political Science Association, September, Washington, D.C.

Grupenhoff, John. 1983. Profile of Congressional Health Legislative Aides. *Mount Sinai Journal of Medicine* 50:1–7.

Haass, Richard N. 1994. Bill Clinton's Adhocracy. *New York Times Magazine,* May 29:40–41.

Hall, Richard, and Frank Wayman. 1990. Buying Time: Moneyed Interests and the Mobilization of Bias in Congressional Committees. *American Political Science Review* 84:797–820.

Hamilton, Alexander, James Madison, and John Jay. 1961. *The Federalist Papers.* New York: New American Library.

Hammond, Thomas, and Jack Knott. 1992. Presidential Power, Congressional Dominance and Bureaucratic Autonomy in a Model of Multi-Institutional Policymaking. Unpublished.

Harris, Richard. 1966. *A Sacred Trust.* New York: New American Library.

Hayes, Michael T. 1978. The Semi-Sovereign Pressure Groups: A Critique of Current Theory and an Alternative Typology. *Journal of Politics* 40:135–61.

———. 1992. *Implementation and Public Policy.* White Plains, N.Y.: Longman.

Health Care Policy Report. 1994. Health, Insurance Industries Boost PACs to Derail Reform, Citizen Action Asserts, 2 (May 30):966–7.

Heclo, Hugh. 1977. *A Government of Strangers.* Washington: Brookings Institution.

———. 1978. Issue Networks and the Executive Establishment. In *The New American Political System,* edited by Anthony King, 87–124. Washington: American Enterprise Institute.

Heinz, John P., Edward O. Laumann, Robert L. Nelson, and Robert H. Salisbury. 1993. *The Hollow Core: Private Interests in National Policy Making.* Cambridge: Harvard University Press.

Heinz, John P., Edward O. Laumann, Robert H. Salisbury, and Robert L. Nelson. 1990. Inner Circles or Hollow Cores? Elite Networks in National Policy Systems. *Journal of Politics* 52:356–90.

Herrick, Rebekah, and Michael K. Moore. 1993. Rethinking Congressional Careers: The Changing Behavioral Implications of Career Path Selection. Paper presented at the annual meeting of the American Political Science Association, September, Washington, D.C.

Hershey, Robert D., Jr. 1994. Everyone Knows a Lobbyist: Now, the U.S. Defines One. *New York Times,* May 11:A-1, A–11.

Hinckley, Barbara. 1983. *Stability and Change in Congress.* New York: Harper and Row.

———. 1990. *The Symbolic Presidency.* New York: Routledge.

Hinds, Michael deCourcy. 1992. U.S. Adds Programs with Little Review of Local Burdens. *New York Times,* Mar. 24:A1, A14.

Holahan, John, Diane Rowland, Judith Feder, and David Heslam. 1993. Explaining Recent Growth in Medicaid Spending. *Health Affairs* 12 (fall):177–93.

Horowitz, David. 1977. *The Courts and Social Policy.* Washington: Brookings Institution.

Hotaling, Gerald T. 1988. *The Sexual Exploitation of Missing Children: A Research Review.* Washington: U.S. Department of Justice, Office of Juvenile Justice and Delinquency Prevention.

Hunt, Albert. 1994. Coelho on Congressional Reform. *Wall Street Journal,* Feb. 3:A15.

Iglehart, John K. 1971. Administration, Congress Struggle for Solution to Health Manpower Shortages. *National Journal,* June 5:1196–219.

———. 1972. Intense Lobbying Drive by Medical Group Dims Prospects for HMO Legislation. *National Journal,* Sept. 2:1404–8.

———. 1973. Executive-Legislative Conflict Looms over Continuation of Health Care Subsidies. *National Journal,* May 5:645–52.

———. 1977. The Hospital Lobby Is Suffering from Self-Inflicted Wounds. *National Journal,* Oct. 1:1526–31.

Ingram, Helen. 1977. Policy Implementation through Bargaining. *Public Policy* 25:449–501.

Ippolito, Dennis. 1981. *Congressional Spending.* Ithaca: Cornell University Press.

Jacobs, Lawrence R. 1993a. *The Health of Nations: Public Opinion and the Making of American and British Health Policy.* Ithaca: Cornell University Press.

———. 1993b. Health Reform Impasse: The Politics of American Ambivalence Toward Government. *Journal of Health Politics, Policy and Law* 18:629–55.

Jacobs, Lawrence R., and Robert Shapiro. 1995. Don't Blame the Public for Failed Health Care Reform. *Journal of Health Politics, Policy and Law* 20:411–23.

Jacobson, Gary C. 1987. *The Politics of Congressional Elections.* 2d ed. Boston: Little, Brown.

Janiskee, Brian. 1995. Bicameralism and Health Legislation in Michigan. Paper presented at the annual meeting of the Midwest Political Science Association, Chicago, Apr. 6–8.

Johnson, Charles A. 1976. Political Culture in American States: Elazar's Formulation Examined. *American Journal of Political Science* 20:491–509.

Johnson, Lyndon Baines. 1971. *The Vantage Point.* New York: Holt, Rinehart and Winston.

Jones, Bryan D., Frank R. Baumgartner, and Jeffery C. Talbert. 1993. The Destruction of Issue Monopolies in Congress. *American Political Scienceview* 87:657–71.

Jones, Charles O. 1994. *The Presidency in a Separated System.* Washington: Brookings Institution.

Jones, Woodrow, and W. Robert Keiser. 1987. Issue Visibility and the Effects of PAC Money. *Social Science Quarterly* 68:170–76.

Kaufman, Herbert. 1977. *Red Tape.* Washington: Brookings Institution.

Kearns, Doris. 1976. *Lyndon Johnson and the American Dream.* New York: Harper and Row.

Keefe, William J. 1984. *Congress and the American People*. 2d ed. Englewood Cliffs, N.J.: Prentice-Hall.

Keiser, K. Robert, and Woodrow Jones Jr. 1986. Do the American Medical Association's Campaign Contributions Influence Health Care Legislation? *Medical Care* 24:761–66.

Kelly, Michael. 1993. David Gergen, Master of the Game. *New York Times Magazine*, Oct. 31:62–71, 80, 94, 97.

Kelman, Steven. 1980. Occupational Safety and Health Administration. In *The Politics of Regulation*, edited by James Q. Wilson, 236–66. New York: Basic Books.

Kernell, Samuel. 1984. The Presidency and the People. In *The Presidency and the Political System*, edited by Michael Nelson. Washington: Congressional Quarterly Press.

———. 1986. *Going Public: New Strategies of Presidential Leadership*. Washington: Congressional Quarterly Press.

———. 1991. Facing an Opposition Congress: The President's Strategic Circumstance. In *The Politics of Divided Government*, edited by Gary Cox and Samuel Kernell. Boulder, Colo.: Westview Press.

Kernell, Samuel, Peter W. Sperlich, and Aaron Wildavsky. 1975. Public Support for Presidents. In *Perspectives on the Presidency*, edited by Aaron Wildavsky, 148–81. Boston: Little, Brown.

Kiewiet, Roderick, and Mathew McCubbins. 1991. *The Spending Power: Congress, the President and the Appropriations Process*. Chicago: University of Chicago Press.

Kingdon, John. 1977. *Congressmen's Voting Decisions*. New York: Harper and Row.

———. 1984. *Agendas, Alternatives and Public Policies*. Boston: Little, Brown.

Kosterlitz, Julie. 1992. Survival Tactics. *National Journal*, Oct. 24:2428–32.

———. 1994. The Big Sell. *National Journal*, May 14:1118–23.

Krauss, Clifford. 1993. Lobbyists of Every Stripe on Health Care Proposal. *New York Times*, Sept. 24:A1, A12.

Kurtz, Howard. 1994. Rolling with the Punches from the Press Corps. *Washington Post National Weekly Edition*, Jan. 24–30:10.

Kurtz, Karl. 1989. State Legislatures in the 1990s. Paper prepared for the Public Affairs Council Handbook on State Government Relations.

———. 1990. The Public Standing of the Legislature. Paper presented at the Eagleton Institute of Politics Symposium on the Legislature in the Twenty-First Century, Williamsburg, Va., Apr. 27–29.

Lambert, David A., and Thomas McGuire. 1990. Political and Economic Determinants of Insurance Regulation in Mental Health. *Journal of Health Politics, Policy and Law* 15:169–89.

Lamm, Richard D. 1990. The Ten Commandments of Health Care. In *The Nation's Health,* edited by P. R. Lee and C. L. Estes, 3d ed., 124–33. Boston: Jones and Bartlett.

"Lawmakers Face Hectic Health Reform Timetable." 1994. *Medicine and Health* 48 (Apr. 11): 1–2.

LeLoup, Lance. 1979. Process versus Policy: The U.S. House Budget Committee. *Legislative Studies Quarterly* 4:227–54.

Lemov, Penelope. 1994. An Acute Case of Health Care Reform. *Governing* 7: 44–50.

Levit, Katharine R., Cathy A. Cowan, Helen C. Lazenby, Patricia A. McDonnell, Arthur L. Sensenia, Jean M. Stiller, and Darleen K. Won. 1994. National Health Spending Trends, 1960–1993. *Health Affairs* 13 (winter):14–31.

Lewin, John. 1992. Promoting an "Everybody Plays" Model. *State Health Notes,* Apr. 20:4, 5, 8.

Lewis, Neil A. 1994. Lobby for Small-Business Owners Puts Big Dent in Health Care Bill. *New York Times,* July 6:A1, A9.

Light, Paul. 1982. *The President's Agenda.* Baltimore: Johns Hopkins University Press.

———. 1984. The Presidential Policy Stream. In *The Presidency and the Political System,* edited by Michael Nelson, 423–48. Washington: Congressional Quarterly Press.

———. 1991. *The President's Agenda: Domestic Policy Choice from Kennedy to Reagan.* Rev. ed. Baltimore: Johns Hopkins University Press.

Long, Norton E. 1949. Power and Administration. *Public Administration Review* 9:257–64.

Loomis, Burdett A. 1984. Congressional Careers and Party Leadership in the Contemporary House of Representatives. *American Journal of Political Science* 28:180–201.

———. 1988. *The New American Politician.* New York: Basic Books.

Lowi, T. J. 1964. American Business, Public Policy, Case-Studies and Political Theory. *World Politics* 16:677–715.

MacKuen, Michael B., and Calvin Mouw. 1992. The Strategic Configuration, Personal Influence and Presidential Power in Congress. *Western Political Quarterly* 45:579–608.

Manley, John. 1965. The House Committee on Ways and Means: Conflict Management in a Congressional Committee. *American Political Science Review* 59:927–39.

Mann, Thomas. 1978. *Unsafe at Any Margin*. Washington: American Enterprise Institute.

Marini, John. 1992. *The Politics of Budget Control: Congress, the Presidency and the Growth of the Administrative State*. Washington: Crane Russak.

Marmor, Theodore. 1970. *The Politics of Medicare*. Chicago: Aldine.

Matlack, Carol, James A. Barnes, and Richard E. Cohen. 1990. Quid without Quo? *National Journal* 22:1473–74, 1479.

Matthews, Donald. 1960. *U.S. Senators and Their World*. New York: Vintage Books.

Mayhew, David. 1974. *Congress: The Electoral Connection*. New Haven: Yale University Press.

———. 1987. The Electoral Connection and the Congress. In *Congress: Structure and Policy*, edited by Mathew McCubbins and Terry Sullivan, 18–29. New York: Cambridge University Press.

McBride, David. 1993. Black America from Community Health Care to Crisis Medicine. *Journal of Health Politics, Policy and Law* 18:319–37.

McCall, Nelda, and Thomas Rice. 1983. Factors Influencing Physician Assignment Decisions Under Medicare. *Inquiry* 20:45–56.

McCubbins, Mathew, and Thomas Schwartz. 1984. Congressional Oversight Overlooked: Police Patrols vs. Fire Alarms. *American Journal of Political Science* 28:165–79.

Meacham, Jon. 1993. Hill Climbers. *Washington Monthly*, June:28–31.

Meier, Kenneth. 1985. *Regulation: Politics, Bureaucracy and Economics*. New York: St. Martin's.

Melnick, R. S. 1983. *Regulation and the Courts: The Case of the Clean Air Act*. Washington: Brookings Institution.

Miller, Gary J. 1993. Formal Theory and the Presidency. In *Researching the Presidency*, edited by George C. Edwards III, John H. Kessel, and Bert A. Rockman, 289–336. Pittsburgh: University of Pittsburgh Press.

Miller, Lisa. 1994. Medical Schools Put Women in Curricula. *Wall Street Journal*, May 24:B1,B7.

Moe, Terry. 1985. The Politicized Presidency. In *The New Direction in American Politics*, edited by John E. Chubb and Paul E. Peterson, 235–71. Washington: Brookings Institution.

Moore, W. John. 1994. Reversal of Fortune. *National Journal* 26 (Nov. 26): 2768–71.

Morgan, Dan. 1994. The Medicaid Time Bomb. *Washington Post National Weekly Edition*, Feb. 7–13:6–8.

Morone, James A. 1990. *The Democratic Wish: Popular Participation and the Limits of American Government*. New York: Basic Books.

—————. 1993. The Health Care Bureaucracy: Small Changes, Big Consequences. *Journal of Health Politics, Policy and Law* 18:723–39.

Morone, James A., and Andrew B. Dunham. 1985. Slouching toward National Health Insurance: The New Health Care Politics. *Yale Journal on Regulation* 2:263–91.

Mosher, Frederick C. 1982. *Democracy and the Public Service.* 2d ed. New York: Oxford University Press.

Mueller, Keith J. 1986. An Analysis of Congressional Health Policy Voting in the 1970s. *Journal of Health Politics, Policy and Law* 11:117–35.

—————. 1992. State Government Policies and Rural Hospitals: Facilitating Change. *Policy Studies Journal* 20:168–81.

Nathan, Richard P. 1983. *The Administrative Presidency.* New York: John Wiley.

—————. 1989. The Role of States in American Federalism. In *The State of the States,* edited by Carl E. Van Horn. Washington: Congressional Quarterly.

—————. 1993. *Turning Promises into Performance.* New York: Twentieth Century Fund.

National Association of County Health Officials (NACHO). 1990. *National Profile of Local Health Departments.* Washington: NACHO.

National Association of State Budget Officers (NASBO). 1992. *State Expenditure Report.* Washington: NASBO.

National Center for Health Statistics. 1993. *Health, United States.* Hyattsville, Md.: U.S. Public Health Service.

National Commission on the Public Service. 1989. *Leadership for America: Rebuilding the Public Service.* Lexington, Mass.: Lexington Books.

National Health Council. 1991. *Congress and Health.* Washington: National Health Council.

—————. 1993. *Health Groups in Washington.* 12th ed. Washington: National Health Council.

Nelson, Barbara. 1978. Setting the Public Agenda: The Case of Child Abuse. In *The Policy Cycle,* edited by Judith May and Aaron Wildavsky, 17–41. Beverly Hills: Sage.

Nelson, Michael. 1982. A Short, Ironic History of American National Bureaucracy. *Journal of Politics* 44:747–78.

Neustadt, Richard E. 1960. *Presidential Power.* New York: John Wiley.

New York Times. 1992. Texas Health Officials Unable to Verify School H.I.V. Cases. *New York Times,* Feb. 27:A20.

Nexon, David. 1987. The Politics of Congressional Health Policy in the Second Half of the 1980s. *Medical Care Review* 44:65–88.

Noah, Timothy. 1993. AMA Lavishly Courts Congressional Staffers Who Will Affect Outcome of Clinton's Health Plan. *Wall Street Journal,* June 30:A16.

O'Leary, Rosemary. 1989. The Impact of Federal Court Decisions on the Policies and Administration of the U.S. Environmental Protection Agency. *Administrative Law Review* 41:549–76.

Oleszek, Walter J. 1989. *Congressional Procedures and the Policy Process.* 3d ed. Washington: Congressional Quarterly Press.

Oliver, Thomas R. 1993. Analysis, Advice, and Congressional Leadership: The Physician Payment Review Commission and the Politics of Medicare. *Journal of Health Politics, Policy and Law* 18:113–74.

Olson, Mancur, Jr. 1968. *The Logic of Collective Action.* New York: Schocken.

Ornstein, Norman J., Thomas E. Mann, and Michael J. Malbin. 1994. *Vital Statistics on Congress, 1993–1994.* Washington: Congressional Quarterly Press.

Palumbo, Dennis. 1990. *Implementation and the Policy Process.* New York: Greenwood.

Parker, Glenn. 1989. *Characteristics of Congress.* Englewood Cliffs, N.J.: Prentice-Hall.

Patterson, Samuel. 1983. Legislators and Legislatures in the American States. In *Politics in the American States,* edited by Virginia Gray, Herbert Jacob, and Kenneth Vines, 4th ed., 135–79. Boston: Little, Brown.

Pear, Robert. 1990. An Office That Has the Capital's Ear. *New York Times,* July 30:A12.

———. 1993a. Drug Industry Gathers a Mix of Voices to Bolster Its Case. *New York Times,* July 7:A1, A6.

———. 1993b. Doctors Rebel over Health Plan in Major Challenge to President. *New York Times,* Sept. 30:A1, A12.

———. 1994a. Clinton Fails to Get Endorsement of Elderly Group on Health Plan. *New York Times,* Feb. 25:A1, A11.

———. 1994b. Report Criticizes the Objectivity of the Federal Watchdog Agency. *New York Times,* Oct. 17:A1.

Pertschuk, Michael. 1986. *Giant Killers.* New York: W. W. Norton.

Peters, B. Guy. 1981. The Problem of Bureaucratic Government. *Journal of Politics* 43:56–82.

Peters, B. G., and B. W. Hogwood. 1985. In Search of the Issue-Attention Cycle. *Journal of Politics* 47:238–53.

Peters, Charles. 1994. Tilting at Windmills. *Washington Monthly* 26 (Jan.–Feb.):5.

Peterson, Mark. 1990. *Legislating Together: The White House and Capitol Hill from Eisenhower to Reagan.* Cambridge: Harvard University Press.

————. 1993. Political Influence in the 1990s: From Iron Triangles to Policy Networks. *Journal of Health Politics, Policy and Law* 18:395–438.

Petracca, Mark. 1992a. The Future of an Interest Group Society. In *The Politics of Interests: Interest Groups Transformed,* edited by Mark Petracca, 345–61. Boulder, Colo.: Westview Press.

————. 1992b. Issue Definitions, Agenda-building and Policymaking. *Policy Currents* 2:1, 4.

Pfiffner, James P. 1987. Political Appointees and Career Executives: The Democracy-Bureaucracy Nexus in the Third Century. *Public Administration Review* 47:57–65.

Piore, Nora, Purlaine Lieberman, and James Linnane. 1977. Financing Local Health Services. In *Health Services: The Local Perspective,* edited by Arthur Levin, 15–28. New York: Academy of Political Science.

Polzer, Karl. 1992. The Role of Federal Standards in Health Systems Reform: How Much Leash Should ERISA Give the States? *Issue Brief 609.* Washington: National Health Policy Forum.

Pressman, Steven. 1984. Physicians' Lobbying Machine Showing Some Signs of Wear. *Congressional Quarterly,* Jan. 17:15–19.

Price, David E. 1971. Professionals and "Entrepreneurs": Staff Orientations and Policy Making on Three Senate Committees. *Journal of Politics* 33:316–36.

————. 1978. Policy Making in Congressional Committees: The Impact of "Environmental" Factors. *American Political Science Review* 72:548–74.

Price, Raymond. 1977. *With Nixon.* New York: Viking Press.

Priest, Dana. 1993. Doctors Attack Efforts to Delegate More Health Care Duties to Nurses. *Washington Post,* Dec. 7:A3.

————. 1994. Kennedy Reminds Washington How It's Done. *Washington Post National Weekly Edition,* May 23–29:13.

Priest, Dana, and David S. Broder. 1994. The Pen as a Mighty Sword. *Washington Post National Weekly Edition,* Jan. 31–Feb. 6:11.

Quirk, Paul. 1981. *Industry Influence in Federal Regulatory Agencies.* Princeton: Princeton University Press.

Rabe, Barry. 1990. Legislative Incapacity: The Congressional Role in Environmental Policy-Making and the Case of Superfund. *Journal of Health Politics, Policy and Law* 15:571–89.

Ratan, Suneel. 1993. How to Really Cut the Budget Deficit. *Fortune,* Oct. 4:101–4.

Rawls, John. 1971. *A Theory of Justice.* Cambridge: Harvard University Press.

Reinhardt, Uwe. 1989. Health Care Spending and American Competitiveness. *Health Affairs* 8 (winter):5–21.

Relman, Arnold. 1980. The New Medical-Industrial Complex. *New England Journal of Medicine* 303 (Oct. 23):963–70.

Reston, James. 1973. *Facing the Lions.* New York: Viking Press.

Rice, Thomas H., and Roberta J. Labelle. 1989. Do Physicians Induce Demand for Medical Services? *Journal of Health Politics, Policy and Law* 14:587–600.

Riker, William H. 1962. *The Theory of Political Coalitions.* New Haven: Yale University Press.

Ripley, Randall B., and Grace A. Franklin. 1986. *Policy Implementation and Bureaucracy.* 2d ed. Chicago: Dorsey Press.

Rivers, Douglas, and Nancy L. Rose. 1985. Passing the President's Program: Public Opinion and Presidential Influence in Congress. *American Journal of Political Science* 29:183–96.

Roberts, Cokie. 1990. Leadership in the Media in the 101st Congress. In *Leading Congress: New Styles, New Strategies,* edited by John J. Kornacki, 85–96. Washington: Congressional Quarterly Press.

Robinson, Chester A. 1991. *The Bureaucracy and the Legislative Process: A Case Study of the Health Care Financing Administration.* Lanham, Md.: University Press of America.

Rochefort, David A., and Roger W. Cobb. 1994. *The Politics of Problem Definition.* Lawrence: University Press of Kansas.

Rockman, Bert. 1984. Legislative-Executive Relations and Legislative Oversight. *Legislative Studies Quarterly* 9:387–440.

Rohde, David. 1990. Divided Government, Agenda Change and Variations in Presidential Support in the House. Paper prepared for a conference in honor of William H. Riker, Rochester, N.Y., Oct. 12–13.

———. 1991. *Parties and Leaders in the Postreform House.* Chicago: University of Chicago Press.

Rohde, David, and Dennis Simon. 1985. Presidential Vetoes and Congressional Response: A Study of Institutional Conflict. *American Journal of Political Science* 29:397–427.

Rohde, David W., Norman J. Ornstein, and Robert L. Peabody. 1985. Political Change and Legislative Norms in the U.S. Senate, 1957–1974. In *Studies of Congress,* edited by Glenn R. Parker, 147–88. Washington: Congressional Quarterly Press.

Romer, Thomas, and James Snyder. 1994. An Empirical Investigation of the Dynamics of PAC Contributions. *American Journal of Political Science* 38: 745–69.

Rosenbaum, David. 1993. For Every Bill There Is the Perfect Lobbyist. *New York Times,* May 5:A1, A12.

Rosenberg, Gerald N. 1991. *The Hollow Hope: Can Courts Bring About Social Change?* Chicago: University of Chicago Press.

Rosenblatt, Rand E. 1993. The Courts, Health Care Reform, and the Reconstruction of American Social Legislation. *Journal of Health Politics, Policy and Law* 18:439–76.

Rosenblatt, Roger. 1994. How Do Tobacco Executives Live with Themselves? *New York Times Magazine*, Mar. 20:34–41, 55, 73–74, 76.

Rosenbloom, David H. 1981. The Judicial Response to the Bureaucratic State. *American Review of Public Administration* 50:29–51.

Rosenheck, R., P. Gallup, and C. A. Leda. 1991. Vietnam Era and Vietnam Combat Veterans among the Homeless. *American Journal of Public Health* 81: 643–46.

Rosenthal, Alan. 1993. *The Third House: Lobbyists and Lobbying in the States.* Washington: Congressional Quarterly Press.

Ross, Sonya. 1994. AARP Members Irate When Leaders Back Bills. *Ann Arbor News*, Aug. 12:A2.

Rourke, Francis. 1984. *Bureaucracy, Politics and Public Policy.* 3d ed. Boston: Little, Brown.

———. 1991. American Bureaucracy in a Changing Political Setting. *Journal of Public Administration Research and Theory* 2:111–29.

Rubin, Alissa. 1993a. Special Interests Stampede To Be Heard on Overhaul. *Congressional Quarterly*, May 1:1081–84.

———. 1993b. With Health Overhaul on Stage, PACs Want a Front Row Seat. *Congressional Quarterly*, July 31:2048–54.

———. 1993c. Generosity of Health PACs Rises as Overhead Approaches. *Congressional Quarterly*, Sept. 25:47–53.

Sabatier, P. A., and H. C. Jenkins-Smith. 1993. *Policy Change and Learning: An Advocacy Approach.* Boulder, Colo.: Westview Press.

Sabato, Larry. 1985. *PAC Power.* New York: W. W. Norton.

Salamon, Lester M., and Alan J. Abramson. 1984. Governance: The Politics of Retrenchment. In *The Reagan Record*, edited by John L. Palmer and Isabel V. Sawhill, 31–68. Washington: Urban Institute Press.

Salisbury, Robert H. 1969. An Exchange Theory of Interest Groups. *Midwest Journal of Political Science* 13:1–32.

———. 1992. *Interests and Institutions: Substance and Structure in American Politics.* Pittsburgh: University of Pittsburgh Press.

Salisbury, Robert, and Kenneth Shepsle. 1981. U.S. Congressman as Enterprise. *Legislative Studies Quarterly* 6:559–76.

Salisbury, Robert H., John P. Heinz, Edward O. Laumann, and Robert L. Nelson.

1987. Who Works with Whom?: Interest Group Alliances and Opposition. *American Political Science Review* 81:1217–34.

Sanford, Terry. 1967. *Storm over the States*. New York: McGraw-Hill.

Schattschneider, E. E. 1935. *Politics, Pressures and the Tariff*. Englewood Cliffs, N.J.: Prentice-Hall.

———. 1960. *The Semi-Sovereign People*. New York: Holt, Rinehart, and Winston.

Schick, Allen. 1980. *Congress and Money*. Washington: Urban Institute Press.

Schlesinger, Joseph A. 1966. *Ambition and Politics*. Chicago: Rand McNally.

Schlozman, Kay L., and John T. Tierney. 1986. *Organized Interests and American Democracy*. New York: Harper and Row.

Schon, Donald A. 1971. *Beyond the Stable State*. New York: Norton.

Schull, Steven A. 1989. *The President and Civil Rights Policy: Leadership and Change*. Westport, Conn.: Greenwood Press.

Scotch, Richard. 1984. *From Good Will to Civil Rights: Transforming Federal Disability Policy*. Philadelphia: Temple University Press.

Scott, Ruth K., and Ronald J. Hrebenar. 1979. *Parties in Crisis*. New York: Wiley and Sons.

Seelye, Katharine Q. 1994. Lobbyists are the Loudest in the Health Care Debate. *New York Times,* Aug. 16:A1, A10.

Segal, David. 1994. A House Divided. *Washington Monthly,* Jan./Feb.:24–32.

Serafini, Marilyn Werber. 1995. Health: Who's In Charge Here? *National Journal,* July 1: 1710–13.

Sharfstein, Joshua M., and Steven S. Sharfstein. 1994. Campaign Contributions from the American Medical Political Action Committee to Members of Congress. *New England Journal of Medicine,* Jan. 6:32–37.

Shear, Jeff. 1994. The Untouchables. *National Journal,* July 16:1681–85.

Shepsle, Kenneth. 1989. Congressional Institutions and Behavior: The Changing Textbook Congress. In *American Political Institutions and the Problems of Our Time,* edited by John E. Chubb and Paul E. Peterson, 238–66. Washington: Brookings Institution.

Shepsle, Kenneth, and Barry Weingast. 1984. Legislative Politics and Budget Outcomes. In *Federal Budget Policy in the 1980s,* edited by Gregory Mills and John Palmer, 343–67. Washington: Urban Institute Press.

———.1987. The Institutional Foundations of Committee Power. *American Political Science Review* 81:85–104.

———. 1991. Penultimate Power: Conference Committees and the Legislative Process. In *Home Style and Washington Work,* edited by Morris P. Fiorina and David W. Rohde, 199–217. Ann Arbor: University of Michigan Press.

Sherer, Renslow. 1990. Heterosexual AIDS: Myth or Epidemic? *Journal of the American Medical Association* 264:1807.

Sigelman, Lee, P. Roder, and C. Sigelman. 1981. Social Service Innovation in the American States: Deinstitutionalization of the Mentally Retarded. *Social Science Quarterly* 62:503–15.

Sigelman, Lee, and Roland E. Smith. 1980. Consumer Legislation in the American States: An Attempt at Explanation. *Social Science Quarterly* 61:58–70.

Silver, George A. 1991. The Route to a National Health Policy Lies through the States. *Yale Journal of Biology and Medicine* 64:443–53.

Simon, Herbert. 1945. *Administrative Behavior: A Study of Decision-Making Processes in Administration Organization.* New York: Free Press.

———. 1960. *The New Science of Management Decision.* New York: Harper and Row.

Sinclair, Barbara. 1989. *The Transformation of the U.S. Senate.* Baltimore: Johns Hopkins University Press.

Skocpol, Theda. 1992. *Protecting Soldiers and Mothers: The Political Origins of Social Policy in the United States.* Cambridge: Harvard University Press.

———. 1995. The Rise and Resounding Demise of the Clinton Plan. *Health Affairs* 14 (spring):67–85.

Smith, Hedrick. 1988. *The Power Game: How Washington Works.* New York: Random House.

Smith, Richard A. 1984. Advocacy, Interpretation and Influence in the U.S. Congress. *American Political Science Review* 78:44–63.

———. 1995. Interest Group Influence in the U.S. Congress. *Legislative Studies Quarterly* 20:89–139.

Smith, Steven, and Christopher Deering. 1990. *Committees in Congress.* 2d ed. Washington: Congressional Quarterly Press.

Smits, H., J. Feder, and W. Scanlon. 1982. Medicare's Nursing-Home Benefit: Variations in Interpretation. *New England Journal of Medicine,* Sept. 30:855–62.

Sparer, Michael, and Lawrence D. Brown. 1993. Between a Rock and a Hard Place: How Public Managers Manage Medicaid. In *Revitalizing State and Local Public Service,* edited by Frank J. Thompson, 279–306. San Francisco: Jossey-Bass.

Spitzer, Robert J. 1983. *The Presidency and Public Policy: The Four Arenas of Presidential Power.* University: University of Alabama Press.

———. 1993. *President and Congress: Executive Hegemony at the Crossroads of American Government.* Philadelphia: Temple University Press.

Squire, Peverill. 1992. Legislative Professionalization and Membership Diversity in State Legislatures. *Legislative Studies Quarterly* 17:69–79.

Starr, Paul. 1982. *The Social Transformation of American Medicine*. New York: Basic Books.

State Health Notes. 1974–95. Washington: Intergovernmental Health Policy Project.

Stillman, Richard J. 1987. *The American Bureaucracy*. Chicago: Nelson-Hall.

Stone, Deborah A. 1988. *Policy Paradox and Political Reason*. Glenview Ill.: Scott, Foresman.

———. 1989. Causal Stories and the Formation of Policy Agendas. *Political Science Quarterly* 104:281–300.

———. 1993. The Struggle for the Soul of Health Insurance. *Journal of Health Politics, Policy and Law* 18:287–317.

Stone, Peter H. 1994. Back Off! *National Journal* 26 (Dec. 3):2840–44.

Stout, Hilary. 1994. In Health-Care Debate, Small Business Benefits At the Expense of Big. *Wall Street Journal*, July 21:A1, A5.

Sullivan, Terry. 1987. Presidential Leadership in Congress: Security Commitments. In *Congress: Structure and Policy*, edited by Mathew McCubbins and Terry Sullivan, 286–308. Cambridge: Cambridge University Press.

———. 1991. The Bank Account Presidency: A New Measure and Evidence on the Temporal Path of Presidential Influence. *American Journal of Political Science*, 35:686–723.

Suro, Robert. 1992. Report of AIDS Unsettles a Town. *New York Times*, Feb. 19: A15.

Suskind, Ron. 1993. Health-Care Reform May Seem Like a Bitter Pill to Localities Sick of Unfunded Federal Mandates. *Wall Street Journal*, Dec. 21, 1993: A14.

Swoboda, Frank, and Martha M. Hamilton. 1994. The War on Workplace Smoke Goes Nationwide. *Washington Post*, Sept. 18:H1.

Tatalovich, Raymond, and Bryon W. Daynes. 1988. *Social Regulatory Policy: Moral Controversies in American Politics*. Boulder, Colo.: Westview Press.

Thaemert, Rita. 1994. Twenty Percent and Climbing. *State Legislatures* 20: 28–32.

Thomas, Clive, and Ronald Hrebenar. 1990. Interest Groups in States. In *Politics in the American States*, edited by Virginia Gray, Herbert Jacob, and Robert Albritton, 5th ed., 123–58. Glenview, Ill.: Scott, Foresman.

Thompson, Frank J. 1983. *Health Policy and the Bureaucracy*. Cambridge: MIT Press.

Tierney, John T. 1987. Organized Interests in Health Politics and Policy-Making. *Medical Care Review* 44:89–118.

Toner, Robin. 1994a. Gold Rush Fever Grips Capital as Health Care Struggle Begins. *New York Times*, Mar. 13:1, 10.

――――. 1994b. For Majority Leader, a Quest for a Health Care Consensus. *New York Times*, July 18:A1, A7.

Torres-Gil, Fernando. 1989. The Politics of Catastrophic and Long-Term Care Coverage. *Journal of Aging and Social Policy* 1:61–86.

Truman, David B. 1951. *The Governmental Process: Political Interests and Public Opinion*. New York: Knopf.

U.S. Congressional Budget Office. 1977. Budget Issue Paper: Long Term Care for the Elderly and Disabled. Washington: Government Printing Office.

U.S. Executive Office of the President, Council on Wage and Price Stability. 1976. The Complex Puzzle of Rising Health Care Costs: Can the Private Sector Fit It Together? Washington: Council on Wage and Price Stability. In Dogmatic Slumbers: American Business and Health Policy, by Lawrence D. Brown. *Journal of Health Politics, Policy and Law* 18:339–57.

――――. 1995. *Budget of the United States*. Washington: Government Printing Office.

U.S. General Accounting Office. 1992. *Access to Health Insurance*. GAO/HRD-92–90. Washington: Government Printing Office.

――――. 1994. *Health Insurance Regulation: Wide Variation in States' Authority, Oversight, and Resources*. GAO/HRD-94–26. Washington: Government Printing Office.

U.S. House of Representatives, Committee on Ways and Means. 1993. *Overview of Entitlement Programs: 1993 Green Book*. Washington: Government Printing Office.

Wagar, Linda. 1994. The Law That Won't Die. *State Government News*, Jan.: 16–19.

Waldo, Dwight. 1955. *The Study of Administration*. New York: Random House.

Walker, David. 1995. *The Rebirth of Federalism*. Chatham, N.J.: Chatham House.

Walker, Jack. 1969. The Diffusion of Innovations among the American States. *American Political Science Review* 63:880–99.

――――. 1991. *Mobilizing Interest Groups in America*. Ann Arbor: University of Michigan Press.

Ward, Daniel. 1993. The Continuing Search for Party Influence in Congress: A View from the Committee. *Legislative Studies Quarterly* 18:211–30.

Weeks, Lewis E., and Howard J. Berman. 1985. *Shapers of American Health Care Policy: An Oral History*. Ann Arbor: Health Administration Press.

Weimer, David L., and Aidan R. Vining. 1992. *Policy Analysis: Concepts and Practice*. 2d ed. Englewood Cliffs, N.J.: Prentice-Hall.

Weingast, Barry, and Mark Moran. 1983. Bureaucratic Discretion or Congressional Control?: Regulatory Policymaking by the Federal Trade Commission. *Journal of Political Economy* 91:765–800.

Weissert, Carol S. 1992. Medicaid in the 1990s: Trends, Innovations, and the Future of the "PAC-Man" of State Budgets. *Publius* 22 (summer):93–109.

———. 1994. Beyond the Organization: The Influence of Community and Personal Values on Street-Level Bureaucrats' Responsiveness. *Journal of Public Administration Research and Theory* 4:225–54.

Weissert, Carol S., Jack H. Knott, and Blair S. Stieber. 1994. Education and the Health Professions: Explaining Policy Choice. *Journal of Health Politics, Policy and Law* 19:361–92.

Weissert, William G. 1972. Bringing Management into Health Care Delivery. Report to the Administrator, Health Services and Mental Health Administration.

———. 1985. Estimating the Long-Term Care Population: Prevalence Rates and Selected Characteristics. *Health Care Financing Review* 6 (summer): 83–91.

———. 1991. A New Policy Agenda for Home Care. *Health Affairs* 10 (summer):67–77.

Weissert, W. G., and C. M. Cready. 1989. Hospital to Nursing Home Discharge Delays: A Pilot Study. *Health Service Research* 23:619–46.

Weissert, W. G., C. M. Cready, and J. E. Pawelak. 1988. The Past and Future of Home and Community Based Long-Term Care. *Milbank Quarterly* 66: 309–88.

Weissert, W. G., T. T. H. Wan, B. Liveratos, and S. Katz. 1980. Effects and Costs of Day Care Services for the Chronically Ill: A Randomized Experiment. *Medical Care* 18:567–84.

Weissert, W. G., T. T. H. Wan, B. Liveratos, and J. Pelligrino. 1980. Cost-Effectiveness of Homemaker Services for the Chronically Ill: An Experimental Study. *Inquiry* 17:230–43.

Weisskopf, Michael. 1991. Writing Laws Is One Thing—Writing Rules Is Something Else. *Washington Post National Weekly Edition,* Sept. 30–Oct. 6:31–32.

———. 1994. Pizzas and Cards Carry the Day. *Washington Post National Weekly Edition,* July 25–31:14–15.

———. 1995. To the Victors Belong the PAC Checks. *Washington Post National Weekly Edition,* Jan. 2–8:13.

Welch, W. P., and Lisa Dubay. 1989. The Impact of Administratively Necessary Days on Hospital Costs. *Medical Care* 27:1117–32.

Wertheimer, Fred. 1983. Common Cause Declares War on Political Action Committees. *Common Cause,* Mar./Apr.:44.

West, William 1984. Structuring Administrative Discretion: The Pursuit of Rationality and Responsiveness. *American Journal of Political Science* 28: 340–60.

West, William, and Joseph Cooper. 1989–90. Legislative Influence v. Presidential Dominance: Competing Models of Bureaucratic Control. *Political Science Quarterly* 104:581–606.

Whiteman, David. 1987. What Do They Know and When Do They Know It?: Health Staff on the Hill. *PS* 20:221–25.

Wildavsky, Aaron. 1966. The Two Presidencies. *Trans-Action* 4:7–14.

———. 1979. *Speaking Truth to Power.* Boston: Little, Brown.

Wilhite, Allen. 1988. Union PAC Contributions and Legislative Voting. *Journal of Labor Research* 9:79–90.

Will, George. 1994. Leaning on the States, *Washington Post*, Apr. 7:A27.

Wilson, James Q. 1973. *Political Organizations.* New York: Basic Books.

———. 1989. *Bureaucracy: What Government Agencies Do and Why They Do It.* New York: Basic Books.

Wilson, Rick. 1992. Review of *Parties and Leaders in the Postreform House* by David Rohde. *American Political Science Review* 86:806–7.

Wilson, Woodrow. 1913. *Congressional Government.* Boston: Houghton Mifflin. Originally published in 1885.

Wines, Michael. 1994. Clinton Puts Onus for Health Care on Republicans. *New York Times*, Aug. 4:A1, A9.

Winn, Mylon. 1987. Competitive Health Care: Assessing an Alternative Solution for Health Care Problems. In *Health Care Issues in Black America: Policies, Problems, and Prospects*, edited by Woodrow Jones Jr. and Mitchell F. Rice, 233–47. Westport, Conn.: Greenwood.

Woodward, B. 1994. *The Agenda: Inside the Clinton White House.* New York: Simon & Schuster.

Wright, J. R. 1985. PACs, Contributions and Roll Calls: An Organizational Perspective. *American Political Science Review* 79:400–14.

———. 1990. Contributions, Lobbying and Committee Voting in the U.S. House of Representatives. *American Political Science Review* 84:417–38.

Wyszewianski, L. 1986. Financially Catastrophic and High-Cost Cases: Definitions, Distinctions and Their Implications for Policy Formulation. *Inquiry* 23:382–94.

Yale Law Journal. 1954. The American Medical Association: Power, Purpose and Politics in Organized Medicine, 63:933–1022.

Young, Garry, and Joseph Cooper. 1993. Multiple Referral and the Transformation of House Decision Making. In *Congress Reconsidered*, edited by

Lawrence C. Dodd and Bruce I. Oppenheimer, 5th ed., 211–34. Washington: Congressional Quarterly Press.

Zachary, G. Pascal. 1994. How Some Schools Get Fat with Federal Pork. *Wall Street Journal,* Apr. 29:B1, B2.

Zimmerman, Joseph. 1991. Federal Preemption under Reagan's New Federalism. *Publius* 21 (winter):7–28.

Index

Library of Congress Cataloging-in-Publication Data
Weissert, Carol S.
   Governing health : the politics of health policy / Carol S. Weissert
and William G. Weissert.
      p.   cm.
   Includes bibliographical references and index.
   ISBN 0-8018-5265-X (hc : alk. paper). — ISBN 0-8018-5266-8
(pbk. : alk. paper)
   1. Medical policy—United States.   I. Weissert, William G.
II. Title
RA395.A3W45   1996
362.1'0973—dc20   95-44487